D0897305

Goodwin and Guze's Psychiatric Diagnosis

Goodwin and Guze's Psychiatric Diagnosis

SEVENTH EDITION

Carol S. North, MD, MPE

Medical Director, The Altshuler Center for Education & Research at Metrocare Services
The Nancy and Ray L. Hunt Chair in Crisis Psychiatry and Professor of Psychiatry
The University of Texas Southwestern Medical Center
Dallas, Texas

Sean H. Yutzy, MD

Adjunct Professor, Department of Psychiatry
Washington University
St. Louis, Missouri

OXFORD
UNIVERSITY PRESS

OXFORD

UNIVERSITY PRESS

Oxford University Press is a department of the University of Oxford. It furthers the University's objective of excellence in research, scholarship, and education by publishing worldwide. Oxford is a registered trade mark of Oxford University Press in the UK and certain other countries.

Published in the United States of America by Oxford University Press
198 Madison Avenue, New York, NY 10016, United States of America.

© Oxford University Press 2019

All rights reserved. No part of this publication may be reproduced, stored in a retrieval system, or transmitted, in any form or by any means, without the prior permission in writing of Oxford University Press, or as expressly permitted by law, by license, or under terms agreed with the appropriate reproduction rights organization. Inquiries concerning reproduction outside the scope of the above should be sent to the Rights Department, Oxford University Press, at the address above.

You must not circulate this work in any other form
and you must impose this same condition on any acquirer.

CIP data is on file at the Library of Congress
ISBN 978-0-19-021546-0

This book is dedicated to those listed on the following pages and to the legions of their assistants and trainees that firmly believed that psychiatry must have a scientific base and who worked diligently to make that belief a reality.

For my wife MB (by S. H. Y)

IN MEMORIUM

ROBERT A. WOODRUFF, JR.
The inspiration for—and co-author of—the first edition of this book

ELI ROBINS
Who, as much as any one person, launched a new era in American psychiatry

SAMUEL B. GUZE
The tough-minded individual who believed that there was only one model of psychiatry: the medical model—which must be part of the mainstream of modern medicine

DON GOODWIN
Gifted writer and co-author of editions two through five

CONTENTS

PREFACE TO THE SEVENTH EDITION

Forty-four years have elapsed since this text was first published. Over this time period, psychiatry has clearly evolved along three noteworthy lines.

First, most psychiatrists have become diagnosticians. The groundwork was set for this in no small part by the authors and collaborators of the early versions of this text, including Eli Robins, Robert A. Woodruff, Donald W. Goodwin, and Samuel B. Guze at Washington University in St. Louis. In particular, their two-pronged philosophical approach to psychiatric illness/diagnosis was to be "agnostic" about the origin of a mental illness and to draw psychiatric conclusions (including diagnostic criteria) based on reliable, reproducible data. The early studies of this group of psychiatric researchers from the 1960s and 1970s eventually produced formal operational criteria sets for the 12 major mental illnesses (adapted from "the Feighner criteria") (11). While this overall approach to psychiatric illness was described as "narrow" by some (and less charitably by others) in mainstream psychiatry at the time, the criteria sets formed the early basis for a common language among psychiatrists. The diagnostic approach used an "atheoretical" basis for the origin of psychiatric illness, drawing conclusions and developing criteria based on scientific evidence. This approach gained much wider acceptance (and general acceptance by the field) after publication of the best-selling *DSM-III* (*Diagnostic and Statistical Manual of Mental Disorders*, 3rd edition, of the American Psychiatric Association) (2) in 1980. The "similarities" between the *DSM-III* and Washington University approaches were not surprising, as the authors noted earlier were among the *DSM-III* taskforce contributors, and one-third of the overall taskforce members had trained at Washington University.

Ultimately, the *DSM-III* solidified a widely acceptable common language and explicit criteria for the major mental illnesses as had long been used in most other areas of medicine. Frustrated by the unknown etiology of most major psychiatric illnesses, young scientifically trained physicians could rely on a published framework as a foundation for communication, research, diagnosis, and treatment. Many well-respected individuals both inside and outside the specialty would attack the approach over the next two decades, but its utility in almost all psychiatric venues remained undeniable.

Of particular interest was that external forces over the ensuing two decades (1980–2000) further solidified psychiatry's use of the diagnostic model. Among other developments, diagnosis became a required practice for reimbursement of services (e.g., diagnostic-related groups, or DRGs), with only specific diagnoses (and not others, especially not Axis II disorders) generating payment; accreditation requirements compelled diagnostic uniformity in general medicine; and communication among treating professionals increased, particularly across medical specialties.

In sum, both internal and external forces have driven psychiatry to accept the diagnostic or medical model as THE approach to major mental illness.

The second noteworthy line of evolution is that continuing critical review over time has clarified this empirically based "approach" to the major psychiatric diagnoses is sustainable and has prevailed. The *DSM-III* has had several subsequent minor revisions (including the *DSM-III*, revised [*DSM-III-R*] in 1987 (3), *DSM-IV* in 1994 (4), and the *DSM-IV*, text revision [*DSM-IV-TR*] (5) in 2000), but most would argue that the process and the findings withstood the test of time to make *DSM-IV/DSM-IV-TR* the most widely accepted psychiatric diagnostic criteria in the world. The stability of this empirical approach first espoused by the original authors of the *Psychiatric Diagnosis* text are a testament to its fundamental inherent strength.

The third line of evolution has been the frank failure of psychiatry to discover the neurobiological underpinnings of the major mental illnesses included in this textbook. New students to psychiatry cannot avoid being confronted with animosity from all quarters toward the latest American diagnostic manual, the *DSM-5* (*Diagnostic and Statistical Manual of Mental Disorders*, 5th edition) (6). The history of what happened is nearly impossible to locate without extensive literature search; thus we briefly review it for instructional purposes.

Following from the successes just noted, psychiatry embarked upon study of the brain as the major imperative for the 1990s. President Bush declared (Proclamation 6158) 1990–2000 to be the "Decade of the Brain," and the search was on for the underlying neurobiology. Tremendous resources were expended. Later, some critics jested that one of the main findings of this initiative was that the brain was much more complicated than imagined. Cellular-level analysis was dealing remotely (extracranially) with 100 billion cells with multitudinous overlapping known and unknown tracks, circuits, and functions as opposed to organs devoted to several metabolic functions. Arising from this early excitement and frank hubris was the notion that neuroscience, imaging, and genetics would yield answers, presumably in short order. The architects of *DSM-5* promised inclusion of these "findings" to support the outstanding questions of validity of the major mental disorders. (Also promised by the Task Force for *DSM-5* was a dimensional approach to psychiatric diagnosis.)

As the scientific findings failed to materialize and complexities of the tasks expanded beyond current capabilities (dimensionalism without reconciling increasing comorbidity risks), various stakeholders began raising questions. Perhaps the most damning criticism—immediately prior to the 2013 introduction of *DSM-5*—was a direct rebuke by the National Institute of Mental Health (NIMH) that not only constituted a major funding source for the *DSM* series but also provided indirect support by requiring *DSM* language in formal NIMH grant applications.

The failure to identify a single basis for any major (or minor) mental illness accompanied *DSM-5*'s departure from the careful iterative style of the *DSM* series (*DSM-III-R* to *DSM-IV-TR*) that introduced abrupt major structural changes, acceptance of poor agreement within criteria, ill-conceived theoretical changes, and overly broadening criteria. These missteps and errors have come to light over the ensuing years with the application of *DSM-5* criteria particularly to issues within government, insurance, clinical practice, research, and society.

Space does not permit comprehensive review of all of the major changes to the criteria in *DSM-5*, but some high points may assist the reader. Perhaps most problematic for the acceptance (and credibility) of *DSM-5* (and, by direct extension, psychiatry) were major structural changes in the approach to diagnoses, particularly removal of the multi-axial system without much empirical basis or guidance. Over the last 33 years, probably 90% of practicing psychiatrists, as well as many more allied health professionals, were educated under the *DSM* system of psychiatric diagnosis. Users of the *DSM-5* were told that the manual had moved to non-axial documentation of diagnosis, by removing Axes I–III, which were "combined," and that impinging social and situational factors and functional impairments should be notated. No elaboration was provided on newly created issues for addressing diagnostic primacy, including definition of primary versus secondary disorders (i.e., first onset versus focus of treatment), formal consideration of how the diagnoses integrate in the *DSM-5* list format, and determination of amount of overall functional impact on the individual— complexities which had been addressed in previous editions of the criteria.

Problematic for research was the poor interrater reliability (whether two examiners of the same case agree or disagree on the diagnosis) of many of the diagnostic criteria in the *DSM-5* field trials. Particularly concerning was the finding that one of the lowest agreements was for one of the most common psychiatric disorders, major depressive disorder.

Somatization disorder (a historically agreed-upon valid and reliable major diagnosis) was "downlisted" and replaced in *DSM-5* with a new major category, somatic symptom disorder. Focusing more on excessive thoughts and feelings related to somatic symptoms, it was opined that the label should also capture most cases of somatization disorder as well as related syndromes. Unfortunately, this new label also captures a large percentage of cancer patients who are "worried" about their disease (and possible death), adding a psychiatric diagnosis to their file.

Concerns for (and by) society centered on the "medicalization" of what some consider normal states and on overdiagnosis. In earlier iterations of the criteria, an exclusion had been included that allowed sadness and grief flowing from the loss of a loved one to be considered within normal for up to two months. This exclusion was removed in *DSM-5* (allowing for a diagnosis of major depression earlier in consideration of pharmacological intervention), causing ongoing rancor within psychiatry even 5 years later. Concerns about the overdiagnosis of attention-deficit/hyperactive disorder (ADHD) creating an unreal "epidemic" of this disorder have been voiced for years by both clinicians and researchers. In 2014, Visser et al. (21) reported that nearly one in five high school boys had been diagnosed with ADHD. Irrespective of this well-known ongoing problem with ADHD diagnosis and the resulting untenable rates, the authors of *DSM-5* sought to broaden the criteria, which would cause the prevalence rates to climb even higher.

Three indisputable facts should be recognized at this point. First, psychiatric illness has existed for thousands of years and it has always represented a descriptive (and treatment) challenge for the "modern medicine" of the time. Second, serious mental illness curiously appears neither to be occurring in epidemics nor disappearing. Third, the machinations of various conceptualizations and unsupported labeling have real potential for harming the credibility that psychiatry has so painstakingly developed over the last 60 years and to directly harm society, the main benefactor of these efforts. We strongly urge readers to maintain focus on the established major diagnoses and the supporting scientifically accumulated evidence (from the last 60 years) which comprises the body of this text.

Two years before his untimely death, Sam Guze asked us (C.S.N. and S.H.Y.) to write the sixth edition of *Psychiatric Diagnosis*. We share his vision of the evolution of the field and agree with his view that although neuroscience has evolved over the decades, the fundamentals of psychiatric diagnosis have remained constant. What we have tried to achieve in this latest seventh edition is to incorporate the relevant new scientific research that, not surprisingly, continues to support the fundamental premise of the primacy of psychiatric diagnosis.

Although we remain steadfast in our position that only about a dozen diagnostic entities warrant inclusion as the major psychiatric disorders (see Preface to the First Edition for this heretical view), the field has been working intensely toward validation of other diagnoses, in particular posttraumatic stress disorder and borderline personality disorder. We include chapters on these two diagnoses because they are of considerable recent interest, and to illustrate the state of the art of the validity and reliability status of these disorders (although not because we consider them to have achieved the same level of validation as the first 12 diagnoses in earlier editions of this text).

We have updated references extensively, replacing many of the citations from original research articles with recent review articles to direct readers to currently accessible sources of the material for further study. Readers pursuing historical study of the original work may find the citations in the earlier editions of this text. The current criteria for these major mental illnesses can be found in the *DSM-5,* except for somatization disorder, which can be found in the *DSM-IV-TR.* The original criteria sets which are the direct forerunners can be found in Feighner J, Robins E, Guze S, Woodruff R, Winokur G, and Munoz R, Diagnostic criteria for use in psychiatric research, *Arch. Gen. Psychiatry,* 26:57–62, 1972.

The current authors remain staunchly aligned with the original goal of *Psychiatric Diagnosis*: to provide a concise compendium of current knowledge in psychiatry, with abundant citations, not much theory, and as little personal opinion as possible.

C. S. N.
Dallas, Texas
S. H. Y.
Tallahassee, Florida

PREFACE TO THE FIRST EDITION

> A rose is a rose is a rose.
> GERTRUDE STEIN

Because it remains a rose.

Classification has two functions: communication and prediction. A rose can be defined precisely. It has pinnate leaves, belongs to the rose family, and so forth. When you say "rose" to a person who knows something about the definition, communication results.

A rose also has a predictable life history: It stays a rose. If it changes into a chrysanthemum, it may not have been a rose in the first place. If roses routinely change into chrysanthemums, like caterpillars into butterflies, well and good. Natural history may include metamorphoses but they must be routine to be "natural."

Classification in medicine is called "diagnosis," and this book is about diagnosis of psychiatric conditions. Diagnostic categories—diseases, illnesses, syndromes—are included if they have been sufficiently studied to be useful. Like roses, they can be defined explicitly and have a more or less predictable course.

In choosing these categories, the guiding rule was: *Diagnosis is prognosis.* There are many diagnostic categories in psychiatry, but few are based on a clinical literature where the conditions are defined by explicit criteria and follow-up studies provide a guide to prognosis. Lacking these features, such categories resemble what sociologists call "labeling." Two examples are "passive-aggressive personality" and "emotionally unstable personality," which, like most personality diagnoses, have been inadequately studied for us to know whether they are useful or not.

Not every patient can be diagnosed by using the categories in this book. For them, "undiagnosed" is, we feel, more appropriate than a label incorrectly implying more knowledge than exists. Terms like "functional" and "psychogenic" and "situational reaction" are sometimes invoked by physicians to explain the unexplained. They usually mean "I don't know," and we try to avoid them.

Because classification in psychiatry is still at a primitive stage, there are reasonable grounds for questioning our choice of categories. It general, we lump rather than split. Hence we have two affective disorders—primary and secondary—rather than the half-dozen affective disorders cited in the official nomenclature. Schizophrenia is divided into "good prognosis" and "bad prognosis" schizophrenia rather than sliced more finely, as some prefer. Our justification for this is "the literature," meaning primarily follow-up studies.

"The follow-up is the great exposer of truth, the rock on which many fine theories are wrecked and upon which better ones can be built," wrote P. D. Scott. "It is to the psychiatrist what the postmortem is to the physician." Not all such studies are perfect, but we feel they are better than no studies. And inevitably there are instances where our "clinical judgment" has prevailed in evaluating the merit of individual studies. No text in psychiatry could be written today without a certain amount of this, but we have tried to limit personal opinion to a minimum. Many if not most assertions have a citation, and the reader can check the references to form his own judgment.

When the term "disease" is used, this is what is meant: A disease is a cluster of symptoms and/or signs with a more or less predictable course. Symptoms are what patients tell you; signs are what you see. The cluster may be associated with physical abnormality or may not. The essential point is that it results in consultation with a physician who specializes in recognizing, preventing, and sometimes, curing diseases.

It is hard for many people to think of psychiatric problems as diseases. For one thing, psychiatric problems usually consist of symptoms—complaints about thoughts and feelings—or behavior disturbing to others. Rarely are there signs—a fever, a rash. Almost never are there laboratory tests to confirm the diagnosis. What people say changes from time to time, as does behavior. It is usually harder to agree about symptoms than about signs. But whatever the psychiatric problems are, they have this in common with "real" diseases—they result in consultation with a physician and are associated with pain, suffering, disability, and death.

Another objection to the disease or medical "model" arises from a misconception about disease. Disease often is equated with physical abnormality. In fact, a disease is a category used by physicians, as "apples" is a category used by grocers. It is a useful category if precise and if the encompassed phenomena are stable over time. Diseases are conventions and may not "fit" anything in nature at all. Through the centuries, diseases have come and gone, some more useful than others, and there is no guarantee that our present "disease"— medical or psychiatric—will represent the same clusters of symptoms and signs a hundred years from now that they do today. On the contrary, as more is learned, more useful clusters surely will emerge.

There are few explanations in this book. This is because for most psychiatric conditions there *are* no explanations. "Etiology unknown" is the hallmark of psychiatry as well as its bane. Historically, once etiology is known, a disease stops being "psychiatric." Vitamins were discovered, whereupon vitamin-deficiency psychiatric disorders no longer were treated by psychiatrists. The spirochete was found, then penicillin, and neurosyphilis, once a major psychiatric disorder, became one more infection treated by nonpsychiatrists.

Little, however, is really known about most medical illnesses. Even infectious diseases remain puzzles in that some infected individuals have symptoms and others do not.

People continue to speculate about etiology, of course, and this is good if it produces testable hypotheses and bad if speculation is mistaken for truth. In this book, speculation largely is avoided, since it is available so plentifully elsewhere.

A final word about this approach to psychiatry. It is sometimes called "organic." This is misleading. A better term, perhaps, is "agnostic." Without evidence, we do not believe pills are better than words. Without evidence, we do not believe chemistry is more important than upbringing. Without evidence, we withhold judgment.

Advocacy is not the purpose of this book. Rather, we hope it will be useful in applying current knowledge to those vexatious problems—crudely defined and poorly understood—that come within the jurisdiction of psychiatry.

D. W. G.
Saint Louis
December 1973

LOOKING FORWARD

PSYCHIATRIC DIAGNOSIS—AN UPDATE AND CONTINUING LOOK FORWARD

Diagnosis is the cornerstone of medicine. It allows physicians to communicate effectively with their patients and other healthcare professionals and serves as a prediction about the future. It is the means by which physicians make treatment decisions and are able to assess whether an intervention has a beneficial effect. In the absence of accurate, reliable and valid diagnosis, medicine becomes a "Tower of Babel" in which clinical information is very difficult to interpret. This lesson has been learned more slowly in psychiatry than in other fields of medicine, but thanks to psychiatrists at Washington University in St. Louis, the field has moved to a reliable, criteria-based system of classification over the past 50 years. Early pioneers included Eli Robins, Sam Guze, George Winokur, and a host of others at Renard Hospital in the 1960s and '70s. Their efforts were highlighted with the publication of a set of criteria for psychiatric diagnoses by John Feighner and colleagues in 1972 (11). Subsequently, Bob Woodruff, Don Goodwin, and Sam Guze published the first edition of this text, *Psychiatric Diagnosis*, in 1974 (22). The book has subsequently undergone several revisions. In 2010, Carol North and Sean Yutzy, former members of the Department of Psychiatry at Washington University, published the sixth edition of this classic text, providing major updates from prior editions and doing a tremendous service for the field of psychiatry. In the latest edition, they have provided us with an outstanding and thoroughly updated version taking into account recent advances in the field.

At the time of the last edition, I wrote a preface discussing a prospective view of psychiatric diagnosis, and described the field as being at an important period in its history. It is now appropriate to take a look at what has happened since that time and how this has influenced psychiatric diagnosis. One of the major developments since the last edition of this text was the publication of *DSM-5* in 2013 (6). *DSM-5* was highly anticipated in 2010 and provided some advances in the criteria for psychiatric illnesses, some new illness classifications, and some changes in how illnesses are categorized. As many in the field thought at the time, *DSM-5* is a thoughtful, but incremental, extension of work that originated with the publication of the Feighner criteria in 1972 (11), the first edition of *Psychiatric Diagnosis* in 1974 (22), and *DSM-III* in 1980 (2). Unfortunately, *DSM-5*, while useful, has not fundamentally altered conceptualization of psychiatric illnesses and may be viewed as a relatively small step forward for the field, remaining consistent with traditional categorical descriptions of disorders. Categorical approaches remain extremely helpful for clinicians, and psychiatric categorical diagnoses can be applied highly reliably, consistent with other recent editions of the *DSM*. As noted in all editions of this book, validation of the major psychiatric syndromes remains problematic and is largely based on clinical criteria initially developed in the 1970s (18). The field continues to lack mechanistic explanations and meaningful biomarkers.

In parallel to *DSM-5*, other attempts have considered psychiatric symptoms from dimensional perspectives, in which specific symptoms and traits are viewed as being continuously distributed in the population with disorders representing far ends of the distribution spectra. The most notable example of this approach is found in the Research Domain Criteria (RDoC) project, launched by the National Institute of Mental Health (NIMH) in 2010 (9). RDoC attempts to relate psychiatric symptoms more closely to advances in brain science and in understanding brain systems that likely underlie these symptoms. This has had a significant impact on research (as would be expected from an NIH-driven initiative), but the impact on psychiatric diagnosis and practice has been much less clear. Nonetheless, a possible marriage of categorical and dimensional approaches remains possible and could have a significant impact going forward, particularly as brain sciences and behavioral genetics continue to evolve.

The past eight years have witnessed major advances in neuroscience and genetics that hold great, but not yet realized potential for psychiatry. In 2009, the first round of the Human Connectome Project (HCP) was launched. This project sought to map functional connectivity neural networks in the normal human adult brain using an array of sophisticated imaging and neuroscience tools, including state-of-the-art functional connectivity magnetic resonance neuroimaging (fcMRI) and sophisticated analytical methods based on graph theory and network analysis (12). HCP provides important information about the brain networks that can be identified in humans, networks that underlie cognition, perception, emotion and motivation, key components of the human mind, and aspects of information processing that are altered in all major psychiatric illnesses. HCP is being extended across the human lifespan and will continue to produce major new insights into how the brain functions in health and illness.

A major challenge going forward concerns how to relate the understanding that has derived from studies of relatively large groups of individuals to the connectomes of individual humans (13), particularly those with psychiatric illnesses. Again, progress is being made in this arena, but it is still not possible to use fcMRI for diagnostic purposes at the level of individual patients. This latter situation could change dramatically before the next editions of *Psychiatric Diagnosis* and the *DSM* are published. Already, significant inroads are being made in using connectivity neuroimaging to subclassify groups of patients with major depression and other illnesses and to make predictions about possible treatments targeted to illness subtypes (10). This work will undoubtedly continue to advance over the next decade and continues to hold great promise for the field.

While advances in human neuroscience have been dramatic over the past eight years, they arguably pale in comparison to the accomplishments in preclinical neuroscience. Neuroscientists now have at their disposal an array of highly sophisticated methodologies to probe the activity of cells and networks of cells in live animals as they perform a variety of behaviors likely related to psychiatric symptoms and syndromes. These techniques include ways to manipulate the expression of specific genes using CRISPR-Cas9 gene editing technology (Clustered Regularly Interspersed Short Palindromic Repeats) (16), the ability to study the anatomy of circuits in exquisite detail using CLARITY methods (7), and the ability to manipulate the activity of neurons and others cells within neural circuits using optogenetics and visible light pulses to activate ion channels and other proteins expressed in specific brain cells (15). This work has advanced greatly in recent years, and studies using these methods are now routinely conducted in major neuroscience laboratories around the world. Studies using these methods have provided new insights into how the mammalian brain processes information, how emotions are coded in the brain, and how specific neural circuits underlie motivated behavior. Coupled with these methods have been advances in animal behavioral studies, including models of animal behavior that may have relevance for psychiatric disorders. As with human neuroscience, studies using these methods and derivatives of these methods are in their infancy, although progress is being made rapidly. How these studies in animals, particularly in rodent models, translate into insights about human disorders and into new treatments remains uncertain, but this is an active sphere of investigation and one that warrants cautious optimism.

We have also witnessed an explosion of information in psychiatric (and complex disease) genetics over the past eight years. The field of psychiatric genetics has long been plagued by identification of genes of small effect size that often have not held up to replication, in part because of under-powered samples.

Advances in genetics including the evolution of more sophisticated analytical methods, coupled with the realization that studies must have very large numbers of participants in order to identify replicable changes, have had a major recent impact. Understanding of numerous psychiatric illnesses, such as autism and schizophrenia, has advanced and provided new insights into the complexity of the genetic structure of these sets of disorders. This includes findings that over 100 genes (likely more) contribute to schizophrenia (1), with perhaps an even higher number of genes being associated with autism. These genes involve complex signaling systems within the brain, including genes that contribute to neuroinflammation, neurodevelopment, and synaptic plasticity, among others (1, 19). Again, it is not certain how this new information will translate into better psychiatric diagnoses, but we can expect increasing use of polygenic risk scores in future studies with the hope of translating this information to the diagnosis and care of individual patients (17).

We are also getting a much clearer understanding of the complexity of psychiatric genetics and recognizing that there is genetic overlap among multiple major psychiatric phenotypes. Phenotypic and genetic pleiotropy will likely become even more complex going forward and could have a major impact on how we think about the diagnostic system. The continuing evolution of sophisticated methods for sequencing genes and for understanding the factors that regulate gene expression, including the important area of epigenetics, will be part of the process. In this latter area lies the critical ability to understand the impact of the environment on gene expression and brain function. Importantly, the cost of studying individual genomes continues to plummet and will be aided by rapidly advancing technologies and analytical methods. Advances in cellular science and the conversion of patient-derived inducible pluripotent stem cells (iPSCs) into neurons and other brain cells, including growth of these cells in organoid models, offer the hope of studying how an individual patient's genetics contribute to changes in brain cell and network function (20).

While advances in neuroscience and genetics have not yet translated into improved diagnosis or validated biomarkers for psychiatric illness, it appears that new treatments are on the horizon, based, at least in part, on sophisticated neuroscience. Eight years ago there was considerable hope about the development of novel pharmacological treatments, including the possibility that ketamine and other antagonists of N-methyl-D-aspartate (NMDA) glutamate receptors could be brought to clinical practice as rapidly acting but transient antidepressants for patients with treatment-resistant major depression. This work has continued to advance and has gained increasing scientific acceptance. While it is still premature to use ketamine in clinical practice and there are concerns about how to maintain the short-term benefits and the possible consequences of long-term use, it appears likely that drugs of this type will be approved and become available over the next few years (23).

The evolution of ketamine marks a major change in the types of drugs that will be available for treating complex psychiatric illnesses. Similarly, other novel agents are in development, again based on advances in neuroscience, including neurosteroids that target gamma aminobutyric acid (GABA) receptors and are at advanced stages of development for treatment of severe postpartum depression, and possibly other forms of depression (14). Newer developments in structural biology using cryo electron microscopy are providing novel insights into how protein structure affects function and how pharmacological agents interact with proteins (8). This latter work offers the hope of identifying much more specific drugs with high therapeutic efficacy and fewer side effects. Another hope going forward is that the combination of functional neuroimaging with neuromodulation methods such as transcranial magnetic stimulation (TMS) can offer more effective treatment strategies with fewer side effects than with current treatments.

In summary, as we enjoy North and Yutzy's insights in this latest edition of *Psychiatric Diagnosis*, psychiatry remains at a critical crossroad. Science will continue to advance and this bodes well for the field and for patients with these devastating and disabling illnesses. North and Yutzy are to be congratulated once again for their efforts in this updated version of *Psychiatric Diagnosis*. Their clarity of thought and tough-minded approach to psychiatry remain a beacon for our field and will serve us well as science advances. It is now up to science to take advantage of its opportunities to provide the next revolution in understanding and treating psychiatric illnesses. Only when that occurs will we be ready for the next edition of the *DSM*.

Charles F. Zorumski, MD
Washington University in St. Louis

REFERENCES

1. [No author listed]. Biological insights from 108 schizophrenia-associated genetic loci. Nature, *511*:421–427, 2014.
2. American Psychiatric Association. *Diagnostic and Statistical Manual of Mental Disorders*, 3rd edition. Washington, DC: Author, 1980.
3. American Psychiatric Association. *Diagnostic and Statistical Manual of Mental Disorders*, 3rd revised edition. Washington, DC: Author, 1987.
4. American Psychiatric Association. *Diagnostic and Statistical Manual of Mental Disorders*, 4th edition. Washington, DC: Author, 1994.
5. American Psychiatric Association. *Diagnostic and Statistical Manual of Mental Disorders*, 4th text revision edition. Washington, DC: Author, 2000.
6. American Psychiatric Association. *Diagnostic and Statistical Manual for Mental Disorders*, 5th edition. Washington, DC: Author, 2013.
7. Chung, K., and Deisseroth, K. CLARITY for mapping the nervous system. Nat. Methods, *10*:508–513, 2013.
8. Costa, T. R. D., Ignatiou, A., and Orlova, E. V. Structural analysis of protein complexes by cryo electron microscopy. Methods Mol. Biol., *1615*:377–413, 2017.
9. Cuthbert, B. N. Research Domain Criteria: toward future psychiatric nosologies. Dialogues Clin. Neurosci., *17*:89–97, 2015.
10. Drysdale, A. T., Grosenick, L., Downar, J., Dunlop, K., Mansouri, F., Meng, Y., Fetcho, R. N., Zebley, B., Oathes, D. J., Etkin, A., Schatzberg, A. F., Sudheimer, K., Keller, J., Mayberg, H. S., Gunning, F. M., Alexopoulos, G. S., Fox, M. D., Pascual-Leone, A., Voss, H. U., Casey, B. J., Dubin, M. J., and Liston, C. Resting-state connectivity biomarkers define neurophysiological subtypes of depression. Nat. Med., *23*:28–38, 2017.
11. Feighner, J. P., Robins, E., Guze, S. B., Woodruff, R. A., Winokur, G., and Muñoz, R. Diagnostic criteria for use in psychiatric research. Arch. Gen. Psychiatry, *26*:57–62, 1972.
12. Glasser, M. F., Coalson, T. S., Robinson, E. C., Hacker, C. D., Harwell, J., Yacoub, E., Ugurbil, K., Andersson, J., Beckmann, C. F., Jenkinson, M., Smith, S. M., and Van Essen, D. C. A multi-modal parcellation of human cerebral cortex. Nature, *536*:171–178, 2016.
13. Gordon, E. M., Laumann, T. O., Gilmore, A. W., Newbold, D. J., Greene, D. J., Berg, J. J., Ortega, M., Hoyt-Drazen, C., Gratton, C., Sun, H., Hampton, J. M., Coalson, R. S., Nguyen, A. L., McDermott, K. B., Shimony, J. S., Snyder, A. Z., Schlaggar, B. L., Petersen, S. E., Nelson, S. M., and Dosenbach, N. U. F. Precision functional mapping of individual human brains. Neuron, *95*:791–807, 2017.
14. Kanes, S., Colquhoun, H., Gunduz-Bruce, H., Raines, S., Arnold, R., Schacterle, A., Doherty, J., Epperson, C. N., Deligiannidis, K. M., Riesenberg, R., Hoffmann, E., Rubinow, D., Jonas, J., Paul, S., and Meltzer-Brody, S. Brexanolone (SAGE-547 injection) in post-partum depression: a randomised controlled trial. Lancet, *390*:480–489, 2017.
15. Kim, C. K., Adhikari, A., and Deisseroth, K. Integration of optogenetics with complementary methodologies in systems neuroscience. Nat. Rev. Neurosci., *18*:222–235, 2017.
16. Komor, A. C., Badran, A. H., and Liu, D. R. CRISPR-based technologies for the manipulation of eukaryotic genomes. Cell, *168*:20–36, 2017.

17. Mistry, S., Harrison, J. R., Smith, D. J., Escott-Price, V., and Zammit, S. The use of polygenic risk scores to identify phenotypes associated with genetic risk of bipolar disorder and depression: a systematic review. J. Affect. Disord., *234*:148–155, 2018.

18. Robins, E., and Guze, S. B. Establishment of diagnostic validity in psychiatric illness: its application to schizophrenia. Am. J. Psychiatry, *126*:983–987, 1970.

19. Sekar, A., Bielar, A. R., de Rivera, H., Davis, A., Hammond, T. R., Kamitaki, N., Tooley, K., Presumey, J., Baum, M., Van Doren, V., Genovese, J., Rose, S. A., Handsaker, R. E., Daly, M. J., Carroll, M. C., Stevens, B., and McCarroll, S. A. Schizophrenia risk from complex variation of complement component 4. Nature, *530*:177–183, 2016.

20. Shinn, M., Knickman, J. R., and Weitzman, B. C. Social relationships and vulnerability to becoming homeless among poor families. Am. Psychol., *46(11)*:1180–1187, 1991.

21. Visser, S. N., Danielson, M. L., Bitsko, R. H., Holbrook, J. R., Kogan, M. D., Ghandour, R. M., Perou, R., and Blumberg, S. J. Trends in the parent-report of health care provider-diagnosed and medicated attention-deficit/hyperactivity disorder: United States, 2003–2011. J. Am. Acad. Child Adolesc. Psychiatry, *53*:34–46, 2014.

22. Woodruff, R. A., Jr., Goodwin, D. W., and Guze, S. B. *Psychiatric Diagnosis*. New York: Oxford University Press, 1974.

23. Zorumski, C. F., and Conway, C. R. Use of ketamine in clinical practice: a time for optimism and caution. JAMA Psychiatry, *74*:405–406, 2017.

Goodwin and Guze's Psychiatric Diagnosis

CHAPTER 1

⌒⌒

Evolution of Psychiatric Diagnosis

The diagnostic approach in psychiatry does not have a long and illustrious tradition in the United States. Historically, Freud and his influential psychoanalytic school in Europe during the late 1800s focused on symptoms that were felt to be of "psychogenic" origin. Subsequently, the fundamental principles of psychoanalysis were imported into the United States, where they predominated for almost three-quarters of the twentieth century.

The American Psychiatric Association (APA) published the first *Diagnostic and Statistical Manual of Mental Disorders* (*DSM*) in 1952 (2), moving American psychiatry incrementally toward a descriptive approach. Although that text included various psychiatric conditions with diagnostic labels, it did not provide explicit criteria, and most symptoms were conceptualized in a framework of a reaction to a situation or stressor. Consistent with the predominating Freudian approach at that time in America, symptoms were considered to originate from underlying dynamic conflicts, representing symbolic meaning. Understanding a patient's symptoms required exploration of that individual's own developmental history and life experiences (35). Problematic to scientific advancement of the field within this approach was the flaw that such prevailing assumptions about the etiology of psychiatric problems were scientifically untestable (45). Further, problems of unreliability plagued symptom interpretation, a process unique to the individual patient and inconsistent from one clinician to the next. Definition of psychiatric problems using these approaches poorly differentiated healthy from ill individuals and hampered communication among clinicians about their cases. In 1968, the APA published the second edition of the diagnostic manual (*DSM-II*) (3), which embraced the disease concept for mental illness—but again without explicit criteria. Diagnostic reliability was not yet a feature of the proffered labels. To find its place among the medical sciences, psychiatry needed to develop an epidemiological system for classifying disease, known as "nosology" (35).

Several European physicians specializing in problems of psychiatry (Kraepelin, Kahlbaum, Bleuler, and others) who predated or were contemporaries of Freud found it more useful to describe the phenomenology of mental illness as clustering in "syndromes" according to their unique symptoms, course, and outcome over time. These physicians followed an earlier and evolving approach to disease initiated by Sydenham in the late 1600s and further developed over the centuries by Koch, Pasteur, Virchow, and others. The relevant assumption by most of these investigators was that identification of a syndrome would lead to a better understanding of the illness and possibly etiology. Kraepelin considered mental disorders to be commensurate with physical diseases. He followed medical traditions of careful observation of many cases to describe overt characteristics of illness, rather than relying on unproven etiological theories. Kraepelin predicted that empirical research would eventually provide evidence of biological origins of mental illness (45, 51).

The classification/diagnostic approach and attendant scientific methods were not systematically applied in American psychiatry until the advent of the "descriptive school" in the latter half of the twentieth century, whose traditions were founded on the earlier work of Sydenham, Kraepelin, and others. During the 1960s and early 1970s, the Washington University group in St. Louis, described as "an outpost of diagnostically oriented thinking" (p. 259) (45), refined the descriptive approach to psychiatry and distinguished themselves as radically different from the prevailing psychoanalytic school. In American psychiatry at that time, the belief that mental disorders were a subset of medical disorders was controversial (45) if not heretical. Members of this group, often referred to as "neo-Kraepelinians," were described by some as "organic" or "biological" in orientation, but their position regarding the origin of symptoms was simply "what the evidence or reproducible data demonstrated."

In 1970, Robins and Guze (44), at Washington University in St. Louis, published their proposal for five phases necessary to establish the validity and reliability of a psychiatric diagnosis. These phases included the following:

1. *Clinical description.* The first step is to describe the clinical picture. Race, sex, age at onset, precipitating factor(s), and other items may be used to define characteristics and occurrence of the disorder. The clinical picture

observed in the United States should be the same as in the United Kingdom, Russia, and elsewhere.

2. *Laboratory studies.* These include any laboratory test of a chemical, physiological, radiological, or anatomical (biopsy or autopsy) nature that could reproducibly demonstrate a finding.

3. *Delimitation from other disorders.* The disorder of interest must be distinguishable from other potentially overlapping disorders.

4. *Follow-up studies.* The initial diagnosis is reconfirmed at follow-up (usually years later), supporting the original diagnosis.

5. *Family studies.* Most psychiatric illnesses have been shown to run in families, whether of genetic or environmental origin. Identification of the illness in the family supports the validity of the diagnosis.

Feighner et al., in 1972 (17), outlined the diagnoses and criteria that met these phases. Included were the following: primary affective disorder (mania/depression), secondary affective disorder, schizophrenia, anxiety neurosis, obsessive-compulsive neurosis, phobic neurosis, hysteria, antisocial personality disorder, alcoholism, drug dependence, mental retardation, organic brain syndrome, anorexia nervosa, and several others. It should be noted that with the possible exception of brain syndrome(s), laboratory studies have still not been developed that reproducibly demonstrate pathological lesions. However, thoughtful and careful completion, with replication, of most of the phases (1, 3, 4, and 5) firmly established the bases for the validity of the major mental illnesses.

To gain a foothold in the published literature, this group published their early work in diagnostic psychiatry in British and other European literature, outside the reach of American hostility to their ideas (Samuel B. Guze, personal communication). In 1974, the first edition of *Psychiatric Diagnosis*, co-authored by Robert A. Woodruff, Jr., Donald W. Goodwin, and Samuel B. Guze, was published by Oxford University Press (50). Although written for the education of medical students, it became an icon for the field. At the time, this text was arguably the most authoritative source of diagnostic psychiatry, as the current diagnostic manual of the APA had not yet incorporated empirically based criteria.

In the late 1970s, Robert Spitzer, with remarkable political finesse, convened meetings of members of the two formal psychiatric schools, psychoanalytic and evidence-based/biological (45), to generate the third edition of the *Diagnostic and Statistical Manual* (*DSM-III*) (4). The text was generally intended to be atheoretical in orientation regarding the origin of most psychopathology. (Of note, to appease an opposition that threatened to block the document's approval, the word *neurosis*, a concept fundamental to Freudian psychoanalysis, was retained parenthetically after the word *disorder* (45). *Neurosis* did not survive the next revision of the diagnostic text.) *DSM-III* was the first of the APA's diagnostic manuals to embrace the Washington University (St. Louis) group's emphasis that medical diagnosis is the keystone of medical practice and research (45). The *DSM-III* text included practically *en bloc* the Feighner criteria for the diagnoses of the major mental illnesses. Unfortunately for validity and reliability considerations, the text also included approximately 365 other "mental disorder" labels developed by expert consensus and with essentially untested criteria (35). Nonetheless, the creation of a common language utilizing valid and reliable psychiatric diagnoses, as well as defining explicit criteria, was an important advance.

Although some considered the advances of *DSM-III* a revolution, many data-oriented psychiatrists saw it as simply a move to align with the substantially evolved general medical model of the time. With *DSM-III*, psychiatric diagnosis became practical and useful to clinicians as well as researchers. Psychiatrists now had psychiatric diagnoses that provided clear boundaries for major psychiatric illnesses within dichotomies rather than dimensions that blurred boundaries between normal and abnormal. These diagnoses were based on documented observations of psychopathology rather than on unsupportable theoretical etiological mechanisms (45). Of particular note was the fact that diagnostic reliability (measured by the *kappa* statistic designed to measure diagnostic concordance or agreement about diagnosis between examinations) of the major diagnoses moved into the good-to-excellent range, equaling the established reliability of medical diagnoses made on clinical grounds. The data-based school continued describing its approach to psychiatric nosology simply as "medical model" (dating back to 1973). This term is broader than "biological" (implying limitation within purely physical processes such as genes and brain chemistry). The medical model is more descriptive of the categorical/diagnostic approach, which encompasses all aspects of illness, including environmental and social aspects, within medical definitions and descriptions.

At first, the academicians involved with the development of *DSM-III* and those embracing the new medical model of psychiatry were alleged to constitute an "invisible college" of professionals trained at Washington University dispersed to leadership positions at the University of Iowa, the University of Minnesota, the University of Kansas, and Columbia University in New York City, among other sites (12). As their numbers and their publications grew and these clinicians/scientists blended into the landscape of American psychiatry under the aegis of *DSM-III* and its predecessors, the invisible college grew into the mainstream institution.

Prevailing forces in medicine and psychiatry at the time facilitated and embraced the changes brought about with *DSM-III* (45). Prior to *DSM-III*, psychiatry had largely fallen outside the mainstream of the science and practice of medicine. Psychologists, social workers, and other mental health professionals threatened to replace psychiatrists. Critics of psychiatry claimed that definitions of mental illnesses did not have objective criteria, some asserting that psychiatric illness did not even exist. *DSM-III* provided objective diagnostic criteria and positioned psychiatric diagnosis within the medical purview. Psychiatry reasserted its place in medicine as a medical specialty. Evolving computer technology contributed substantially to the investigation of empirical aspects of disease. Advances in diagnosis provided powerful incentives to the pharmaceutical industry and independent researchers to develop new medications and other treatments targeted for treatment of specific disorders. Insurance companies sought diagnostic structure to guide reimbursement for treatment of validated disorders with demonstrable evidence of specified treatments for them. The achievement of diagnostic reliability led to new research opportunities and directions (45).

Subsequent versions of the APA textbook (*DSM-III-R* (5), *DSM-IV* (6), and *DSM-IV-TR* (7)) further solidified and reaffirmed the transformation of American psychiatry to an empirically based system of classification of diagnosis that *DSM-III* initiated (45). They also, however, further increased and expanded the number of labeled mental disorders (6, 7). Unfortunately, the new labels promulgated have not met the five phases outlined by Robins and Guze, which over time have become the "gold standard" for establishing validity and reliability of a psychiatric diagnosis. In sum, the vast majority of diagnostic labels in the latest version (*DSM-5*) have not met the diagnostic gold standard. Not surprisingly, research on many of the coded non-major "mental disorders" or labels during the 1990s and later have led to significant questions about comorbidity (i.e., problems with delimitation). (For specific examples of these problems, see also Chapters 5 and 10 on posttraumatic stress disorder and borderline personality disorder, respectively.)

The effects of the medical model movement in psychiatry have been substantial. The National Institute of Mental Health (NIMH) embraced the *DSM-III* (27). Shortly after the publication of *DSM-III*, students and physicians from American medical schools and residency programs were expected to pass qualifying examinations based on APA diagnostic criteria. Scholarly journals and federal research-granting agencies similarly assumed conformation to current diagnostic conventions as delineated in

APA criteria. Colleagues in different locales, even different countries, could finally collaborate using a common diagnostic language (45).

Through this history, the *Psychiatric Diagnosis* textbook stayed alive. Accumulated data in support of the valid major mental illnesses over half a century were slowly and painstakingly gathered into the second, third, fourth, fifth, sixth, and now seventh editions. The original authors have all passed away: first Bob Woodruff (1976), later Don Goodwin (1999), and finally Sam Guze (2000). The text's current authors were trained by the original members of the Washington University group, Eli Robins and Sam Guze, and, as students, read *Psychiatric Diagnosis* along with the hundreds and thousands of other students educated with this text over the years.

The subsequent chapters in this text review the accumulated wealth of data over the years relevant to the diagnoses included in it. The information is not meant to comprise a cutting-edge review of the latest findings in research. Rather, it is meant to provide fundamental and time-tested evidence for psychiatric disorders to teach and support the principles of psychiatric diagnosis so eloquently constructed through established empirical research.

This chapter would not be complete without addressing and placing in proper perspective the major trends that are currently buffeting the field of psychiatry. Medicine, and particularly psychiatry, has come under significant pressure to assess pathology in short time frames and develop outcome measures to justify an intervention. Expectations to collect large amounts of data rapidly and inexpensively, under pressures to limit costs in the face of inadequate resources, have encouraged the substitution of brief screening instruments and self-report questionnaires for identification of psychiatric disorders in lieu of more burdensome and costly full diagnostic assessment—in both research and clinical settings. These shortcuts, however, cannot substitute for carefully establishing a psychiatric diagnosis.

Although some screening tools may have utility for other limited purposes, such as following symptom levels over time, they do not rely on or yield adequate information for a formal diagnosis. Screening instruments may be appropriate and useful for identifying a high-risk subgroup when the population of interest is too large to permit full diagnostic assessment of all its members and to identify a subset of individuals at high risk for illness who can then be further assessed using the full diagnostic criteria. Screening instruments without formal interview, however, should not be relied on for assigning a psychiatric diagnosis that provides the basis for treatment decisions. Further, screening instruments are inadequate for assessing general-population prevalence rates of psychopathology.

Unfortunately, the research literature is fraught with examples of studies inappropriately using screening instruments to diagnose cases and estimate population prevalence. In addition, short time frames for completion of clinical and research contacts and assessments without benefit of collateral information such as medical records (which are becoming more difficult to obtain because of systems complexities and shorter holding times before destruction), inability to locate and interview family members who can provide relevant history, and inability to complete appropriate testing all contribute to diagnostic imprecision.

Evolving developments in biological and radiological technology are increasingly providing new directions for scientific exploration. Many such leads, holding the promise of fundamental advances in the understanding of psychopathology, have disappointingly not delivered as anticipated. A classic example is the dexamethasone suppression test, introduced in the early 1980s, which was hoped to be psychiatry's first laboratory test (14). This putative marker generated great interest and hundreds of articles; however, low sensitivity of the test limited its clinical utility (9), although it has remained a useful research tool. Efforts are continuously ongoing to develop a biological or imaging test or procedure that can identify any psychiatric illness.

Psychiatric genetics is another area that was hoped to translate into nosological insights that could further revolutionize conceptualization and utility of psychiatric diagnosis. It has been predicted that increasing elucidation of genotype–phenotype relationships may eventually force the abandonment of traditional Kraepelinian dichotomy in the classification of psychiatric illness (15). Continuing research, however, has yielded growing frustration and no indications that genetic research findings will fundamentally alter empirically based classification of psychiatric illness any time soon. First, no "Mendelian-like" genes have been found for the major psychiatric disorders, and it is generally recognized that none will be found. Second, efforts to carve nature at its joints are not destined to cleave psychiatric disorders using purely genetic tools, because the psychiatric phenotype is more than a product of its genes. Kendler (29) concluded in 2006 that even genes known to be involved in the generation of psychopathology cannot provide the basis for construction of psychiatric diagnoses. He predicted that molecular genetics, like traditional genetics, will offer disappointingly little in terms of advancing conceptualization of psychiatric diagnosis. As this text goes to press, continually advancing genetics methodologies, including genome-wide linkage and candidate and genome association, have yet to provide definitive answers, as can be seen in the subsequent chapters.

Advances in biological science continually challenge the field of psychiatry to evolve. An empirical approach to classification in psychiatry was revolutionary in the 1970s when, as previously noted, a small group of academicians and their text, *Psychiatric Diagnosis,* were instrumental in changing the field. Formal criteria (Research Diagnostic Criteria, RDC) were incorporated into the *DSM-III* and subsequent editions of the classification system, using a dichotomous approach to diagnosis with criteria and scientific evidence basis for incremental change. This approach was generally accepted for many years, but subsequent pressures to change arose during a period of exponential growth in research, particularly after publication of the *DSM-III-R* in 1987. Not surprisingly, critics of the *DSM* classification system have replayed and amplified suggestions of past eras for a "dimensional construction" of diagnostic concepts.

Critics of the categorical diagnostic approach rightfully pointed to the inflation of the number of recognized psychiatric diagnoses as problematic (36). Other critics were troubled by the inability to classify symptomatic individuals not meeting diagnostic criteria as supporting the promotion of concepts of "partial" or "spectrum" diagnoses. Continuing concerns about lack of clear demarcation between diagnostic cases and others (37) had not recognized the original specification that the system was imperfect and that approximately one out of five cases assessed in the Washington University tradition were not cross-sectionally classifiable in the diagnostic structure. Uncertainties in estimation of boundaries had been built into the Feighner diagnostic classification process to circumvent otherwise unsolvable problems of diagnostic decision-making.

Nonetheless, in response to some of the aforementioned criticisms (and others), in 2002, Kupfer et al. wrote in *A Research Agenda for DSM-V,* produced jointly by the APA and NIMH, that "a slavish adoption of DSM-IV definitions may have hindered research in the etiology of mental disorders" (p. xix) (33). Substantive consideration was to be given to a paradigm change. In 2006, David Kupfer (Chair of Task Force for *DSM-V*) and Darrel Reiger (Vice Chair) were named, and in 2007 and 2008, the members of the *DSM-5* Task Force and the 13 Work Groups were nominated and approved (8). (Note the change in formatting of the criteria edition number from Roman numeral to Arabic between the time of the planning phases and publication of *DSM-5*.) According to the APA (8), the priorities were to include the following: 1) add dimensional measures to enhance diagnosis, 2) include etiological and neurobiological research in the definitions and criteria, 3) align the *DSM* series with the International Classification of Diseases (ICD), and, finally, 4) improve clinical utility.

Regardless of whether this effort in retrospect may have been grandiose is debatable, the academic concerns escalating to outright attack on the process (11, 18, 22, 31, 39–42, 48) began well before publication of the *DSM-5* and have continued for years on many aspects of the current criteria (19, 20, 24, 30, 32, 46, 49). Recognizing that the field of psychiatry is not immune to vigorous academic debate, this particular debate was unexpectedly intense (21). Problematic were the facts that the first two of the APA priorities listed for *DSM-5* did not materialize, the individual Work Groups rejected most of the dimensional measures (53), and neurobiological and genetic evidence remained elusive (38). Clinical utility of the posited criteria was called into question because of major alterations to the long-accepted structure of the criteria, including removal of the multi-axial system and the Global Assessment of Functioning (GAF) scale (43). Additionally, a large number of proponents (and users) of the *DSM* series, both researchers and clinicians, were troubled by changes to various criteria sets (47, 52)—as exemplified by "a rancorous battle" (p. 7) (53) over the personality disorder criteria. Not surprisingly, the battles spilled into the mass media.

At the launch of *DSM-5* in 2013, calls were made by the former *DSM-IV* Task Force Chairman Alan Frances (23) to use *DSM-5* "cautiously if at all" (p. 222) and by former director Thomas Insel of the NIMH (who partly funded the project) to directly move away from the tenets of the *DSM-5*, further contributing to the chaos (27). Contemporaneous with direct concerns about the development and direction of the *DSM-5*, along with the early failure of genetic and neurobiological evidence to map the major diagnostic labels, was publication in 2010 by Insel (27) of the NIMH promoting the Research Domain Criteria (RDoC). Directly citing the seminal work of Robins and Guze in the 1970s which directly folded into the Research Diagnostic Criteria (and later into the *DSM-III* as noted above), Insel raised the issue of trying to move forward a research paradigm to establish a new nosological framework to better integrate upcoming anticipated neurobiological and genetics findings into diagnostic criteria. Such a classification scheme would have the clearly identified goal of better treatment outcomes (28).

Cuthbert and Insel (16) further elaborated the RDoC structure, encouraging research around five major domains: 1) Negative Valence Systems (pushing reactions to aversive stimuli), 2) Positive Valence Systems (moving reactions to positive stimuli), 3) Cognitive Systems (including mental processes), 4) Social Processes (responsible for interpersonal behavior and cognition), and 5) Arousal and Regulatory Systems (involved in context-based homeostatic systems and neurological systems). In theory, the purpose would be to organize these items as they evolve into a new diagnostic nosology. (This material was later expanded and made available on the NIMH website (1).) Review of the research literature completed by Carconne (13) identified, of most import, the finding that work was proceeding on this new construct.

Naturally, significant concerns have been raised on a number of fronts, including preferential NIMH funding directed to this paradigm, limitations of technology which may simply not exist to allow this research to proceed, and finally, the research may be "oversold" (p. 47) (25). Noteworthy and forgotten by some was the fact that Insel clearly identified at the outset (2013) that the paradigm may not work in clinical settings (28).

These last two major events and their aftermath may underscore what some opine is, or should be, a crisis in psychiatric diagnosis (10, 16, 34). It is easy in retrospect to criticize the frankly failed attempt at a paradigm shift to dimensionalism in *DSM-5* and a complex theoretical neuroscience research paradigm, which the authors admitted may never bear clinical fruit in the decades to come; however, it is a problem to dismiss the entire dimensionalism theory. Many research authors have been in support of adding this paradigm to the diagnostic nomenclature for many reasons, but with the main goals of better capturing and defining cases. Further, and persuasive, is the fact that historically, in the original paradigm shift away from psychoanalysis by Robins and Guze, the dichotomous approach to major mental disorder yielded problems with diagnosing a "substantial minority of patients" (p. 51) (26) using the major valid categories set forth. The *DSM* series maintained the Atypical/Not Otherwise Specified categories to avoid excluding people with mental illness who did "not meet the criteria." Clearly, these residual categories were repositories for substantial numbers of individuals with mental illness who did not fit perfectly. Dimensionalism theory may succeed in part in the future if it can be a crosswalk more directly to clinical application (25) or indirectly through a valid research paradigm. Until one of these pathways is introduced and generally accepted, reservations by the field as a whole will probably remain.

In summary, psychiatric diagnosis remains of paramount medical and psychiatric importance. There is no shortcut to diagnosis using screening tools to estimate likelihood within individual patients or entire populations. Further, while dimensional aspects of illness may add to our understanding of psychiatric disorders, they currently cannot replace psychiatric diagnosis. For the foreseeable future, psychiatrists and other medical doctors must continue to rely on established psychiatric diagnoses and gathering information the old-fashioned way—through clinical interviews with patients—to guide assessment and treatment decisions.

Finally, the current edition of this text flows from the original and seminal work by its predecessors to establish and validate psychiatric diagnoses that support the mainstream activities of medical practice and research. We do not entertain the recently popular screening tools, notions of "partial" or "spectrum" diagnosis, dimensional classifications, or disorders outside those considered sufficiently validated and useful within empirical traditions of psychiatric diagnosis. Clearly the diagnostic traditions based on empirical findings over approximately five decades—sufficiently revised in this text to accommodate new knowledge and the changing field—will instruct future generations of students in the fundamental concepts of psychiatric diagnosis.

REFERENCES

1. [No authors listed]. Development of the RDoC Framework. National Institute of Mental Health, 2016. Last accessed 3/5/18. https://www.nimh.nih.gov/research-priorities/rdoc/development-of-the-rdoc-framework.shtml.
2. American Psychiatric Association. *Diagnostic and Statistical Manual: Mental Disorders*, 1st edition. Washington, DC: Author, 1952.
3. American Psychiatric Association. *Diagnostic and Statistical Manual of Mental Disorders*, 2nd edition. Washington, DC: Author, 1968.
4. American Psychiatric Association. *Diagnostic and Statistical Manual of Mental Disorders*, 3rd edition. Washington, DC: Author, 1980.
5. American Psychiatric Association. *Diagnostic and Statistical Manual of Mental Disorders*, 3rd revised edition. Washington, DC: Author, 1987.
6. American Psychiatric Association. *Diagnostic and Statistical Manual of Mental Disorders*, 4th edition. Washington, DC: Author, 1994.
7. American Psychiatric Association. *Diagnostic and Statistical Manual of Mental Disorders*, 4th text revision edition. Washington, DC: Author, 2000.
8. American Psychiatric Association. From planning to publication: developing the DSM-5 (fact sheet). American Psychiatric Association, 2013. Last accessed 3/7/18. https://www.psychiatry.org/File%20Library/Psychiatrists/Practice/DSM/APA_DSM-Development-of-DSM-5.pdf.
9. American Psychiatric Association Task Force on Laboratory Tests in Psychiatry. The dexamethasone suppression test: an overview of its current status in psychiatry. Am. J. Psychiatry, *144*:1253–1262, 1987.
10. Aragona, M. The role of comorbidity in the crisis of the current psychiatric classification system. Philos. Psychiatr. Psychol., *16*:1–11, 2009.
11. Batstra, L., and Frances, A. Diagnostic inflation: causes and a suggested cure. J. Nerv. Ment. Dis., *200*:474–479, 2012.
12. Blashfield, R. K. Feighner et al., invisible colleges, and the Matthew effect. Schizophr. Bull., *8*:1–12, 1982.
13. Carcone, D., and Ruocco, A. C. Six years of research on the National Institute of Mental Health's Research Domain Criteria (RDoC) initiative: a systematic review. Front Cell Neurosci., *11*:46, 2017.

14. Carroll, B. J. The dexamethasone test for melancholia. Br. J. Psychiatry, 140:292–304, 1982.

15. Craddock, N., O'Donovan, M. C., and Owen, M. J. Genes for schizophrenia and bipolar disorder? Implications for psychiatric nosology. Schizophr. Bull., 32:9–16, 2006.

16. Cuthbert, B. N., and Insel, T. R. Toward the future of psychiatric diagnosis: the seven pillars of RDoC. BMC Med., 11:126, 2013.

17. Feighner, J. P., Robins, E., Guze, S. B., Woodruff, R. A., Winokur, G., and Muñoz, R. Diagnostic criteria for use in psychiatric research. Arch. Gen. Psychiatry, 26:57–62, 1972.

18. First, M. B. Paradigm shifts and the development of the Diagnostic and Statistical Manual of Mental Disorders: past experiences and future aspirations. Can. J. Psychiatry, 55:692–700, 2010.

19. First, M. B. Diagnostic and Statistical Manual of Mental Disorders, 5th edition, and clinical utility. J. Nerv. Ment. Dis., 201:727–729, 2013.

20. First, M. B. The importance of developmental field trials in the revision of psychiatric classifications. Lancet Psychiatry, 3:579–584, 2016.

21. First, M. B. The DSM revision process: needing to keep an eye on the empirical ball. Psychol. Med., 47:19–22, 2017.

22. First, M. B., Pincus, H. A., Levine, J. B., Williams, J. B., Ustun, B., and Peele, R. Clinical utility as a criterion for revising psychiatric diagnoses. Am. J. Psychiatry, 161:946–954, 2004.

23. Frances, A. The new crisis of confidence in psychiatric diagnosis. Ann. Intern. Med., 159:221–222, 2013.

24. Frances, A. The past, present and future of psychiatric diagnosis. World Psychiatry, 12:111–112, 2013.

25. Frances, A. RDoC is necessary, but very oversold. World Psychiatry, 13:47–49, 2014.

26. Guze, S. B. *Why Psychiatry Is a Branch of Medicine*. New York: Oxford University Press, 1992.

27. Insel, T. Transforming diagnosis. National Institute of Mental Health, 2013. Last accessed 3/5/18. https://www.nimh.nih.gov/about/directors/thomas-insel/blog/2013/transforming-diagnosis.shtml.

28. Insel, T., Cuthbert, B., Garvey, M., Heinssen, R., Pine, D. S., Quinn, K., Sanislow, C., and Wang, P. Research domain criteria (RDoC): toward a new classification framework for research on mental disorders. Am. J. Psychiatry, 167:748–751, 2010.

29. Kendler, K. S. Reflections on the relationship between psychiatric genetics and psychiatric nosology. Am. J. Psychiatry, 163:1138–1146, 2006.

30. Kendler, K. S. A history of the DSM-5 Scientific Review Committee. Psychol. Med., 43:1793–1800, 2013.

31. Kendler, K. S., and First, M. B. Alternative futures for the DSM revision process: iteration v. paradigm shift. Br. J. Psychiatry, 197:263–265, 2010.

32. Kendler, K. S., and Solomon, M. Expert consensus v. evidence-based approaches in the revision of the DSM. Psychol. Med., 46:2255–2262, 2016.

33. Kupfer, F. K., First, M. B., and Regier, D. A. *A Research Agenda for DSM-V*. Washington, DC: American Psychiatric Association, 2002.

34. Markon, K. E. Epistemological pluralism and scientific development: an argument against authoritative nosologies. J. Pers. Disord., 27:554–579, 2013.

35. Mayes, R., and Horwitz, A. V. DSM-III and the revolution in the classification of mental illness. J. Hist. Behav. Sci., 41:249–267, 2005.

36. Mullen, P. E. A modest proposal for another phenomenological approach to psychopathology. Schizophr. Bull., 33:113–121, 2007.
37. Neese, R. M., and Jackson, E. D. Evolution: psychiatric nosology's missing biological foundation. Clin. Neuropsychiatry, 3:121–131, 2006.
38. Nemeroff, C. B., Weinberger, D., Rutter, M., MacMillan, H. L., Bryant, R. A., Wessely, S., Stein, D. J., Pariante, C. M., Seemuller, F., Berk, M., Malhi, G. S., Preisig, M., Brune, M., and Lysaker, P. DSM-5: a collection of psychiatrist views on the changes, controversies, and future directions. BMC Med., 11:202, 2013.
39. Phillips, J., Frances, A., Cerullo, M. A., Chardavoyne, J., Decker, H. S., First, M. B., Ghaemi, N., Greenberg, G., Hinderliter, A. C., Kinghorn, W. A., LoBello, S. G., Martin, E. B., Mishara, A. L., Paris, J., Pierre, J. M., Pies, R. W., Pincus, H. A., Porter, D., Pouncey, C., Schwartz, M. A., Szasz, T., Wakefield, J. C., Waterman, G. S., Whooley, O., and Zachar, P. The six most essential questions in psychiatric diagnosis: a pluralogue part 1: conceptual and definitional issues in psychiatric diagnosis. Philos. Ethics Humanit. Med., 7:3, 2012.
40. Phillips, J., Frances, A., Cerullo, M. A., Chardavoyne, J., Decker, H. S., First, M. B., Ghaemi, N., Greenberg, G., Hinderliter, A. C., Kinghorn, W. A., LoBello, S. G., Martin, E. B., Mishara, A. L., Paris, J., Pierre, J. M., Pies, R. W., Pincus, H. A., Porter, D., Pouncey, C., Schwartz, M. A., Szasz, T., Wakefield, J. C., Waterman, G. S., Whooley, O., and Zachar, P. The six most essential questions in psychiatric diagnosis: a pluralogue part 2: issues of conservatism and pragmatism in psychiatric diagnosis. Philos. Ethics Humanit. Med., 7:8, 2012.
41. Phillips, J., Frances, A., Cerullo, M. A., Chardavoyne, J., Decker, H. S., First, M. B., Ghaemi, N., Greenberg, G., Hinderliter, A. C., Kinghorn, W. A., LoBello, S. G., Martin, E. B., Mishara, A. L., Paris, J., Pierre, J. M., Pies, R. W., Pincus, H. A., Porter, D., Pouncey, C., Schwartz, M. A., Szasz, T., Wakefield, J. C., Waterman, G. S., Whooley, O., and Zachar, P. The six most essential questions in psychiatric diagnosis: a pluralogue part 3: issues of utility and alternative approaches in psychiatric diagnosis. Philos. Ethics Humanit. Med., 7:9, 2012.
42. Phillips, J., Frances, A., Cerullo, M. A., Chardavoyne, J., Decker, H. S., First, M. B., Ghaemi, N., Greenberg, G., Hinderliter, A. C., Kinghorn, W. A., LoBello, S. G., Martin, E. B., Mishara, A. L., Paris, J., Pierre, J. M., Pies, R. W., Pincus, H. A., Porter, D., Pouncey, C., Schwartz, M. A., Szasz, T., Wakefield, J. C., Waterman, G. S., Whooley, O., and Zachar, P. The six most essential questions in psychiatric diagnosis: a pluralogue part 4: general conclusion. Philos. Ethics Humanit. Med., 7:14, 2012.
43. Regier, D. A., Kuhl, E. A., and Kupfer, D. J. The DSM-5: classification and criteria changes. World Psychiatry, 12:92–98, 2013.
44. Robins, E., and Guze, S. B. Establishment of diagnostic validity in psychiatric illness: its application to schizophrenia. Am. J. Psychiatry, 126:983–987, 1970.
45. Rogler, L. H. Making sense of historical changes in the Diagnostic and Statistical Manual of Mental Disorders: five propositions. J. Health Soc. Behav., 38:9–20, 1997.
46. Wakefield, J. C. DSM-5, psychiatric epidemiology and the false positives problem. Epidemiol. Psychiatr. Sci., 24:188–196, 2015.
47. Wakefield, J. C. Diagnostic issues and controversies in DSM-5: return of the false positives problem. Annu. Rev. Clin. Psychol., 12:105–132, 2016.
48. Wakefield, J. C., and First, M. B. Placing symptoms in context: the role of contextual criteria in reducing false positives in Diagnostic and Statistical Manual of Mental Disorders diagnoses. Compr. Psychiatry, 53:130–139, 2012.

49. Wakefield, J. C., and First, M. B. Clarifying the boundary between normality and disorder: a fundamental conceptual challenge for psychiatry. Can. J. Psychiatry, *58*:603–605, 2013.

50. Woodruff, R. A., Jr., Goodwin, D. W., and Guze, S. B. *Psychiatric Diagnosis.* New York: Oxford University Press, 1974.

51. Young, A. *The Harmony of Illusions: Inventing Post-traumatic Stress Disorder.* Princeton, NJ: Princeton University Press, 1996.

52. Zachar, P., and Kendler, K. S. The philosophy of nosology. Annu. Rev. Clin. Psychol., *13*:49–71, 2017.

53. Zachar, P., Krueger, R. F., and Kendler, K. S. Personality disorder in DSM-5: an oral history. Psychol. Med., *46*:1–10, 2016.

ᴏᴧᴐ

Mood (Affective) Disorders

There is a pitch of unhappiness so great that the goods of nature may be entirely forgotten, and all sentiment of their existence vanish from the mental field. For this ex-
tremity of pessimism to be reached, something more is needed than observation of life
and reflection upon death. The individual must in his own person become the prey of
pathological melancholy. . . . Such sensitiveness and susceptibility to mental pain is a
rare occurrence where the nervous constitution is entirely normal; one seldom finds it in
a healthy subject even where he is the victim of the most atrocious cruelties of outward
fortune . . . it is positive and active anguish, a sort of psychical neuralgia wholly unknown
to healthy life.

William James
The Varieties of Religious Experience: A Study in Human Nature (pp. 237–238) (95)

Depression and euphoria are the primary symptoms of mood disorders,
but not the only ones. Associated with low moods are such symptoms
as insomnia, anorexia, suicidal thoughts, and feelings of worthlessness or
of being a burden to others; associated with euphoria are such symptoms
as hyperactivity, decreased need for sleep, and flight of ideas. The extent
of depression or euphoria is often inappropriate to the patient's life situation, a fact sometimes as obvious to patients as to their relatives and
friends. Previously known as "affective disorders," these conditions were
renamed "mood disorders" in the 1987 edition of the American Psychiatric
Association's diagnostic manual, *DSM-III-R* (5).

Whatever the name, the definition remains unchanged. It refers to a
group of disorders characterized by prolonged disturbances of mood
accompanied by several symptoms as just described. Mood disorders have

been divided and subdivided endlessly as investigators endeavor to distinguish "normal" from "abnormal" mood and to create clinical clusters with distinct natural histories, familial prevalence, course and prognoses, and response to treatment. After more than a century there is still disagreement about the most satisfactory classification.

Amid all this diversity, there is a common theme: Mood disorders are primarily characterized by depressed mood, elevated mood (mania), or alternations of depressed and elevated moods. Severe depression is diagnosed as major depressive disorder. The building blocks for defining mood disorders are mood episodes, which represent a distinct and persistent change from a person's typical mood with accompanying symptoms, lasting 2 weeks for a major depressive episode and 1 week for a manic episode. The most recent classification of mood disorders is provided by *DSM-5*, published by the American Psychiatric Association in 2013 (6).

Manic episodes are characterized by persistent high or irritable mood along with increased energy and/or activity, accompanied by at least three (four, if the mood is only irritable) other symptoms, such as decreased need for sleep, racing thoughts, talking excessively, grandiosity, and hypersexuality. Depressive episodes are characterized by persistent depressed mood and/or loss of interest or pleasure, with at least five symptoms including disturbances of sleep, appetite, energy, and concentration; feeling worthless or guilty; and suicidal ideation or suicide attempts.

Manic and major depressive episodes by themselves do not constitute diagnoses, because a patient with a mood disorder may experience different types of mood episodes over the course of a single illness, and the different episodes would not be diagnosed as separate disorders. This is illustrated by the classical term for manic mood disorder, "manic depressive illness," reflecting the presence of both manic and major depressive episodes as part of the disorder. A newer term, "bipolar disorder," also expresses this same central feature of the disorder. The two terms are interchangeable.

Mood disorders are defined as bipolar when mania occurs, regardless of whether depressive episodes occur. When the disorder involves solely depression, the term "unipolar" or "major" depression is used. A natural initial impression of the terms "bipolar" and "unipolar" is that bipolar implies a history of both mania and depression, whereas unipolar implies a history of one or the other alone. "Bipolar" actually refers to a history of mania regardless of whether depression has also been present. "Unipolar" refers to episodes of depression without mania.

As many as 40% of patients meeting criteria for bipolar disorder have episodes with "mixed features," referring to manic or depressive episodes in which both depressive and manic symptoms are present. Bipolar illness with four or more mood episodes (mania, hypomania, or depression) within 12 months is specified as "rapid cycling."

Milder depressive syndromes are called "dysthymia"; milder forms of mania are called "hypomania." Milder expressions of bipolar disorder with both hypomanic and depressive episodes in the absence of manic or psychotic episodes are diagnosed as bipolar II disorder if the depressive episodes meet full criteria for a major depressive episode and cyclothymia if they do not. For all of these terms, more than disturbed mood is required. There must be a syndrome, a group of characteristic clinical features that distinguish one disorder from another.

HISTORICAL BACKGROUND

Descriptions of mood disorders began with Hippocrates. The term "melancholia" is usually attributed to him, as is the notion that it results from the influence of black bile and phlegm on the brain "darkening the spirit and making it melancholy" (p. 204) (93).

About 500 years later, Aretaeus of Cappadocia recognized and recorded an association between melancholia and mania early in the second century A.D. (pp. 299–300) (2):

> Those affected with melancholia are not every one of them affected according to one particular form; they are either suspicious of poisoning or flee to the desert from misanthropy, or turn superstitious, or contract a hatred of life. If at any time a relaxation takes place, in most cases hilarity supervenes . . . the patients are dull or stern, dejected or unreasonably torpid, without any manifest cause . . . they also become peevish, dispirited, sleepless, and start up from a disturbed sleep. Unreasonable fear also seizes them, if the disease tends to increase . . . they complain of life, and desire to die.

Aretaeus observed that depression was often episodic but also occurred in a chronic, unremitting form. Like Hippocrates, he attributed the cause to a humoral imbalance: "If it [black bile] be determined upwards to the stomach and diaphragm, it forms melancholy, for it produces flatulence and eructations of the fetid and fishy nature, and it sends rumbling wind downwards and disturbs the understanding" (p. 41) (23).

The nineteenth-century French physician Falret described an episodic variety of depression with remissions and attacks of increasing duration, an illness occurring more frequently among women than men, sometimes associated with precipitating events, and sometimes alternating with mania (*la folie circulaire*). Falret and his contemporary Baillarger (who also described recurring attacks of mania and melancholia) probably influenced Kraepelin's later concept of manic depressive psychosis.

In 1896 Kraepelin made his major contribution to psychiatry by separating the functional psychoses into two groups, dementia praecox and manic depressive psychosis. Dementia praecox was chronic and un-remitting with a generally poor prognosis. Manic depressive psychosis, on the other hand, did not usually end in chronic invalidism. After publishing the sixth edition of his textbook in 1896, Kraepelin continued to define the limits of dementia praecox narrowly, but he expanded those of manic depressive psychosis to include almost all abnormalities of mood. Chronic depression was included as well as episodic illness; mania was included as well as depression (109).

Kraepelin had insisted that manic depressive psychosis was generally independent of social and psychological forces, that the cause of the illness was "innate." Freud and the psychoanalysts assumed the opposite. Freud in *Mourning and Melancholia*, published in 1917, outlined his theories of the psychodynamic genesis of depression (60). He hypothesized that de-pression had in common with the process of mourning a response to the loss of a "love-object," that is, the loss of something greatly valued. Grief, a healthy response, differed from melancholia in that the latter involved direction of unresolved, negative feelings inward, resulting in despair, a sense of worthlessness, thoughts of self-harm, and other depressive symptoms.

Since early in the twentieth century there has been considerable con-troversy over the distinction between "endogenous" depression and "reactive" depression. This controversy had its origin partially in the differing viewpoints of the Kraepelinians and Freudians toward mental phenomena in general. Kraepelin and his followers searched for the limits of pathological behavior by describing the symptoms of syndromes in keeping with the traditions of nineteenth-century German medi-cine. Freud and his pupils searched for mental mechanisms that might be most obvious in pathological states but were not limited to those states. Such differences in attitude were augmented by the fact that Kraepelinian psychiatrists dealt chiefly with severely ill, hospitalized patients, whereas Freudian psychiatrists tended to treat mildly ill, nonhospitalized patients.

Reactive depression was held to be a direct result of precipitating events or unique individual responses of social and psychological stress, and equated with neurosis. ("Neurosis" is a psychoanalytic term referring to chronic states of unhappiness and distress hypothesized to result from intrapsychic conflicts, encompassing depressive and anxious syndromes. This term was removed from American diagnostic criteria for mental disorders in 1980.) Endogenous depression, in contrast, was equated with psychosis. Reactive depression was considered to be less responsive to somatic therapies and milder than endogenous forms of depression, although empirical research has not confirmed these assumptions (104). The current diagnostic classification of depressive disorders in *DSM-5* does not mention reactive/endogenous subtypes.

The separation of mood disorders into unipolar and bipolar subtypes was first proposed by Leonhard et al. in 1962 (114). Support for the separation has emerged from several decades of research evidence from studies in Europe and the United States pointing to important clinical and epidemiological differences between the two types of disorders (139, 165, 218, 219). Compared to unipolar disorders, bipolar disorders tend to have an earlier age of onset, cyclical depressions, a higher frequency of postpartum onsets, and a greater tendency for suicide attempts. Unipolar cases have a somewhat older age of onset, are more likely to have single episodes, and have longer episodes. Bipolar disorder cases are more likely to be psychotic and to manifest psychomotor retardation and anhedonia. Unipolar cases more often have agitated depressions and accompanying anxiety and somatization. Unipolar depression, unlike bipolar depression, has a distinct female preponderance. There is a greater prevalence of mood disorder among relatives of bipolar patients than among relatives of unipolar patients (19, 75, 146).

Many questions about the classification of mood disorders remain unresolved. An abiding problem is an old question of how to separate the experience of bereavement from that of depression. *DSM-5* leaves in the hands of the clinician the decision of whether to diagnose major depressive disorder in the context of a significant loss (224).

EPIDEMIOLOGY

Estimates of the prevalence of major depressive disorder depend on the sample or population studied and on the definition of the illness. The Epidemiologic Catchment Area study, a national household study of psychiatric disorders using structured diagnostic interviews conducted nearly 40 years ago, provided a 5% lifetime prevalence of major depressive disorder in the US general population (211). A much higher rate of

17% was reported by a more recent national household study of psychiatric disorders, the National Comorbidity Survey, which used a different diagnostic instrument, provided memory cues, and studied a younger sample (105, 210). Methodological differences in these studies make it difficult to know which statistics are more accurate. A systematic review of 18 population prevalence studies determined pooled lifetime prevalence rates to be 6.7% for major depression and 0.8% for bipolar disorder (209). The authors of this review were unable to account for all of the variability across studies on the basis of common methodological differences.

Most studies show that mood disorders are more common in women than in men. However, this may apply only to unipolar disorder, with women outnumbering men by about two to one (50, 75, 105, 111, 157, 211). Apparently, men and women about equally share the risk of bipolar disorder (50, 75, 211). Among patients with bipolar disorder, some, but not all, studies have found that women have more depressive episodes and men have more manic episodes (50).

Studies in humans and animals have concluded that early life trauma and adverse environments may confer vulnerability to depression later in life. Presumably, these results are mediated through effects on the hypothalamic-pituitary-adrenal (HPA) axis (8, 65, 132, 150).

Heightened productivity in bipolar affective disorder could lead to transient gains in occupational or educational achievement (75); however, studies have demonstrated lower socioeconomic status in bipolar patients compared to the rest of the population (51, 75, 76, 78). Their unaffected relatives may also have a socioeconomic advantage (112). Therefore, bipolar traits appear to confer some occupational advantage, but when those traits occur as part of full-blown bipolar illness, they are occupationally detrimental (112).

Awareness of an association between artistic genius and temperamental moodiness dates to the time of Aristotle (16). Modern research has demonstrated an association of creativity with bipolar disorder and an overrepresentation of creative professions among individuals with bipolar disorder, and these characteristics have been observed in their unaffected relatives as well (78, 202).

The prevalence of depressive and bipolar disorders is higher in urban than in rural settings, in developing than in developed countries, and in regions with military conflict (55, 110, 163, 204). Reviews of population studies internationally have reported that prevalence rates of both unipolar and bipolar disorder are highest in European studies and lowest in Asian studies (55–57).

CLINICAL PICTURE

The chief complaints of patients with a depressive episode are usually psychological: feelings of worthlessness, despair, or ideas of self-harm. But it is also common for depressed patients to complain chiefly of pains, tachycardia, breathing difficulty, gastrointestinal dysfunction, headache, or other somatic disturbances (7, 85, 178).

The dysphoric mood experienced by patients with depressive illness is usually characterized as sadness or despondency, but some patients describe themselves as feeling hopeless, irritable, fearful, worried, or simply discouraged. A few patients presenting with what seems to be major depressive disorder report only minimal feelings of dysphoria. Such patients may complain primarily of insomnia and anorexia. They may even cry profusely while telling the examining physician that they do not feel sad. These patients are unusual, but not unknown to psychiatrists. Regardless, a patient with depressive illness may have no symptoms of sadness or low mood if anhedonia is predominant during the episode (6). It may seem counterintuitive that major depressive disorder can present without depressed mood, but recognition of this possibility can help the clinician identify cases like these, which may present more often in medical settings.

Other characteristic symptoms of depression are anorexia with weight loss; insomnia; early morning awakening; loss of energy, described as general tiredness or fatigability; agitation or (its opposite) psychomotor retardation; loss of interest in usual activities, including loss of interest in sex; feelings of self-reproach or guilt, which may be delusional in intensity; inability to focus one's thoughts, often with a simultaneous awareness of slowed thinking; and recurrent thoughts of death or suicide.

It is common for patients with major depressive disorder to say, "Something is wrong with my mind." Patients will often tell their physician that they fear they are losing their mind or have a sense of emotions out of control. It is also common for depressed patients to have a low expectancy of recovery. Such a pessimistic outlook should serve as a warning that the patient may be depressed. Medically ill patients seldom give up all hope of improvement, even if they are seriously ill.

In some depressed patients, agitation is so overwhelming that other symptoms go almost unnoticed. These patients are brought to physicians when they are found by relatives or friends to be pacing, wringing their hands, bemoaning their fate, clinging to anyone who will listen. They ask for reassurance, they beg for help, yet nothing satisfies them.

In other patients, psychomotor retardation is prominent. There may be marked slowing of both thought and motor behavior. Tasks that once took minutes may require hours. These patients may be so slowed that it is painful to listen to their conversation. Psychomotor retardation can be so severe that a patient becomes mute or even stuporous (59, 215).

Paranoid symptoms can occur as part of major depressive disorder. There are usually exaggerated ideas of reference associated with notions of worthlessness. Characteristic delusions of patients with depression are those of a hypochondriacal or nihilistic type. Some severely ill depressed patients seem to feel they are so guilty and evil that they have become the focus of universal abhorrence or even that the world is disintegrating because of their terrible inadequacies and failures.

Hallucinations may also occur in major depressive disorder. These commonly involve accusatory voices or visions of deceased relatives associated with feelings of guilt. Delusions and hallucinations occurring in major depressive disorder are usually "mood congruent" with content that is consistent with the person's dominant mood. Delusions and hallucinations occurring during major depressive disorder commonly involve themes of guilt, disease, poverty, death, or deserved punishment. Delusions and hallucinations occurring as part of mania are often of inflated worth, power, or special relationship to a deity or famous person.

The *DSM-5* criteria include mood congruence as a specifier for psychotic features in mood disorders. Mood-*in*congruent psychotic features are more often seen in schizophrenia, in which, for example, the patient may seem cheerful and relaxed while describing terrifying, delusional experiences. The importance of mood congruence is based more on general clinical impressions than on systematic studies.

Depressed patients may or may not mention events that they consider important in producing their illness. When a precipitating event is described, it is sometimes surprisingly trivial and difficult for the examining physician to take seriously. Furthermore, some symptoms may have actually begun before the so-called precipitating event. This suggests that some patients who begin to feel depressed search for reasons to explain their depression, unable or unwilling to believe they could feel as they do for no apparent reason.

Stressful events frequently mentioned by women as precipitants of depression are pregnancy and childbirth. A study of women with mood disorders found that the first episode of depression occurred during pregnancy or postpartum in 37% of bipolar and 17% of unipolar cases (98). In particular, a postpartum onset of depression is a strong indicator of eventual conversion to bipolar disorder (146).

A change in drinking habits often accompanies depressive illness (93, 194). Middle-aged individuals with no previous history of alcoholism who begin to drink heavily may be suffering from depression. On the other hand, some individuals drink less than usual when depressed.

A physician (168) has written movingly about how it feels to have depressive illness:

> Firstly, it is very unpleasant: depressive illness is probably more unpleasant than any disease except rabies. There is constant mental pain and often psychogenic physical pain too. If one tries to get such a patient to titrate other pains against the pain of his depression one tends to end up with a description that would raise eyebrows even in a medieval torture chamber.
>
> Naturally, many of these patients commit suicide. They may not hope to get to heaven but they know they are leaving hell. Secondly, the patient is isolated from family and friends, because the depression itself reduces his affection for others and he may well have ideas that he is unworthy of their love or even that his friendship may harm them. Thirdly, he is rejected by others because they cannot stand the sight of his suffering.
>
> There is a limit to sympathy. Even psychiatrists have protective mechanisms for dealing with such cases: the consultant may refer the patient to an outpatient clinic; he may allow too brief a consultation to elicit the extent of the patient's suffering; he may, on the grounds that the depression has not responded to treatment, alter his diagnosis to one of personality disorder—comforting, because of the strange but widespread belief that patients with personality disorders do not suffer.
>
> Fourthly, and finally, the patient tends to do a great cover-up. Because of his outward depression he is socially unacceptable, and because of his inward depression he feels even more socially unacceptable than he really is. He does not, therefore, tell others how bad he feels.
>
> Most depressives, even severe ones, can cope with routine work— initiative and leadership are what they lack. Nevertheless, many of them can continue working, functioning at a fairly low level, and their deficiencies are often covered up by colleagues. Provided some minimal degree of social and vocational functioning is present, the world leaves the depressive alone and he battles on for the sake of his god or his children, or for some reason which makes his personal torment preferable to death.

The cardinal features of mania are euphoria, hyperactivity, and flight of ideas. Not all manic moods are euphoric; some are irritable instead. Flight of ideas is a rapid digression from one idea to another. A common response to a patient with mania is that of sympathetic amusement. In fact, experienced clinicians who find themselves amused by a patient immediately consider the possibility that the patient's condition is either mania or hypomania.

Flight of ideas, unlike the incoherence and tangentiality of schizophrenia, is usually understandable, even though some connections between ideas may be tenuous. (Comedians often use a well-controlled flight of ideas to amuse audiences.) Attention may be called to this symptom by a push of speech, that is, speech in which a great deal is said in a short period of time. Such speech may exhibit rhyming, punning, and jocular associations.

Psychotic symptoms may also occur in mood disorders: persecutory and grandiose delusions, hallucinations, and ideas of reference. They are usually mood congruent. Some patients exhibit depression and mania simultaneously. They may cry while speaking euphorically or show other unusual combinations of symptoms.

Psychologist Kay Jamison described the emotional suffering of her own experience with bipolar depression (p. 114) (96):

> Profound melancholia is a day-in, day-out, night-in, night-out, almost arterial level of agony. It is a pitiless unrelenting pain that affords no window of hope, no alternative to a grim and brackish existence, and no respite from the cold undercurrents of thought and feeling that dominate the horribly restless nights of despair.

Jamison also described her experience of mania (p. 212) (96):

> . . . the seductiveness of these unbridled and intense moods is powerful; and the ancient dialogue between reason and the senses is almost always more interestingly and passionately resolved in favor of the senses. The milder manias have a way of promising—and, for a very brief while, delivering—springs in the winter and epochal vitalities. In the cold light of day, however, the reality and destructiveness of rekindled illness tend to dampen the evocativeness of such selective remembered, wistful, intense, and gentle moments. Any temptation that I now may have to recapture such moods by altering my medication is quickly hosed down by the cold knowledge that a gentle intensity soon becomes first a frenetic one and then, finally, an uncontrolled insanity.

Mood disorders have been described in children. Some children have episodes of depression that resemble major depressive disorder in adulthood: crying, social withdrawal, hypersensitivity, and behavioral problems (129, 212). Even though the symptom presentation in children and adolescents is similar to that of adult major depressive disorder (129, 212), it is not clear whether such episodes are an early manifestation of primary depressive disorder. Two observations suggest that they may not be: 1) unlike adult depression, childhood depression is not more common in females

(212); 2) even though children with major depressive disorder subjectively describe sleep difficulties much like those of adults with this disorder, polysomnographic (electroencephalographic) studies of these children's sleep have not found consistent changes in sleep architecture paralleling those in adult depression (i.e., sleep discontinuities, reduced total sleep and deep sleep stages, and increased rapid eye movement sleep) (12, 171, 214).

These findings suggest either that sleep disturbance makes a rather abrupt appearance within the depressive syndrome, or that the depressive disorders of children and adults differ in important ways. Because human growth hormone (HGH) is excreted mostly during sleep, sleep has an additional function in children not present in adults and it may be more protected in children. Very young children demonstrate the greatest levels of deepest (stage 4) sleep and are highly resistant to being awakened from deep sleep, phenomena that decrease gradually with increasing age (171). Regardless, it appears that sleep abnormalities are less associated with childhood depression than with depressive illness in later years.

The pediatric diagnosis of bipolar disorder, especially in very young children such as preschoolers, remains controversial. Bipolar disorder in children has historically been considered to be rare (175). The frequency of diagnosis of bipolar disorder in children has risen rapidly in recent decades in the United States (73, 74), but not in European countries (79). Pediatric bipolar disorder, especially in older children, has many similarities to adult bipolar disorder when the same diagnostic criteria are used. Pediatric presentations, however, tend to have episodes that are less discrete, shorter, more frequent, more often mixed, changing polarity more rapidly, and associated with more hyperactivity and psychiatric comorbidity (73, 74, 79, 175). Current challenges to the validity of pediatric bipolar disorder as a syndrome are reflected in difficulties differentiating it from its highly prevalent comorbidities and determining consistent long-term outcomes (131, 175).

BIOLOGICAL FINDINGS

The monoamine model of depression emerged in the mid-1960s. Arising from pharmacological research demonstrating monoaminergic effects of the early monoamine oxidase inhibitors and tricyclic antidepressants to be effective for the treatment of depression (58, 130), this theory implicated central nervous system depletion of norepinephrine and serotonin neurotransmitters. The development of the monoamine theory helped to advance biological research into psychiatric disorders for more than two decades (86, 143). Subsequently, other neurotransmitter systems have also been implicated in both mania and depression: dopamine, glutamate, and gamma-aminobutyric acid (GABA) (58, 86).

Despite directions suggested by these theoretical neurotransmission models, abnormalities in monoamine and other neurotransmitter systems have not proven fundamental to understanding the etiology of mood disorders (86). The strongest evidence against the monoamine hypothesis in the etiology of depression is the well-established incomplete (60%–70%) response to antidepressant medications that target abnormalities in this system (58, 142). Monoamine abnormalities could possibly represent downstream effects of other more primary dysfunctions in mood disorders (86). It has become apparent that the neuropathology of depression is far more complex than what the monoamine theory can explain (58, 130). The clinically and etiologically heterogeneous nature of depression currently defies explanations of its origins by any unified hypothesis (86, 142). Considerable evidence has accumulated for potential contributions of dysregulation of the HPA axis (58, 130, 206), inflammatory cytokine dysfunction (86, 206), insufficient neurotrophin production (nerve growth factor [NGF] and brain-derived neurotrophic factor [BDNF]) (206), abnormalities of the gut microbiome and delivery of gastrointestinal signaling peptides (206), and circadian rhythm abnormalities (86).

Functional and structural neuroimaging studies and postmortem brain pathology studies have demonstrated abnormalities in brain activity, volume, and architecture in lateral prefrontal and anterior cingulate cortex, basal ganglia, and hippocampus and amygdala in depression (54, 58, 86). Reduced hippocampal volume has been found to be proportional to depressive illness duration (86). This is consistent with the possibility that untreated depression may lead to hippocampal volume loss, possibly through processes of impaired neuroplasticity and hippocampal neurogenesis or through glucocorticoid and glutamatergic neurotoxicity (86). Recent network-based brain research has advanced the understanding of depression as a complex disorder that involves disruptions of neural circuitry across interconnected brain regions (54, 86, 142).

Few studies have directly compared the neurobiology of unipolar and bipolar depression. No consistent replicable evidence of biological differences between unipolar and bipolar depression has emerged (40, 123). Functional, structural, and metabolic changes in mood disorder have been found especially in the prefrontal cortex, hippocampus, and amygdala and in the interconnections of these brain structures. Reduced neurotrophic factors and cytokine abnormalities have also been identified in bipolar illness (48, 123).

NATURAL HISTORY

The natural history of mood disorders is variable. The age of risk extends throughout life. Together with the usual episodic nature of the illness, the age of risk distinguishes mood disorders from most other psychiatric illnesses.

The average age of onset of major depressive disorder has been measured in the mid-20s (26, 193, 211), but there is some evidence that the onset could be shifting to earlier ages, including the late teen years (176). For bipolar disorder, the average age of onset is around 18 years (138, 211). Age of onset has been found to be correlated in family members with bipolar illness (18, 118). In 5%–10% or more of patients presenting with a depressive episode, the illness will eventually declare itself as bipolar (27, 68, 173), with an annual conversion rate of about 1% from unipolar depression to bipolar disorder (11).

The length of individual episodes of major depressive disorder is quite variable, ranging from a few days to many years. About half of depressive episodes will remit within 6 months and 80% by 2 years. By 10 years, more than 90% of episodes will have ended, but recovery is unlikely thereafter (176). The period of highest risk for relapse is shortly after remission. Patients who have residual symptoms have an excess of five times the likelihood of relapse compared to patients with minimal or no residual symptoms (100). The longer the patient remains well, the lower the current risk of relapse.

Between episodes of major depressive disorder, residual symptoms are not uncommon. Analysis of data from the NIMH National Collaborative Depression Study demonstrated that patients may experience some symptoms more than half of the time when not experiencing full depressive episodes (100). A 23-year follow-up study found that an average of 15% of the time (41 months) was spent in a depressive episode (222).

Major depressive disorder is a recurring disorder: Three out of four patients can be expected to experience a subsequent depressive episode (176, 193, 222). The median time to first recurrence is about three years, and the time to subsequent recurrence is successively shorter with each episode. The likelihood of recurrence increases on average by 16% with each depressive episode (176). Risk of relapse is associated with greater duration and number of prior depressive episodes, baseline severity of depression, earlier age of onset, female sex, never-married status, inadequate social support, and psychiatric comorbidity (176, 193).

Bipolar disorder exhibits similar patterns: Most patients with a manic episode will have multiple recurrences of depression and/or mania (71).

Patients continue to have residual symptoms about half the time between episodes, experiencing episodes of illness approximately one-third of the time (191). Patients with bipolar disorder spend approximately three times as much time in depressive phases as in manic phases of illness (18, 30), more so among women (50). With treatment, episodes are substantially diminished in frequency and intensity. Many patients with bipolar disorder return to healthy functioning between episodes of illness (72, 199).

COMPLICATIONS

Major depressive disorder and suicide are clearly connected: 50%–70% of individuals who commit suicide can be found retrospectively to have had symptoms characteristic of depression. A review of 17 studies of suicide found that 15% of patients with major depression will eventually die by suicide (82). However, the patients studied were severe cases in inpatient settings, and not necessarily representative of all depressed patients, who may have substantially lower rates (177). The specific suicide rate in relation to mood disorders is elevated 10 to 30 times the rate in the general population (10, 156).

Although a large proportion of people who commit suicide have made previous suicide attempts, only a fraction of attempters eventually kill themselves. Prior suicide attempts have been found to be associated with subsequent suicide (87). About 1 out of 10 or 20 attempters will be found dead by suicide within 5 to 10 years after an attempt (66, 158, 197). The period of highest risk appears to be during the first 2 follow-up years (66, 197). The first few weeks after discharge from inpatient psychiatric care represent a time of heightened suicide risk (87). The medical seriousness of the attempt is a weak predictor at best; medically trivial attempts are sometimes followed by eventual suicide. Suicide risk appears to decrease after initiation of antidepressants or psychotherapy for major depressive disorder (87).

The risk of suicide is not necessarily correlated with symptom severity. Suicide risk is associated with psychiatric illness, age greater than 65 years, being male, living alone, recent stressors (especially major losses), access to firearms, hopelessness, prior attempts, and communication of suicidal intent (69). Suicidal communication must be considered in light of the diagnosis. The disorders most frequently associated with suicide are mood and substance use disorders, but schizophrenia and personality disorders are also disorders prominently represented in completed suicides (22, 87, 94, 200). Among patients with bipolar disorder, a history of suicide in a close family member is significantly associated with suicide risk (184); depressive episodes and mixed mood states also confer increased suicide risk in bipolar disorder (183).

Folklore that patients who talk of suicide do not commit suicide is untrue. Suicidal communication may impart increased risk. However, those who are serious about completing the act often do not convey intent to others in their final days (94).

Mortality risk is increased eight times for patients with major depressive disorder. Most of this excess mortality is from unnatural causes, especially suicide, which accounts for 55% of excess deaths in major depressive disorder. Patients with mood disorders also have excess mortality from causes other than suicide (94). Deaths from natural causes occur 1.3 times more than expected in the general population, with infections, mental, cardiovascular, and respiratory system disorders accounting for most of the excess risk (84). Total life expectancy is reduced by 19 years in major depressive disorder and 17 years in bipolar disorder (3).

Alcohol and drug use disorders may be a complication of mood disorders. This is particularly evident when a person begins to drink heavily in mid- or late life. Alcohol and drug use disorders not comorbid with a mood disorder usually begin earlier in life.

Poor judgment that often emerges during mood disorder episodes can lead to social and personal complications. Impulsivity, spending sprees, and unrealistic decisions are characteristic of manic episodes. Bad decisions also commonly accompany depressive episodes. Decisions to leave a job, move to a different city, or separate from a spouse may result from the restless dissatisfaction of depression. Clinicians often advise depressed patients not to make major life decisions until they are clearly in remission.

Studies of psychiatric illness in the postpartum period indicate that in women with bipolar disorder, episodes of depression or mania are more likely to occur during the puerperium than at other times in their lives. Having had a postpartum episode of depression, the likelihood that a woman with bipolar illness will have another episode after a subsequent pregnancy is high. Studies have demonstrated episodes of puerperal mania or psychosis in 20%–30% of women with bipolar illness after delivery; a family history of puerperal psychosis increases the rate to more than 50% after delivery (33, 99).

Three studies have demonstrated that major depressive disorder is significantly related to poor academic performance, including college dropout (9, 92, 136). In one study at a large university, diagnosed depression was associated with a drop of half a letter grade point average, but those who received treatment for depression evidenced a nearly equivalent gain in grade point average (92). In another study at a major university, students who withdrew from school because of depression did not fare as well on return to classes as other returning students who did not have depression (136).

Cognitive testing in major depressive disorder may show impaired attention, deficits in explicit verbal and visual memory (but implicit memory appears to be preserved), impairment in executive functioning, and slowing in motor and cognitive domains. Severity of depression is associated with degree of cognitive impairment (128). These abnormalities are more pronounced in the elderly (141).

The memory impairment with depression can be so profound that a mistaken diagnosis of dementia is made. The true identity of the problem is revealed when memory returns to normal after recovery from the depression. This memory impairment owing to depression has been called "pseudodementia." Occasionally, depressive symptoms in the elderly can herald the onset of a dementing disorder. Cognitive control dysfunction in elderly patients with depression predicts poor response to antidepressant treatment (141).

Cognitive difficulties have been observed in manic as well as depressive phases of bipolar illness (75, 117, 123, 159). Reversal of cognitive impairments in mood disorders may not always accompany recovery from the mood episode (75, 117, 126, 127). The cognitive impairments in bipolar disorder may represent trait markers that are also somewhat state modulated. During bipolar episodes, cognitive impairment may be as severe as that observed in schizophrenia, but outside of mood episodes, cognitive functioning in patients with bipolar disorder is superior to that of patients with schizophrenia (162, 170).

FAMILY AND GENETIC STUDIES

Family studies from the 1960s and earlier demonstrated that mood disorders tend to be inherited in families (220). More recent studies differentiating unipolar and bipolar mood disorders concluded that bipolar patients have bipolar relatives and unipolar patients have unipolar relatives (38, 54, 70, 86, 190). Family studies have consistently found a higher risk for bipolar illness in relatives of patients with bipolar illness but not in relatives of patients with unipolar depression. However, relatives of patients with unipolar depression and relatives of patients with bipolar illness have substantially elevated risk for unipolar depression (38, 54, 70, 83, 117).

Data from twin studies have provided strong evidence for the role of genetic factors in mood disorders (38, 54, 70, 86). Numerous twin studies of mood disorders have been conducted, beginning as early as 1928 (190). Twin studies of both bipolar disorder and unipolar depression have consistently found far higher rates of concordance among monozygotic than among dizygotic twin pairs (70, 83, 190). Importantly, the difference between monozygotic twin concordance and 100% points to the contribution of nongenetic factors to these disorders (38, 70, 155). The heritability of unipolar depression has been estimated at 30%–50% (53, 54, 61, 83, 86), and the heritability estimates for bipolar disorder are considerably higher, 70%–90% (28, 38, 61, 155, 190). Thus, bipolar illness appears to be more strongly influenced by genetic factors than unipolar illness. Findings from family studies support conceptual distinctions between unipolar and bipolar mood disorders as genetically separate diseases (83).

Adoption studies provide the most powerful method for testing the relative contributions of genetic and environmental factors to heredity by comparing rates of disorders in biological and adoptive family members (138, 190). The few adoption studies that have been conducted on mood disorders have demonstrated significant associations between unipolar depression in adoptees and their biological but not their adoptive relatives; some evidence for a similar pattern was found for bipolar disorder (38, 138, 190).

Early research into the genetics of psychiatric disorders consisted of linkage studies of a few large affected family pedigrees in a search for rare genetic mutations (38). The genetic analysis methods at the time limited genetic research to pursuit of selected candidate genes hypothesized as implicated in the neurobiology of depression (such as serotonin and dopamine receptors) in small numbers of individuals (53). Genetic linkage studies examined co-segregation of phenotypes with DNA markers or chromosomal regions. Genetic association studies examined associations of diseases with common genetic variation in alleles known as single nucleotide polymorphisms (SNPs).

A major problem with this earlier research was that large samples (hundreds to thousands of patients) were needed to provide sufficient statistical power to detect genetic associations with disease, but the methods available were prohibitively expensive and cumbersome. Thus, studies were inevitably underpowered, and replication of the findings was not possible (155). Ultimately, no simple Mendelian genetic patterns of inheritance of psychiatric illness have been identified (53, 70). The current understanding is that the mode of genetic transmission of psychiatric disorders is non-Mendelian and almost certainly polygenic (38, 70, 155).

Subsequent technological advances enabled high-speed genetic analysis, leading to successful mapping of the entire human genome and identification of SNPs, in turn providing understanding of common human genetic variation (38). These technological advances enabled genotyping of larger samples of unrelated individuals to detect genetic associations at the population level across the entire human genome and development of genome-wide association studies (GWAS) involving hundreds of thousands of SNPs in thousands of people (38, 70, 155). GWAS research has the advantage that it does not rely on prior hypotheses, making it an unbiased, agnostic approach (38, 53, 70). It also has the advantage that it enables analysis of a million or more genetic variants across the entire genome (53).

GWAS was applied to bipolar disorder in research published for the first time in 2007 (70), and the first depression GWAS study was published in 2009 (53). Over the next decade, more than 2,000 GWAS articles were published in the academic literature, of which 14 examined depressive disorders and at least 7 focused on bipolar disorder (53, 70). Unfortunately, GWAS also needs very large samples to yield statistical power to detect a signal in the data (38), because statistical correction for multiple tests (a million in GWAS) requires a p value <0.00000005 threshold for statistical significance. This means that sample sizes of at least 10,000 are needed (53). For bipolar disorder, genome-wide significant findings to date explain no more than a few percent of the overall heritability, but estimates that at least 25% of its overall heritability might be explained by common variants have demonstrated a need for much larger GWAS sample sizes than currently possible, possibly tens of thousands (70). This has led to combining data across various research studies. The Psychiatric Genomics Consortium (PGC) was established in 2007 as an international collaborative effort to amass sufficient sample sizes for effective GWAS research (53, 70).

To date, 27 genetic variants have been implicated in major depressive disorder. These relate to serotonin synthesis, dopamine and drug metabolism, calcium signaling, binding and salivary secretion, embryonic development, cellular stress response and blood coagulation, and heart function. For bipolar disorder, 65 genetic variants have been implicated, involving cell activation and proliferation and signal transduction, apoptosis and chromatin modification, chemokine signaling, glutamate signaling and regulation, immunological response, cell adhesion and migration, neurotransmitter degradation, and tumor suppression (61).

An important limitation of GWAS is that it does not account for environmental effects that are well established to interact with genetic factors in the contribution of risk for disease (53). Gene–environment (G×E) epigenetic research has examined biological relationships with DNA methylation and histone modifications in association with environmental stressors, although this research has been limited by small samples (97, 121). A study by Caspi et al. (31) generated much initial interest with their finding that a serotonin transporter gene polymorphism appears to moderate the effect of stress on depression susceptibility. Numerous studies attempting to replicate these findings have been inconclusive (53, 97).

In summary, not only do mood disorders likely result from several genes acting simultaneously, but it is also likely that these disorders result from the effects of several genes interacting with one another and interacting with environmental factors (70, 155). Additionally, genetic abnormalities in mood disorders have increasingly been demonstrated in recent research to overlap with other disorders such as schizophrenia (38, 70, 103, 155).

DIFFERENTIAL DIAGNOSIS

Making the distinction between grief and major depressive disorder can be difficult. Bereaved people may present with symptoms of both grief and depression (188, 189, 224). During the first few months after the loss of a loved one, depressive symptoms are common (187); the diagnosis of a depressive disorder may be deferred (224). A diagnosis of major depressive disorder is appropriate at any time if the symptom picture involves markedly impaired functioning, preoccupations of worthlessness, suicidality, psychosis, or psychomotor retardation (224). Because depressive episodes are so disruptive, distressing, and costly, and confer increased risk for suicide regardless of the context of bereavement, diagnosis of depression following loss of a loved one can facilitate initiation of treatment and improved outcomes (67, 189, 224). Grief symptoms are not generally responsive to antidepressant treatment, but depressive symptoms in the context of bereavement are (188, 189, 224).

Differential diagnosis of anxiety disorders and major depressive disorder can be difficult, because anxiety symptoms often occur during major depressive episodes and depressive symptoms are often seen in anxiety disorders (113). Symptoms that are better considered to be explained by another disorder are not diagnosed as a separate disorder but are rather considered part of the other disorder. This system of hierarchical diagnosis was replaced in *DSM-III-R* and subsequent editions of the criteria, with all disorders meeting diagnostic criteria being diagnosed independently. Research has demonstrated that anxiety disorders more often begin earlier in life than depressive disorders (113). The longitudinal course of major depressive disorder is more favorable than that for anxiety disorders, and comorbidity of major depressive disorder with an anxiety disorder is associated with a worse long-term course (164).

Patients with major depressive disorder often report somatic symptoms. Mood symptoms are reported by many patients who meet criteria for somatization disorder. Many patients with major depressive disorder may report many somatic symptoms, but these symptoms are seldom spread throughout the system review, unlike the multisymptomatic, multisyndromic pattern characteristic of patients with somatization disorder. The hallmark combination of conversion symptoms (unexplained neurological symptoms) and medically unexplained reproductive symptoms observed in somatization disorder occurs only infrequently in major depressive disorder.

Obsessions are common in major depressive disorder. If obsessions and compulsions antedate depressive symptoms and meet criteria for obsessive-compulsive disorder, a diagnosis of major depressive disorder is not made unless depressive episodes are distinct from the course of the obsessional illness.

Distinguishing between schizophrenia and mood disorders is usually not a problem. Schizophrenia, a chronic illness of insidious onset, does not follow the remitting course that is typical of mood disorders. Patients with major depressive disorder do not develop the formal thought disorder that is characteristic of schizophrenia. Occasionally, the distinction between mania and schizophrenia may be difficult. Bizarre and dramatic hallucinations, delusions, and other abnormalities of mental content like those seen in schizophrenia may occur in mania. A previous history of episodic illness with remission or the presence of euphoria, hyperactivity, or flight of ideas indicates that the diagnosis may be mania rather than schizophrenia. Although schizophrenia and bipolar disorder are well documented to segregate separately in families, overlap of these two disorders in some families is observed (28, 36, 122, 162), especially in psychotic forms of bipolar illness. A family history of bipolar disorder in a patient presenting with psychosis should encourage the clinician to consider the possibility of a mood disorder in the differential diagnosis, although it does not necessarily rule against schizophrenia.

For patients with symptoms suggesting both schizophrenia and a mood disorder, clinicians have the option of a diagnosis of schizoaffective disorder, which occupies a diagnostic space somewhere between schizophrenia and bipolar illness. The diagnosis of schizoaffective disorder was first introduced in the American psychiatric nomenclature in 1980 to accommodate diagnosis in patients presenting with a psychotic disorder together with prominent manic and/or depressive symptoms (122, 217).

In earlier editions of the criteria, schizoaffective illness was a subtype of schizophrenia (122, 217). Characteristics of schizoaffective disorder are intermediate between the more severe and chronic features of schizophrenia and the more episodic course associated with a better prognosis of bipolar disorder (125, 201). Extensive research has failed to establish acceptable diagnostic reliability and longitudinal stability of schizoaffective disorder, raising questions about the validity of this diagnosis (108, 122, 147, 181, 182, 217). This diagnosis has been overused and misapplied in clinical practice (122, 217), further degrading the meaning of this term. These problems have prompted some experts to recommend a return to the Kraepelinian dichotomization of schizophrenia and mood disorders with abandonment of the diagnosis of schizoaffective disorder (108, 122). Consistent with Kraepelin's dichotomy, patients with good-prognosis features (sudden onset, good premorbid functioning, and lack of flat affect) appear to have family histories and course more consistent with mood disorders, and those without good-prognosis features appear to have family histories and a course more consistent with schizophrenia. Today, schizoaffective psychosis is classified as part of schizophrenia-related psychotic disorders rather than with the mood disorders (201).

Depression may accompany chronic and acute brain syndromes. As many as 30%–50% of patients with dementia have depressive symptoms, especially in earlier stages of dementia. Comorbid major depressive disorder can be diagnosed in more than 10% of patients with Alzheimer's dementia and 50% of patients with cerebrovascular dementia (116). Cerebrovascular depression is especially pernicious, being more disabling and resulting in poorer outcomes than in other kinds of depression (179). Patients with depression of clearly cerebrovascular origins do not have the associated family history of major depressive disorder observed in patients with major depressive disorder (179). Memory impairment that occasionally presents in severely depressed and elderly patients may create diagnostic dilemmas in determining the primary source of the problem—the depression or the dementia (116, 179). Differential diagnosis may be aided by consideration of age of onset, rate and course of cognitive change, subjective memory complaints, and sleep/wake cycle disturbances (116, 179).

Psychiatric symptoms can result from side effects of certain drugs. It has long been known that steroids can precipitate psychotic, manic, and depressive states (160). Other medications implicated in the emergence of depressive syndromes are antihypertensive agents, lipid-lowering drugs (statins), and estrogen-receptor modulators (107, 160). Available evidence implicates interferon-alpha, interleukin-2, gonadotropin-releasing hormone agonists, mefloquine, progestin-releasing contraceptives, and propranolol in the occurrence of depressive-like symptoms. The role of these agents in generating major depressive disorder, however, is not established in diagnostic studies (107, 160).

Bipolar disorder should always be considered in the differential diagnosis of patients with unipolar depression, because half or more of the first episodes of bipolar disorder are depressive episodes, and the illness proceeds to manifest with a subsequent manic episode (173). Bipolar disorder must be differentiated from substance use disorders and personality disorders, and, in children, from conduct disorder and attention-deficit/hyperactivity disorder (73, 175).

CLINICAL MANAGEMENT

The management of major depressive disorder always involves supportive psychotherapy (7). Many clinicians believe that *insight-directed* psychotherapy, involving examination of motives and deep feelings, is not wise because it tends to increase the patient's feelings of guilt. Available evidence, however, indicates that certain types of psychotherapy may be useful for mild or moderate depression. The treatment studies are of three types: 1) psychotherapy alone compared with control group, 2) psychotherapy compared with antidepressant drugs, and 3) combined psychotherapy and drugs compared with psychotherapy alone and drugs alone. Five main types of psychotherapy examined in this research are 1) cognitive therapy, 2) behavioral therapy, 3) interpersonal therapy, 4) psychodynamic therapy, and 5) supportive therapy (43, 44, 102, 216).

The goal of *cognitive therapy* (often referred to as cognitive-behavioral or behavioral-cognitive therapy) is to identify existing negative cognitions and replace them with more positive functionally adaptive ones (90, 216), and mindfulness-based meditation techniques have become popular in conjunction with cognitive therapy. In *behavior therapy*, the patient learns new behavioral and interpersonal skills to achieve desired responses from others (90). Behavioral activation therapy specifically involves scheduling of activities to develop positive, rewarding interactions to replace avoidance and stagnancy (90). *Interpersonal psychotherapy* facilitates return to healthy functioning by focusing on the present rather than the past and interpersonal rather than intrapsychic processes; goals are development of coping, problem-solving, and social and interpersonal skills (90). In *psychodynamic therapy*, the therapist and patient explore recurrent relationship conflicts, including experiences beginning in childhood, and through understanding of historical relationship patterns, conflicts can be resolved to facilitate change (216). *Supportive therapy* is nondirective therapy primarily involving listening and empathy, allowing ventilation of the patient's emotions and experiences (216).

Several comprehensive reviews of studies comparing psychotherapy, pharmacotherapy, and/or combinations of psychotherapy and pharmacotherapy for the treatment of less severe forms of major depressive disorder have determined that psychotherapy alone and pharmacotherapy alone are both efficacious and superior to no treatment (41, 44, 46, 203, 208, 216). Thus, both psychotherapy and pharmacotherapy may be considered first-line treatments in mild to moderate depression in outpatient medical and mental health practice (35, 102, 208). Medication provides benefits of rapid and robust response (102). Psychotherapy appears to help keep patients engaged in therapy and reduce relapse, especially after medication discontinuation (42, 80, 102). Psychotherapy also appears to be associated with gains in interpersonal skills, social adjustment, well-being, and treatment satisfaction not provided by pharmacotherapy alone (91, 102). The type of psychotherapy that has been most researched is cognitive-behavioral therapy (41, 44, 216). The different types of therapy have generally been found to have comparable efficacy (13), but there is some evidence of slight superiority of cognitive-behavioral therapy (41, 43). Reviews of studies comparing combinations of treatment with pharmacotherapy and psychotherapy have concluded that combined pharmacotherapy and psychotherapy appears to have small but consistent advantages over either type of treatment alone, especially for more severe depression (41–44, 80, 102, 207, 216).

Some patients may not be good candidates for one therapy or another. Pregnancy and intolerable side effects may deter the use of medications (4, 80, 148, 195, 198, 208). Some patients may resist psychotherapy, and others may not accept medications (133, 216). Fortunately, research indicates that patients with less severe depression can generally be offered the treatment alternative they find most suitable, because outcomes of pharmacotherapy and psychotherapy for them are generally similar (80). It is generally agreed that in selecting treatment, it is important take into account patient preference (45, 80, 102, 133, 208, 216). Among patients with severe depression, however, combined pharmacotherapy and psychotherapy is recommended (43, 80).

The two major somatic approaches to the management of depressive episodes are pharmacotherapy and electrotherapy. The first antidepressant medications were of the monoamine oxidase inhibitor-A (MAO-A) inhibitor class (120). Initially developed for the treatment of tuberculosis, these medications were found to have energizing effects. Monoamine oxidase inhibitors (MAOIs) have potentially serious side effects. Foods and beverages containing tyramine (a pressor substance)—particularly cheese, some wines, and beer—should be avoided because of the danger of a hypertensive crisis. To avoid hypertensive crises, patients taking MAOIs should also not take drugs containing amphetamines or sympathomimetic substances. Over the years, safety concerns have limited the broad use of MAOI antidepressants (198, 203).

Selegiline, approved by the U.S. Food and Drug Administration (FDA) for the treatment of depression in 2006, is an MAOI packaged in a transdermal system. It is a selective MAO-B inhibitor at low doses, but at higher doses it also inhibits MAO-A (39). The tyramine dietary modifications are not needed at lower doses (up to 6 mg per 24 hours), but more experience is needed before recommending higher doses without tyramine avoidance. The main side effects of the transdermal preparation are dermal reactions and insomnia. Classic MAOI side effects such as sexual dysfunction and excessive weight gain are fortunately uncommon with selegiline (39).

For many years, tricyclic antidepressants (e.g., imipramine and amitriptyline) supplanted MAOIs as the mainstay of pharmacotherapy for depression (213). Tricyclic antidepressants have several unpleasant side effects: dry mouth, orthostatic hypotension, tremor, oversedation, and weight gain. Cardiac arrhythmias are less common but potentially serious side effects (198, 213).

Individuals vary widely in their ability to metabolize tricyclic antidepressants; as much as a 40-fold difference has been reported between fast and slow metabolizers. Cytochrome P450 polymorphisms, particularly in the CYP2D6 and CYP3C19 enzymes, affect antidepressant metabolism (88, 89, 198). What a prescriber assumes to be a therapeutic dose may actually produce toxic plasma levels or, alternatively, subtherapeutic levels of the drug. Therefore, genetic testing for these enzymes may assist in the initial dosing of these medications. Monitoring plasma levels of tricyclics is advised for rapid metabolizers and when seemingly therapeutic doses produce either no improvement or significant side effects (88).

In the late 1980s, a new class of antidepressants became available. The selective serotonin-uptake inhibitors (SSRIs) were developed because of evidence of involvement of serotonin in depression (203). This class of antidepressants includes fluoxetine, sertraline, paroxetine, and citalopram, and many others. Subsequently, other antidepressants were developed with dual actions to block not only serotonin but also norepinephrine (venlafaxine) or dopamine (bupropion) (203). These "second-generation" antidepressant medications have become very popular in clinical practice, far exceeding the use of the older classes of antidepressants (198).

The newer antidepressant medications have fewer side effects and more favorable safety profiles, especially lower lethality with overdose (198, 213). It was initially thought that cardiotoxicity was not an issue with the second-generation medications, but QT prolongation and arrhythmias such as torsade de points were later identified to represent a real risk, warranting an FDA black box warning (198). Other adverse effects of these medications include risk for falls; potential for hyponatremia, especially in the first 6 weeks of treatment; risk for upper gastrointestinal bleeding, particularly during use of nonsteroidal anti-inflammatory drugs; medication discontinuation syndromes; and serotonin syndrome (a potentially fatal condition presenting with hyperthermia, altered mental status, and tremor or clonus) (198). Common side effects of these medications include sexual dysfunction, gastrointestinal disturbances, and weight gain (198). All antidepressant medications, regardless of class, must be administered for at least several weeks and sometimes even months before significant antidepressant effects can be anticipated (198).

Choosing the most suitable antidepressant for a particular patient is informed by science, but it is also an art. The effectiveness of various antidepressants is essentially comparable; therefore, the choice of antidepressant is based on the drug's side-effect profile (198, 208, 213). Antidepressant medications vary in side-effect profiles, allowing the clinician to tailor the side effects to the patient's specific situation. For example, bupropion has an energizing effect and may interfere with sleep. Mirtazapine may cause sedation in lower doses and activation in higher doses, a feature that may be useful in the treatment of depression associated with sleeplessness or agitation. Mirtazapine may significantly increase body weight, and bupropion may be associated with weight loss. When weight gain is undesirable and alertness is desirable, bupropion may be a reasonable choice. For treatment of depression in emaciated or apprehensive cancer patients, the weight gain and sedation associated with mirtazapine favor this drug as a treatment option.

Following symptom remission in depression, there is believed to be a period of increased risk of symptom recurrence. Because there is no way to determine the length of this period, it is common practice to continue antidepressant medication for at least 6 months after the remission of acute symptoms.

No randomized controlled studies have compared the efficacy of lithium to a modern antidepressant in unipolar depression, precluding definitive conclusions about the usefulness of lithium in unipolar depression (18). Studies that have been done have not established efficacy of lithium monotherapy for unipolar depression (1, 18). Addition of lithium has been well documented, however, as effective in augmenting the therapeutic effects of antidepressant medication in unipolar illness (1, 17, 18, 149). The likelihood of unipolar depression response to lithium is greater for patients with a positive family history for bipolar illness or pure familial depressive disorder (1, 52).

Some patients experience depression during certain times of the year, especially around the winter solstice, when the days are shortest (137). The *DSM-5* criteria for major depressive disorder include a seasonal specifier for recurrent major depressive episodes that follow a pattern of onset at a particular time of the year, such as fall or winter (but it can be a summertime phenomenon) (6). Suspected contributors to this type of illness include circadian rhythm disturbance, imbalance of serotonin and melatonin, and vitamin D insufficiency (137). Available treatments for seasonal depression include antidepressant medications, psychotherapy and lifestyle counseling, vitamin D supplementation, and bright-light therapy (137, 172, 180, 194). Melatonin has been tried to prevent seasonal depression, but its efficacy for this indication is not established (101).

The academic literature is replete with warnings against combining alcohol with psychotropic medications used in treatment of depression (198). In the case of alcohol and barbiturates, the combination may be lethal. There is less additive effect between alcohol and benzodiazepine tranquilizers. Combining alcohol with tricyclic antidepressants increases sedative effects of both (32). Acute alcohol ingestion increases plasma concentrations of tricyclic antidepressants, increasing the likelihood of fatal poisoning (32, 196). In the presence of alcohol use disorder, however, antidepressant medications are metabolized at an accelerated rate, resulting in lower blood levels (196).

Antidepressant drugs—demonstrated in controlled studies to shorten depressive episodes, reduce the intensity of symptoms, and possibly prevent recurrence—have not demonstrably reduced suicide among patients with mood disorders (25, 37). There has been some evidence of increased risk of suicidality during the early course of recovery from depression with antidepressant treatment, especially with SSRIs and in adolescents (81). The mechanism for this phenomenon is unclear, however, and these findings do not warrant rejection of antidepressants for the treatment of depression out of concern for precipitating suicide attempts. Suicide-prevention centers, established in many cities during the 1960s, had no apparent effect on the suicide rate. In contrast, treatment with lithium has been demonstrated to yield a distinct advantage for reduction of suicides and of deaths from any cause (1, 34, 149, 198).

Unfortunately, many patients with major depressive disorder fail to achieve and sustain symptomatic remission (135). This means that the clinician will need to find other solutions, such as switching the antidepressant to another or adding adjunctive treatment. Although a popular strategy among clinicians, the practice of combining antidepressants has not been supported by evidence of superiority over monotherapy in controlled trials (135). The most evidence of efficacy among strategies to address initial antidepressant failure is by augmentation with second-generation antipsychotic medications such as aripiprazole, quetiapine, or risperidone (135, 192). This strategy is not without a negative side, however. First, use of these antipsychotic medications as adjunctive agents has been found to be associated with all the known potential adverse effects of these antipsychotic medications, especially movement disorders, sedation, weight gain, and metabolic syndrome (192). Clinicians have been cautioned to interpret these findings carefully because of identified methodological shortcomings in many of these studies that may have resulted in inflated apparent benefits of treatment and minimized the apparent incidence of adverse effects (192). Other evidence has supported augmentation of antidepressant medication with lithium or thyroid hormone, but the evidence is mixed for augmentation of antidepressants with stimulant medications (135). Controlled trials have demonstrated support for augmentation with other modalities as well, including cognitive behavioral therapy, exercise, and especially neurostimulatory modalities (135).

In 2000, a small crossover study serendipitously found that a subanesthetic dose of ketamine, an *N*-methyl-D-aspartate (NMDA) receptor antagonist, appeared to improve symptoms of depression, especially sadness, helplessness, and suicidality. The benefit was apparent within a few hours, but unfortunately dissipated after a few days (151, 221). The possibility of establishing a treatment for depression that is both fast-acting and robust emerging from this research stimulated a great deal of interest (223). A number of small studies followed to investigate ketamine for treatment of depression. These studies demonstrated rapid remission of depression after a single dose (144, 221). Cautions surrounding use of ketamine for depression in clinical practice have arisen from established side effects (prominent psychotomimetic and dissociative effects), safety concerns (risk for neurotoxicity with repeated dosing), and addiction and abuse liability (151, 223). These problems with ketamine suggest that its use for treatment of depression might need to be limited to patients with the most dire needs, such as patients with treatment-resistant depression or suicidality, and to clinical settings that allow close patient monitoring, such as the emergency department (223).

Electroconvulsive therapy (ECT) is considered the most effective form of treatment available for depression and one of the most efficacious of all medical treatments, with documented efficacy rates as high as 70%–90% (106, 119, 161, 205). The use of ECT declined after effective medications for the treatment of depression became accessible. For a time, this treatment was generally reserved for patients who do not respond to antidepressants or who are so ill that they cannot be treated outside a hospital. This approach was eventually challenged by data demonstrating the high effectiveness and established safety of this treatment modality (14, 161, 205). In part, the reluctance to utilize this treatment more readily is because of unfavorable public perception and continuing negative media depiction of the practice (161, 205). When ECT was first introduced into clinical practice in the early 1940s, it frequently caused vertebral and other fractures. As advances in the medical modification of electrotherapy have been made, the treatment has evolved into a technologically sophisticated procedure with a proven track record of safety (119). Now the procedure is less frightening to patients and is less commonly associated with complications. Patients are anesthetized briefly with a very rapid-acting barbiturate and then given a muscle relaxant, usually succinylcholine. Electrodes are placed in the frontotemporal regions and a small, measured amount of electricity is passed between them (161).

The most troublesome side effect of ECT is memory loss (161). This undesirable aspect of the treatment is typically limited to memory loss for the treatment interval, a brief period before initiating treatment, and several weeks after the course. Most patients do not find this to be a problem (77, 161). Delivering unilateral ECT to the nondominant side of the brain minimizes this side effect (77, 161).

ECT is generally considered the safest procedure when performed under general anesthesia (161). Risk of death following ECT is increased with recent myocardial infarction or states of elevated intracranial pressure. These concerns should be weighed against the risk of not treating severe depression in patients with these medical issues. Electroconvulsive therapy may be the safest and most effective treatment of mood disorders for women in their first trimester of pregnancy, postoperatively, and for severely depressed patients with various medical illnesses (161). It is safely used in children under age 18 and in the elderly (64, 161, 169).

First-line treatment with ECT should be considered when risks of the psychiatric illness are greater than the risks of the procedure, especially in the context of life-threatening psychiatric situations such as those involving suicidality or severe nutritional compromise (161). Additionally, because response to ECT is generally more rapid and robust than to antidepressant medication, it should be considered when fast response is important (124, 161). It should also be considered first for patients with a history of poor medication response and good ECT response, and for patients expressing a preference for ECT (161).

Repetitive transcranial magnetic stimulation (rTMS), a procedure that applies alternating electromagnetic fields to stimulate brain cortex without producing seizures, has been investigated for the treatment of major depressive disorder, and it received FDA approval in 2008 for this indication. Statistically significant therapeutic effects of rTMS have been demonstrated for both unipolar and bipolar depression (20, 21), but this treatment has not achieved the exceptional level of effectiveness of ECT (20). Other brain stimulation treatments that have shown promise for mood disorders include vagal nerve stimulation, which received FDA approval in 2008; deep brain stimulation; magnetic seizure therapy; and transcranial direct current stimulation, which uses weak direct currents without producing a seizure (119).

Lithium carbonate has historically been the drug of choice in the treatment of mania (18, 29, 63, 102, 140, 154, 167, 185). For acute manic episodes, addition of an antipsychotic medication to a classic mood stabilizer such as lithium or valproate may enhance treatment effectiveness, especially for patients with hyperactivity or agitation (63). Some clinicians begin to treat mania with both an antipsychotic agent and lithium, stopping the antipsychotic after 4 or 5 days when lithium has begun to take effect (18, 63, 102). Full lithium effectiveness may not be achieved until at least 2 or 3 weeks of treatment (18). The greatest utility of lithium is for maintenance therapy, to prevent recurrence of manic and depressive symptoms, stabilize mood, and improve functioning (18, 63, 75, 140, 185). Mixed, rapid-cycling, secondary, and comorbid mania are not as responsive as pure mania is to lithium. Predictors of a positive response to lithium are a classic episodic course with remission between mood episodes, lack of mood-incongruent psychotic features, and a family history of bipolar disorder, especially if there is also a family history of favorable lithium response (18, 167).

Optimal lithium serum levels for effective maintenance therapy of bipolar disorder are 0.8–1.0 mMol/L, but side effects and risk of renal toxicity make a more realistic serum level window in the range of 0.6–0.8 mMol/L (18, 29, 186). Serum levels less than 0.4 mMol/L may allow subthreshold symptoms to persist but may be effective in preventing depressive episodes. For acute mania, levels up to 1.2 mMol/L may be needed (18, 29). Generally, total doses of 1,200–2,400 mg of lithium per day in divided form (300 to 600 mg per dose) are required to achieve such serum levels (29). Once-daily dosing has been found to produce no adverse effects on prophylactic efficacy or side effects and may result in better patient adherence (29). Patients must be titrated to adequate serum levels on a divided dosage schedule because lithium levels are based on divided dosing with serum drawn 12 hours after the last dose. After successful titration, conversion to once-daily dosing can be undertaken (29).

Because lithium is a potentially toxic drug, its use must be monitored by repeatedly checking serum levels, particularly early in treatment. Most patients experience a fine tremor of the hands at therapeutic levels of lithium (0.8–1.5 mMol/L). At higher levels, ataxia, disorientation, somnolence, seizures, and finally circulatory collapse may occur. Toxicity begins at levels above 1.5 mMol/L, and life-threatening complications occur above 2.0 mMol/L (29).

The usefulness of lithium is not limited to the treatment of mania. Lithium is effective at preventing bipolar depressive as well as manic episodes (18, 75). There is considerable evidence that lithium reduces morbidity and may have specific anti-suicide properties in bipolar illness (18, 34, 47, 75, 115).

Two anticonvulsant medications, valproate and carbamazepine, have mood-stabilizing properties and are well documented to be effective for the treatment of mania (18). Both are FDA approved for this indication; carbamazepine was the first to receive FDA approval, in 2004 (18). Carbamazepine is rarely prescribed as a first-line agent for mania because of problems with slow onset of action (5–28 days), side effects (nausea, dizziness, fatigue, diplopia, and ataxia) necessitating a lengthy titration process, safety concerns (agranulocytosis, hepatotoxicity, and rashes, requiring close clinical and laboratory monitoring), and interactions with other medications (as a CYP450 enzyme inducer) (18, 75).

Valproate is regularly used for the treatment of mania, and it has also been proven useful for mixed, rapid-cycling, and psychotic bipolar episodes (18, 75). It appears to have efficacy similar to lithium and similar time to effectiveness, but fewer troublesome side effects. It can be rapidly titrated within a few days, from a typical starting dose of 750 mg up to 1,500 mg or more, targeting a serum valproate level of at least 95 μg/mL needed for effectiveness but not over 125 μg/mL, which is associated with side effects. Side effects include nausea, diarrhea, tremor, and sedation (18). Risks for mild thrombocytopenia and hepatotoxicity also increase at serum levels above about 125 μg/mL. Valproate and carbamazepine are both teratogenic and are thus not recommended for women of childbearing age (18, 75).

Other anticonvulsants have been investigated for bipolar illness, including lamotrigine, oxcarbazepine, topiramate, and gabapentin. Their efficacy for treatment of mania has not been established, however (18). Lamotrigine has been found to confer modest benefit for both treatment and prevention of bipolar depression episodes, with more prominent effectiveness in patients with more severe depression (18, 62, 63, 174).

Antipsychotic medications provide rapid benefit for psychosis and agitation in mania, especially for the majority of patients with mania who have psychotic symptoms (75). Second-generation antipsychotics are preferentially used for the treatment of acute mania, because of ease of administration, rapidity of onset, and more favorable side-effect profiles, but first-generation antipsychotics are no less effective (18, 75). Second-generation antipsychotic agents with documented efficacy for acute mania include risperidone, olanzapine, quetiapine, ziprasidone, aripiprazole, and asenapine. Antipsychotic dosing for mania is similar to that for schizophrenia (18). Compared to lithium, antipsychotics have a faster onset of action and greater potency for the treatment of acute mania (18, 63), but reliance on a stabilizer of mood such as lithium is a more suitable plan for primary maintenance therapy in patients with bipolar disorder (63).

When treatment with a single agent fails, two or more medications may be used in combination. The most evidence has been established for the combination of lithium or valproate with a second-generation antipsychotic agent (63, 75, 140). The side-effect burden is substantially greater, however, when combinations of medications are used (18, 167).

Despite the well-appreciated utility of antidepressants for treatment of unipolar depression, these medications do not appear to be particularly beneficial for bipolar depression and may actually be deleterious for treatment and prevention of episodes (134, 145, 152, 153). Antidepressants can precipitate mania in patients with bipolar depression and may induce mixed episodes (with simultaneous features of mania and depression) and rapid cycling between states of mania and depression (15, 145, 166). This risk is greater among juveniles and patients with a family history of bipolar disorder (15). It is therefore recommended that, when possible, antidepressants be discontinued during the maintenance phase of bipolar disorder, or at least be used in conjunction with a mood stabilizer, which may help prevent switching to mania (145, 166).

High-potency benzodiazepines, especially clonazepam and lorazepam, are commonly used in the treatment of acute mania by providing sedation and reducing anxiety (18, 24). Because sleep disturbance may predispose to manic episodes, judicious short-term use of benzodiazepines may help prevent episodes.

As with unipolar depression, ECT is considered a very effective treatment for bipolar depression (49, 161). It is also useful in the treatment for mania, especially for treatment-resistant illness (49, 161).

REFERENCES

1. Abou-Saleh, M. T., Muller-Oerlinghausen, B., and Coppen, A. J. Lithium in the episode and suicide prophylaxis and in augmenting strategies in patients with unipolar depression. Int. J. Bipolar Disord., 5:11, 2017.

2. Adams, F. The extant works of Aretaeus the Cappadocian. In *On the Causes and Symptoms of Chronic Diseases, Book 1*. London: Sydenham Society, 1856.

3. Ajetunmobi, O., Taylor, M., Stockton, D., and Wood, R. Early death in those previously hospitalised for mental healthcare in Scotland: a nationwide cohort study, 1986-2010. BMJ Open, 3, 2013.

4. Alwan, S., Friedman, J. M., and Chambers, C. Safety of selective serotonin reuptake inhibitors in pregnancy: a review of current evidence. CNS Drugs, 30:499–515, 2016.

5. American Psychiatric Association. *Diagnostic and Statistical Manual of Mental Disorders*, 3rd revised edition. Washington, DC: Author, 1987.

6. American Psychiatric Association. *Diagnostic and Statistical Manual for Mental Disorders*, 5th edition. Washington, DC: Author, 2013.

7. American Psychiatric Association. Practice guideline for the treatment of patients with major depressive disorder (revision). Am. J. Psychiatry, 157:1–45, 2000.

8. Anacker, C., O'Donnell, K. J., and Meaney, M. J. Early life adversity and the epigenetic programming of hypothalamic-pituitary-adrenal function. Dialogues Clin. Neurosci., 16:321–333, 2014.

9. Andrews, B., and Wilding, J. M. The relation of depression and anxiety to life-stress and achievement in students. Br. J. Psychol., 95:509–521, 2004.

10. Angst, J., Angst, F., and Stassen, H. H. Suicide risk in patients with major depressive disorder. J. Clin. Psychiatry, 60(Suppl 2):57–62, 1999.

11. Angst, J., Sellaro, R., Stassen, H. H., and Gamma, A. Diagnostic conversion from depression to bipolar disorders: results of a long-term prospective study of hospital admissions. J. Affect. Disord., 84:149–157, 2005.

12. Augustinavicius, J. L., Zanjani, A., Zakzanis, K. K., and Shapiro, C. M. Polysomnographic features of early-onset depression: a meta-analysis. J. Affect. Disord., 158:11–18, 2014.

13. Baardseth, T. P., Goldberg, S. B., Pace, B. T., Wislocki, A. P., Frost, N. D., Siddiqui, J. R., Lindemann, A. M., Kivlighan, D. M., III, Laska, K. M., Del Re, A. C., Minami, T., and Wampold, B. E. Cognitive-behavioral therapy versus other therapies: redux. Clin. Psychol. Rev., 33:395–405, 2013.

14. Bailine, S., Fink, M., Knapp, R., Petrides, G., Husain, M. M., Rasmussen, K., Sampson, S., Mueller, M., McClintock, S. M., Tobias, K. G., and Kellner, C. H. Electroconvulsive therapy is equally effective in unipolar and bipolar depression. Acta Psychiatr. Scand., 121:431–436, 2010.

15. Baldessarini, R. J., Faedda, G. L., Offidani, E., Vazquez, G. H., Marangoni, C., Serra, G., and Tondo, L. Antidepressant-associated mood-switching and transition

from unipolar major depression to bipolar disorder: a review. J. Affect. Disord., *148*:129–135, 2013.

16. Barnes, J. *The Complete Works of Aristotle: The Revised Oxford Translation, One-Volume Digital Edition*. Princeton, NJ: Princeton University Press, 1984.

17. Bauer, M., Bschor, T., Kunz, D., Berghofer, A., Strohle, A., and Muller-Oerlinghausen, B. Double-blind, placebo-controlled trial of the use of lithium to augment antidepressant medication in continuation treatment of unipolar major depression. Am. J. Psychiatry, *157*:1429–1435, 2000.

18. Bauer, M., and Gitlin, M. *The Essential Guide to Lithium Treatment*. New York: Springer, 2016.

19. Benazzi, F. Is there a continuity between bipolar and depressive disorders? Psychother. Psychosom., *76*:70–76, 2007.

20. Berlim, M. T., Van den Eynde, F., and Daskalakis, Z. J. Efficacy and acceptability of high frequency repetitive transcranial magnetic stimulation (rTMS) versus electroconvulsive therapy (ECT) for major depression: a systematic review and meta-analysis of randomized trials. Depress. Anxiety, *30*:614–623, 2013.

21. Berlim, M. T., Van den Eynde, F., Tovar-Perdomo, S., and Daskalakis, Z. J. Response, remission and drop-out rates following high-frequency repetitive transcranial magnetic stimulation (rTMS) for treating major depression: a systematic review and meta-analysis of randomized, double-blind and sham-controlled trials. Psychol. Med., *44*:225–239, 2014.

22. Bertolote, J. M., Fleischmann, A., De Leo, D., and Wasserman, D. Psychiatric diagnoses and suicide: revisiting the evidence. Crisis, *25*:147–155, 2004.

23. Blazer, D. G. *The Age of Melancholy: "Major Depression" and Its Social Origins*. New York: Routledge, 2005.

24. Bobo, W. V., Reilly-Harrington, N. A., Ketter, T. A., Brody, B. D., Kinrys, G., Kemp, D. E., Shelton, R. C., McElroy, S. L., Sylvia, L. G., Kocsis, J. H., McInnis, M. G., Friedman, E. S., Singh, V., Tohen, M., Bowden, C. L., Deckersbach, T., Calabrese, J. R., Thase, M. E., Nierenberg, A. A., Rabideau, D. J., Schoenfeld, D. A., Faraone, S. V., and Kamali, M. Complexity of illness and adjunctive benzodiazepine use in outpatients with bipolar I or II disorder: results from the Bipolar CHOICE study. J. Clin. Psychopharmacol., *35*:68–74, 2015.

25. Braun, C., Bschor, T., Franklin, J., and Baethge, C. Suicides and suicide attempts during long-term treatment with antidepressants: a meta-analysis of 29 placebo-controlled studies including 6,934 patients with major depressive disorder. Psychother. Psychosom., *85*:171–179, 2016.

26. Bromet, E., Andrade, L. H., Hwang, I., Sampson, N. A., Alonso, J., de Girolamo G., de Graf, R., Demyttenaere, K., Hu, C., Iwata, N., Karam, A. N., Kaur, J., Kostyuchenko, S., Lepine, J. P., Levinson, D., Matschinger, H., Mora, M. E., Browne, M. O., Posada-Villa, J., Viana, M. C., Williams, D. R., and Kessler, R. C. Cross-national epidemiology of DSM-IV major depressive episode. BMC Med., *9*:90, 2011.

27. Bukh, J. D., Andersen, P. K., and Kessing, L. V. Rates and predictors of remission, recurrence and conversion to bipolar disorder after the first lifetime episode of depression—a prospective 5-year follow-up study. Psychol. Med., *46*:1151–1161, 2016.

28. Cardno, A. G., and Owen, M. J. Genetic relationships between schizophrenia, bipolar disorder, and schizoaffective disorder. Schizophr. Bull., *40*:504–515, 2014.

29. Carter, L., Zolezzi, M., and Lewczyk, A. An updated review of the optimal lithium dosage regimen for renal protection. Can. J. Psychiatry, *58*:595–600, 2013.

30. Carvalho, A. F., McIntyre, R. S., Dimelis, D., Gonda, X., Berk, M., Nunes-Neto, P. R., Cha, D. S., Hyphantis, T. N., Angst, J., and Fountoulakis, K. N. Predominant polarity as a course specifier for bipolar disorder: a systematic review. J. Affect. Disord., *163*:56–64, 2014.

31. Caspi, A., Sugden, K., Moffitt, T. E., Taylor, A., Craig, I. W., Harrington, H., McClay, J., Mill, J., Martin, J., Braithwaite, A., and Poulton, R. Influence of life stress on depression: moderation by a polymorphism in the 5-HTT gene. Science, *301*:386–389, 2003.

32. Chan, L. N., and Anderson, G. D. Pharmacokinetic and pharmacodynamic drug interactions with ethanol (alcohol). Clin. Pharmacokinet., *53*:1115–1136, 2014.

33. Chaudron, L. H., and Pies, R. W. The relationship between postpartum psychosis and bipolar disorder: a review. J. Clin. Psychiatry, *64*:1284–1292, 2003.

34. Cipriani, A., Hawton, K., Stockton, S., and Geddes, J. R. Lithium in the prevention of suicide in mood disorders: updated systematic review and meta-analysis. BMJ, *346*:f3646, 2013.

35. Clark, D. M. Implementing NICE guidelines for the psychological treatment of depression and anxiety disorders: the IAPT experience. Int. Rev. Psychiatry, *23*:318–327, 2011.

36. Cosgrove, V. E., and Suppes, T. Informing DSM-5: biological boundaries between bipolar I disorder, schizoaffective disorder, and schizophrenia. BMC Med., *11*:127, 2013.

37. Coupland, C., Hill, T., Morriss, R., Arthur, A., Moore, M., and Hippisley-Cox, J. Antidepressant use and risk of suicide and attempted suicide or self harm in people aged 20 to 64: cohort study using a primary care database. BMJ, *350*:h517, 2015.

38. Craddock, N., and Sklar, P. Genetics of bipolar disorder. Lancet, *381*:1654–1662, 2013.

39. Cristancho, M. A., and Thase, M. E. Critical appraisal of selegiline transdermal system for major depressive disorder. Expert. Opin. Drug Deliv., *13*:659–665, 2016.

40. Cuellar, A. K., Johnson, S. L., and Winters, R. Distinctions between bipolar and unipolar depression. Clin. Psychol. Rev., *25*:307–339, 2005.

41. Cuijpers, P., Berking, M., Andersson, G., Quigley, L., Kleiboer, A., and Dobson, K. S. A meta-analysis of cognitive-behavioural therapy for adult depression, alone and in comparison with other treatments. Can. J. Psychiatry, *58*:376–385, 2013.

42. Cuijpers, P., De Wit, L., Weitz, E., Andersson, G., and Huibers, M. J. H. The combination of psychotherapy and pharmacotherapy in the treatment of adult depression: a comprehensive meta-analysis. J. Evid. Based Psychother., *15*:147–168, 2015.

43. Cuijpers, P., Ebert, D. D., Acarturk, C., Andersson, G., and Cristea, I. A. Personalized psychotherapy for adult depression: a meta-analytic review. Behav. Ther., *47*:966–980, 2016.

44. Cuijpers, P., Karyotaki, E., Weitz, E., Andersson, G., Hollon, S. D., and van, S. A. The effects of psychotherapies for major depression in adults on remission, recovery and improvement: a meta-analysis. J. Affect. Disord., *159*:118–126, 2014.

45. Cuijpers, P., Sijbrandij, M., Koole, S. L., Andersson, G., Beekman, A. T., and Reynolds, C. F., III. The efficacy of psychotherapy and pharmacotherapy in treating depressive and anxiety disorders: a meta-analysis of direct comparisons. World Psychiatry, *12*:137–148, 2013.

46. Cuijpers, P., Turner, E. H., Mohr, D. C., Hofmann, S. G., Andersson, G., Berking, M., and Coyne, J. Comparison of psychotherapies for adult depression to pill placebo control groups: a meta-analysis. Psychol. Med., *44*:685–695, 2014.

47. da Costa, S. C., Alencar, A. P., Nascimento Neto, P. J., dos Santos, M. S., da Silva, C. G., Pinheiro, S. F., Silveira, R. T., Bianco, B. A., Pinheiro, R. F., Jr., de Lima, M. A., Reis, A. O., and Rolim Neto, M. L. Risk factors for suicide in bipolar disorder: a systematic review. J. Affect. Disord., *170*:237–254, 2015.
48. de Sá, A. S., Campos, C., Rocha, N. B., Yuan, T. F., Paes, F., Arias-Carrion, O., Carta, M. G., Nardi, A. E., Cheniaux, E., and Machado, S. Neurobiology of bipolar disorder: abnormalities on cognitive and cortical functioning and biomarker levels. CNS Neurol. Disord. Drug Targets, *15*:713–722, 2016.
49. Dierckx, B., Heijnen, W. T., van den Broek, W. W., and Birkenhager, T. K. Efficacy of electroconvulsive therapy in bipolar versus unipolar major depression: a meta-analysis. Bipolar Disord., *14*:146–150, 2012.
50. Diflorio, A., and Jones, I. Is sex important? Gender differences in bipolar disorder. Int. Rev. Psychiatry, *22*:437–452, 2010.
51. Duarte, W., Becerra, R., and Cruise, K. The relationship between neurocognitive functioning and occupational functioning in bipolar disorder: a literature review. Eur. J. Psychol., *12*:659–678, 2016.
52. Duffy, A., Grof, P., Robertson, C., and Alda, M. The implications of genetics studies of major mood disorders for clinical practice. J. Clin. Psychiatry, *61*:630–637, 2000.
53. Dunn, E. C., Brown, R. C., Dai, Y., Rosand, J., Nugent, N. R., Amstadter, A. B., and Smoller, J. W. Genetic determinants of depression: recent findings and future directions. Harv. Rev. Psychiatry, *23*:1–18, 2015.
54. Fakhoury, M. New insights into the neurobiological mechanisms of major depressive disorders. Gen. Hosp. Psychiatry, *37*:172–177, 2015.
55. Ferrari, A. J., Charlson, F. J., Norman, R. E., Flaxman, A. D., Patten, S. B., Vos, T., and Whiteford, H. A. The epidemiological modelling of major depressive disorder: application for the Global Burden of Disease Study 2010. PLoS One, *8*:e69637, 2013.
56. Ferrari, A. J., Somerville, A. J., Baxter, A. J., Norman, R., Patten, S. B., Vos, T., and Whiteford, H. A. Global variation in the prevalence and incidence of major depressive disorder: a systematic review of the epidemiological literature. Psychol. Med., *43*:471–481, 2013.
57. Ferrari, A. J., Stockings, E., Khoo, J. P., Erskine, H. E., Degenhardt, L., Vos, T., and Whiteford, H. A. The prevalence and burden of bipolar disorder: findings from the Global Burden of Disease Study 2013. Bipolar Disord., *18*:440–450, 2016.
58. Ferrari, F., and Villa, R. F. The neurobiology of depression: an integrated overview from biological theories to clinical evidence. Mol. Neurobiol., *54*:4847–4865, 2017.
59. Francis, A. Catatonia: diagnosis, classification, and treatment. Curr. Psychiatry Rep., *12*:180–185, 2010.
60. Freud, S. Mourning and Melancholia. In *The Complete Psychological Works of Sigmund Freud*, Strachey, J. (ed.). London: Hogarth Press, pp. 237–259, 1957.
61. Gatt, J. M., Burton, K. L., Williams, L. M., and Schofield, P. R. Specific and common genes implicated across major mental disorders: a review of meta-analysis studies. J. Psychiatr. Res., *60*:1–13, 2015.
62. Geddes, J. R., Calabrese, J. R., and Goodwin, G. M. Lamotrigine for treatment of bipolar depression: independent meta-analysis and meta-regression of individual patient data from five randomised trials. Br. J. Psychiatry, *194*:4–9, 2009.
63. Geddes, J. R., and Miklowitz, D. J. Treatment of bipolar disorder. Lancet, *381*:1672–1682, 2013.
64. Geduldig, E. T., and Kellner, C. H. Electroconvulsive therapy in the elderly: new findings in geriatric depression. Curr. Psychiatry Rep., *18*:40, 2016.

65. Gershon, N. B., and High, P. C. Epigenetics and child abuse: modern-day Darwinism—the miraculous ability of the human genome to adapt, and then adapt again. Am. J. Med. Genet. C. Semin. Med. Genet., *169*:353–360, 2015.

66. Gibb, S. J., Beautrais, A. L., and Fergusson, D. M. Mortality and further suicidal behaviour after an index suicide attempt: a 10-year study. Aust. N. Z. J. Psychiatry, *39*:95–100, 2005.

67. Gilman, S. E., Breslau, J., Trinh, N. H., Fava, M., Murphy, J. M., and Smoller, J. W. Bereavement and the diagnosis of major depressive episode in the National Epidemiologic Survey on Alcohol and Related Conditions. J. Clin. Psychiatry, *73*:208–215, 2012.

68. Gilman, S. E., Dupuy, J. M., and Perlis, R. H. Risks for the transition from major depressive disorder to bipolar disorder in the National Epidemiologic Survey on Alcohol and Related Conditions. J. Clin. Psychiatry, *73*:829–836, 2012.

69. Gliatto, M. F., and Rai, A. K. Evaluation and treatment of patients with suicidal ideation. Am. Fam. Physician, *59*:1500–1506, 1999.

70. Goes, F. S. Genetics of bipolar disorder: recent update and future directions. Psychiatr. Clin. North Am., *39*:139–155, 2016.

71. Goldberg, J. F., Garno, J. L., and Harrow, M. Long-term remission and recovery in bipolar disorder: a review. Curr. Psychiatry Rep., 7:456–461, 2005.

72. Goldberg, J. F., and Harrow, M. Consistency of remission and outcome in bipolar and unipolar mood disorders: a 10-year prospective follow-up. J. Affect. Dis., *81*:123–131, 2004.

73. Goldstein, B. I. Recent progress in understanding pediatric bipolar disorder. Arch. Pediatr. Adolesc. Med., *166*:362–371, 2012.

74. Goldstein, B. I., and Birmaher, B. Prevalence, clinical presentation and differential diagnosis of pediatric bipolar disorder. Isr. J. Psychiatry Relat. Sci., *49*:3–14, 2012.

75. Grande, I., Berk, M., Birmaher, B., and Vieta, E. Bipolar disorder. Lancet, *387*:1561–1572, 2016.

76. Grande, I., Goikolea, J. M., de, D. C., Gonzalez-Pinto, A., Montes, J. M., Saiz-Ruiz, J., Prieto, E., and Vieta, E. Occupational disability in bipolar disorder: analysis of predictors of being on severe disablement benefit (PREBIS study data). Acta Psychiatr. Scand., *127*:403–411, 2013.

77. Greenberg, R. M., and Kellner, C. H. Electroconvulsive therapy: a selected review. Am. J. Geriatr. Psychiatry, *13*:268–281, 2005.

78. Greenwood, T. A. Positive traits in the bipolar spectrum: the space between madness and genius. Mol. Neuropsychiatry, 2:198–212, 2017.

79. Grimmer, Y., Hohmann, S., and Poustka, L. Is bipolar always bipolar? Understanding the controversy on bipolar disorder in children. F1000Prime Rep., 6:111, 2014.

80. Guidi, J., Tomba, E., and Fava, G. A. The sequential integration of pharmacotherapy and psychotherapy in the treatment of major depressive disorder: a meta-analysis of the sequential model and a critical review of the literature. Am. J. Psychiatry, *173*:128–137, 2016.

81. Gupta, S., Gersing, K. R., Erkanli, A., and Burt, T. Antidepressant regulatory warnings, prescription patterns, suicidality and other aggressive behaviors in major depressive disorder and anxiety disorders. Psychiatr. Q., *87*:329–342, 2016.

82. Guze, S. B., and Robins, E. Suicide and primary affective disorders. Br. J. Psychiatry, *117*:437–438, 1970.

83. Hamet, P., and Tremblay, J. Genetics and genomics of depression. Metabolism, *54*:10–15, 2005.

84. Harris, E. C., and Barraclough, B. Excess mortality of mental disorder. Br. J. Psychiatry, 173:11–53, 1998.

85. Harshaw, C. Interoceptive dysfunction: toward an integrated framework for understanding somatic and affective disturbance in depression. Psychol. Bull., 141:311–363, 2015.

86. Hasler, G. Pathophysiology of depression: do we have any solid evidence of interest to clinicians? World Psychiatry, 9:155–161, 2010.

87. Hawton, K., Casanas, I. C., Haw, C., and Saunders, K. Risk factors for suicide in individuals with depression: a systematic review. J. Affect. Disord., 147:17–28, 2013.

88. Hicks, J. K., Sangkuhl, K., Swen, J. J., Ellingrod, V. L., Muller, D. J., Shimoda, K., Bishop, J. R., Kharasch, E. D., Skaar, T. C., Gaedigk, A., Dunnenberger, H. M., Klein, T. E., Caudle, K. E., and Stingl, J. C. Clinical Pharmacogenetics Implementation Consortium guideline (CPIC) for CYP2D6 and CYP2C19 genotypes and dosing of tricyclic antidepressants: 2016 update. Clin. Pharmacol. Ther., 2016. doi: 10.1002/cpt.597

89. Hicks, J. K., Swen, J. J., Thorn, C. F., Sangkuhl, K., Kharasch, E. D., Ellingrod, V. L., Skaar, T. C., Muller, D. J., Gaedigk, A., and Stingl, J. C. Clinical Pharmacogenetics Implementation Consortium guideline for CYP2D6 and CYP2C19 genotypes and dosing of tricyclic antidepressants. Clin. Pharmacol. Ther., 93:402–408, 2013.

90. Hofmann, S. G., Asmundson, G. J., and Beck, A. T. The science of cognitive therapy. Behav. Ther., 44:199–212, 2013.

91. Hundt, N. E., Mignogna, J., Underhill, C., and Cully, J. A. The relationship between use of CBT skills and depression treatment outcome: a theoretical and methodological review of the literature. Behav. Ther., 44:12–26, 2013.

92. Hysenbegasi, A., Hass, S. L., and Rowland, C. R. The impact of depression on the academic productivity of university students. J. Ment. Health Policy Econ., 8:145–151, 2005.

93. Ingram, R. E., Scott, W., and Siegle, G. Depression: social and cognitive aspects. In Oxford Textbook of Psychopathology, Millon, T., Blaney, P. H., Davis, R. D. (eds.). New York: Oxford, pp. 203–226, 1999.

94. Isometsä, E. T. Psychological autopsy studies—a review. Eur. Psychiatry, 16:379–385, 2001.

95. James, W. Lectures VI and VII: the sick soul. In The Varieties of Religious Experience: A Study in Human Nature. Melbourne, Australia: LimpidSoft, pp. 211–270, 1902.

96. Jamison, K. An Unquiet Mind. New York: Knopf, 1995.

97. Januar, V., Saffery, R., and Ryan, J. Epigenetics and depressive disorders: a review of current progress and future directions. Int. J. Epidemiol., 44:1364–1387, 2015.

98. Johnson, G. F. S., and Leeman, M. M. Onset of illness in bipolar manic-depressives and their affectively ill first-degree relatives. Biol. Psychiatry, 12:733–741, 1977.

99. Jones, I., and Craddock, N. Familiality of the puerperal trigger in bipolar disorder: results of a family study. Am. J. Psychiatry, 158:913–917, 2001.

100. Judd, L. L. Dimensional paradigm of the long-term course of unipolar major depressive disorder. Depress. Anxiety, 29:167–171, 2012.

101. Kaminski-Hartenthaler, A., Nussbaumer, B., Forneris, C. A., Morgan, L. C., Gaynes, B. N., Sonis, J. H., Greenblatt, A., Wipplinger, J., Lux, L. J., Winkler, D., Van Noord, M. G., Hofmann, J., and Gartlehner, G. Melatonin and agomelatine for preventing seasonal affective disorder. Cochrane Database Syst. Rev., CD011271, 2015.

102. Karyotaki, E., Smit, Y., Holdt, H. K., Huibers, M. J., Robays, J., de Beurs, D., and Cuijpers, P. Combining pharmacotherapy and psychotherapy or monotherapy for major depression? A meta-analysis on the long-term effects. J. Affect. Disord., 194:144–152, 2016.

103. Kavanagh, D. H., Tansey, K. E., O'Donovan, M. C., and Owen, M. J. Schizophrenia genetics: emerging themes for a complex disorder. Mol. Psychiatry, 20:72–76, 2015.

104. Kessing, L. V. Epidemiology of subtypes of depression. Acta Psychiatr. Scand. Suppl., 115(433):85–89, 2007.

105. Kessler, R. C., Berglund, P., Demler, O., Jin, R., Koretz, D., Merikangas, K. R., Rush, A. J., Walters, E. E., and Wang, P. S. The epidemiology of major depressive disorder: results from the National Comorbidity Survey Replication (NCS-R). JAMA, 289:3095–3105, 2003.

106. Kolar, D. Current status of electroconvulsive therapy for mood disorders: a clinical review. Evid. Based Ment. Health, 20:12–14, 2017.

107. Kotlyar, M., Dysken, M., and Adson, D. E. Update on drug-induced depression in the elderly. Am. J. Geriatr. Psychiatry, 3:288–300, 2005.

108. Kotov, R., Leong, S. H., Mojtabai, R., Erlanger, A. C., Fochtmann, L. J., Constantino, E., Carlson, G. A., and Bromet, E. J. Boundaries of schizoaffective disorder: revisiting Kraepelin. JAMA Psychiatry, 70:1276–1286, 2013.

109. Kraepelin, E. *Manic Depressive Insanity and Paranoia.* Edinburgh: E.S. Livingstone, 1921.

110. Kroon, J. S., Wohlfarth, T. D., Dieleman, J., Sutterland, A. L., Storosum, J. G., Denys, D., de Haan, L., and Sturkenboom, M. C. Incidence rates and risk factors of bipolar disorder in the general population: a population-based cohort study. Bipolar Disord., 15:306–313, 2013.

111. Kuehner, C. Why is depression more common among women than among men? Lancet Psychiatry, 4:146–158, 2017.

112. Kyaga, S., Lichtenstein, P., Boman, M., and Landen, M. Bipolar disorder and leadership—a total population study. Acta Psychiatr. Scand., 131:111–119, 2015.

113. Lamers, F., van, O. P., Comijs, H. C., Smit, J. H., Spinhoven, P., van Balkom, A. J., Nolen, W. A., Zitman, F. G., Beekman, A. T., and Penninx, B. W. Comorbidity patterns of anxiety and depressive disorders in a large cohort study: the Netherlands Study of Depression and Anxiety (NESDA). J. Clin. Psychiatry, 72:341–348, 2011.

114. Leonhard, K., Korff, I., and Shulz, H. Die Temperamente in den Familien der monopolaren und bipolaren Phasichen. Psychosen Psychiatr. Neurol., 143:416–434, 1962.

115. Lewitzka, U., Severus, E., Bauer, R., Ritter, P., Muller-Oerlinghausen, B., and Bauer, M. The suicide prevention effect of lithium: more than 20 years of evidence—a narrative review. Int. J. Bipolar Disord., 3:32, 2015.

116. Leyhe, T., Reynolds, C. F., III, Melcher, T., Linnemann, C., Kloppel, S., Blennow, K., Zetterberg, H., Dubois, B., Lista, S., and Hampel, H. A common challenge in older adults: classification, overlap, and therapy of depression and dementia. Alzheimers Dement., 13:59–71, 2017.

117. Lim, C. S., Baldessarini, R. J., Vieta, E., Yucel, M., Bora, E., and Sim, K. Longitudinal neuroimaging and neuropsychological changes in bipolar disorder patients: review of the evidence. Neurosci. Biobehav. Rev., 37:418–435, 2013.

118. Lin, P. I., McInnis, M. G., Potash, J. B., Willour, V., MacKinnon, D. F., DePaulo, J. R., and Zandi, P. P. Clinical correlates and familial aggregation of age at onset in bipolar disorder. Am. J. Psychiatry, 163:240–246, 2006.

119. Loo, C., Katalinic, N., Mitchell, P. B., and Greenberg, B. Physical treatments for bipolar disorder: a review of electroconvulsive therapy, stereotactic surgery and other brain stimulation techniques. J. Affect. Disord., 132:1–13, 2011.

120. Lopez-Munoz, F., and Alamo, C. Monoaminergic neurotransmission: the history of the discovery of antidepressants from 1950s until today. Curr. Pharm. Des., 15:1563–1586, 2009.

121. Ludwig, B., and Dwivedi, Y. Dissecting bipolar disorder complexity through epigenomic approach. Mol. Psychiatry, 21:1490–1498, 2016.

122. Malaspina, D., Owen, M. J., Heckers, S., Tandon, R., Bustillo, J., Schultz, S., Barch, D. M., Gaebel, W., Gur, R. E., Tsuang, M., Van, O. J., and Carpenter, W. Schizoaffective disorder in the DSM-5. Schizophr. Res., 150:21–25, 2013.

123. Maletic, V., and Raison, C. Integrated neurobiology of bipolar disorder. Front Psychiatry, 5:98, 2014.

124. Maletzky, B. M. The first-line use of electroconvulsive therapy in major affective disorders. J. ECT, 20:112–117, 2004.

125. Mancuso, S. G., Morgan, V. A., Mitchell, P. B., Berk, M., Young, A., and Castle, D. J. A comparison of schizophrenia, schizoaffective disorder, and bipolar disorder: results from the Second Australian National Psychosis Survey. J. Affect. Disord., 172:30–37, 2015.

126. Martinez-Aran, A., Vieta, E., Colom, F., Torrent, C., Sanchez-Moreno, J., Reinares, M., Benabarre, A., Goikolea, J. M., Brugue, E., Daban, C., and Salamero, M. Cognitive impairment in euthymic bipolar patients: implications for clinical and functional outcome. Bipolar Disord., 6:224–232, 2004.

127. Martinez-Aran, A., Vieta, E., Reinares, M., Colom, F., Torrent, C., Sanchez-Moreno, J., Benabarre, A., Goikolea, J. M., Comes, M., and Salamero, M. Cognitive function across manic or hypomanic, depressed, and euthymic states in bipolar disorder. Am. J. Psychiatry, 161:262–270, 2004.

128. Marvel, C. L., and Paradiso, S. Cognitive and neurological impairment in mood disorders. Psychiatr. Clin. North Am., 27:19–36, vii–viii, 2004.

129. Maslow, G. R., Dunlap, K., and Chung, R. J. Depression and suicide in children and adolescents. Pediatr. Rev., 36:299–308, 2015.

130. Massart, R., Mongeau, R., and Lanfumey, L. Beyond the monoaminergic hypothesis: neuroplasticity and epigenetic changes in a transgenic mouse model of depression. Philos. Trans. R. Soc. Lond. B Biol. Sci., 367:2485–2494, 2012.

131. McClellan, J., Kowatch, R., and Findling, R. L. Practice parameter for the assessment and treatment of children and adolescents with bipolar disorder. J. Am. Acad. Child Adolesc. Psychiatry, 46:107–125, 2007.

132. McCrory, E., De Brito, S. A., and Viding, E. The link between child abuse and psychopathology: a review of neurobiological and genetic research. J. R. Soc. Med., 105:151–156, 2012.

133. McHugh, R. K., Whitton, S. W., Peckham, A. D., Welge, J. A., and Otto, M. W. Patient preference for psychological vs pharmacologic treatment of psychiatric disorders: a meta-analytic review. J. Clin. Psychiatry, 74:595–602, 2013.

134. McInerney, S. J., and Kennedy, S. H. Review of evidence for use of antidepressants in bipolar depression. Prim. Care Companion CNS Disord., 16: 10.4088/PCC.14r01653, 2014.

135. McIntyre, R. S., Filteau, M. J., Martin, L., Patry, S., Carvalho, A., Cha, D. S., Barakat, M., and Miguelez, M. Treatment-resistant depression: definitions, review of the evidence, and algorithmic approach. J. Affect. Disord., *156*:1–7, 2014.

136. Meilman, P. W., Manley, C., Gaylor, M. S., and Turco, J. H. Medical withdrawals from college for mental health reasons and their relation to academic performance. J. Am. Coll. Health, *40*:217–223, 1992.

137. Melrose, S. Seasonal affective disorder: an overview of assessment and treatment approaches. Depress. Res. Treat., *2015*:178564, 2015.

138. Merikangas, K. R., and Low, N. C. The epidemiology of mood disorders. Curr. Psychiatry Rep., 6:411–421, 2004.

139. Mitchell, P. B., and Malhi, G. S. Bipolar depression: phenomenological overview and clinical characteristics. Bipolar Disord., 6:530–539, 2004.

140. Miura, T., Noma, H., Furukawa, T. A., Mitsuyasu, H., Tanaka, S., Stockton, S., Salanti, G., Motomura, K., Shimano-Katsuki, S., Leucht, S., Cipriani, A., Geddes, J. R., and Kanba, S. Comparative efficacy and tolerability of pharmacological treatments in the maintenance treatment of bipolar disorder: a systematic review and network meta-analysis. Lancet Psychiatry, *1*:351–359, 2014.

141. Morimoto, S. S., Kanellopoulos, D., Manning, K. J., and Alexopoulos, G. S. Diagnosis and treatment of depression and cognitive impairment in late life. Ann. N. Y. Acad. Sci., *1345*:36–46, 2015.

142. Mulders, P. C., van Eijndhoven, P. F., Schene, A. H., Beckmann, C. F., and Tendolkar, I. Resting-state functional connectivity in major depressive disorder: a review. Neurosci. Biobehav. Rev., *56*:330–344, 2015.

143. Mulinari, S. Monoamine theories of depression: historical impact on biomedical research. J. Hist. Neurosci., *21*:366–392, 2012.

144. Muller, J., Pentyala, S., Dilger, J., and Pentyala, S. Ketamine enantiomers in the rapid and sustained antidepressant effects. Ther. Adv. Psychopharmacol., *6*:185–192, 2016.

145. Muneer, A. Treatment of the depressive phase of bipolar affective disorder: a review. J. Pak. Med. Assoc., *63*:763–769, 2013.

146. Munk-Olsen, T., Laursen, T. M., Meltzer-Brody, S., Mortensen, P. B., and Jones, I. Psychiatric disorders with postpartum onset: possible early manifestations of bipolar affective disorders. Arch. Gen. Psychiatry, *69*:428–434, 2012.

147. Murru, A., Manchia, M., Tusconi, M., Carpiniello, B., Pacchiarotti, I., Colom, F., and Vieta, E. Diagnostic reliability in schizoaffective disorder. Bipolar Disord., *18*:78–80, 2016.

148. Muzik, M., and Hamilton, S. E. Use of antidepressants during pregnancy? What to consider when weighing treatment with antidepressants against untreated depression. Matern. Child Health J., *20*:2268–2279, 2016.

149. Nelson, J. C., Baumann, P., Delucchi, K., Joffe, R., and Katona, C. A systematic review and meta-analysis of lithium augmentation of tricyclic and second generation antidepressants in major depression. J. Affect. Disord., *168*:269–275, 2014.

150. Nemeroff, C. B., Bremner, J. D., Foa, E. B., Mayberg, H. S., North, C. S., and Stein, M. B. Posttraumatic stress disorder: a state-of-the-science review. J. Psychiatr. Res., *40*:1–21, 2006.

151. Newport, D. J., Carpenter, L. L., McDonald, W. M., Potash, J. B., Tohen, M., and Nemeroff, C. B. Ketamine and other NMDA antagonists: early clinical trials and possible mechanisms in depression. Am. J. Psychiatry, *172*:950–966, 2015.

152. Nierenberg, A. A. An analysis of the efficacy of treatments for bipolar depression. J. Clin. Psychiatry, *69(Suppl 5)*:4–8, 2008.

153. Nierenberg, A. A. Effective agents in treating bipolar depression. J. Clin. Psychiatry, 69:e29, 2008.
154. Nivoli, A. M., Murru, A., Goikolea, J. M., Crespo, J. M., Montes, J. M., Gonzalez-Pinto, A., Garcia-Portilla, P., Bobes, J., Saiz-Ruiz, J., and Vieta, E. New treatment guidelines for acute bipolar mania: a critical review. J. Affect. Disord., 140:125–141, 2012.
155. Offord, J. Genetic approaches to a better understanding of bipolar disorder. Pharmacol. Ther., 133:133–141, 2012.
156. O'Leary, D., Paykel, E., Todd, C., and Vardulaki, K. Suicide in primary affective disorders revisited: a systematic review by treatment era. J. Clin. Psychiatry, 62:804–811, 2001.
157. Otte, C., Gold, S. M., Penninx, B. W., Pariante, C. M., Etkin, A., Fava, M., Mohr, D. C., and Schatzberg, A. F. Major depressive disorder. Nat. Rev. Dis. Primers, 2:16065, 2016.
158. Owens, D., Horrocks, J., and House, A. Fatal and non-fatal repetition of self-harm. Systematic review. Br. J. Psychiatry, 181:193–199, 2002.
159. Ozerdem, A., Ceylan, D., and Can, G. Neurobiology of risk for bipolar disorder. Curr. Treat. Options Psychiatry, 3:315–329, 2016.
160. Patten, S. B., and Barbui, C. Drug-induced depression: a systematic review to inform clinical practice. Psychother. Psychosom., 73:207–215, 2004.
161. Payne, N. A., and Prudic, J. Electroconvulsive therapy: part I. A perspective on the evolution and current practice of ECT. J. Psychiatr. Pract., 15:346–368, 2009.
162. Pearlson, G. D. Etiologic, phenomenologic, and endophenotypic overlap of schizophrenia and bipolar disorder. Annu. Rev. Clin. Psychol., 11:251–281, 2015.
163. Peen, J., Schoevers, R. A., Beekman, A. T., and Dekker, J. The current status of urban–rural differences in psychiatric disorders. Acta Psychiatr. Scand., 121:84–93, 2010.
164. Penninx, B. W., Nolen, W. A., Lamers, F., Zitman, F. G., Smit, J. H., Spinhoven, P., Cuijpers, P., de Jong, P. J., van Marwijk, H. W., van der Meer, K., Verhaak, P., Laurant, M. G., de Graff, R., Hoogendijk, W. J., van der Wee, N., Ormel, J., van Dyck, R., and Beekman, A. T. Two-year course of depressive and anxiety disorders: results from the Netherlands Study of Depression and Anxiety (NESDA). J. Affect. Disord., 133:76–85, 2011.
165. Perris, C. The importance of Karl Leonhard's classification of endogenous psychoses. Psychopathology, 23:282–290, 1990.
166. Phillips, M. L., and Kupfer, D. J. Bipolar disorder diagnosis: challenges and future directions. Lancet, 381:1663–1671, 2013.
167. Post, R. M., Ostacher, M. J., and Singh, V. Controversies in the psychopharmacology of bipolar disorder. J. Clin. Psychiatry, 75:e30, 2014.
168. Price, J. S. Chronic depressive illness. Br. Med. J., 1:1200–1201, 1979.
169. Puffer, C. C., Wall, C. A., Huxsahl, J. E., and Frye, M. A. A 20 year practice review of electroconvulsive therapy for adolescents. J. Child Adolesc. Psychopharmacol., 26:632–636, 2016.
170. Quraishi, S., and Frangou, S. Neuropsychology of bipolar disorder: a review. J. Affect. Dis., 72:209–226, 2002.
171. Rao, U. Sleep disturbances in pediatric depression. Asian J. Psychiatry, 4:234–247, 2011.
172. Rastad, C., Ulfberg, J., and Lindberg, P. Improvement in fatigue, sleepiness, and health-related quality of life with bright light treatment in persons with

seasonal affective disorder and subsyndromal SAD. Depress. Res. Treat., *2011*:543906, 2011.

173. Ratheesh, A., Cotton, S. M., Betts, J. K., Chanen, A., Nelson, B., Davey, C. G., McGorry, P. D., Berk, M., and Bechdolf, A. Prospective progression from high-prevalence disorders to bipolar disorder: exploring characteristics of pre-illness stages. J. Affect. Disord., *183*:45–48, 2015.

174. Reid, J. G., Gitlin, M. J., and Altshuler, L. L. Lamotrigine in psychiatric disorders. J. Clin. Psychiatry, 74:675–684, 2013.

175. Renk, K., White, R., Lauer, B. A., McSwiggan, M., Puff, J., and Lowell, A. Bipolar disorder in children. Psychiatry J., *2014*:928685, 2014.

176. Richards, D. Prevalence and clinical course of depression: a review. Clin. Psychol. Rev., *31*:1117–1125, 2011.

177. Rihmer, Z., and Kiss, K. Bipolar disorders and suicidal behaviour. Bipolar Disord., 4(*Suppl 1*):21–25, 2002.

178. Rijavec, N., and Grubic, V. N. Depression and pain: often together but still a clinical challenge: a review. Psychiatr. Danub., 24:346–352, 2012.

179. Robinson, R. G., and Jorge, R. E. Post-stroke depression: a review. Am. J. Psychiatry, 173:221–231, 2016.

180. Rohan, K. J., Mahon, J. N., Evans, M., Ho, S. Y., Meyerhoff, J., Postolache, T. T., and Vacek, P. M. Randomized trial of cognitive-behavioral therapy versus light therapy for seasonal affective disorder: acute outcomes. Am. J. Psychiatry, 172:862–869, 2015.

181. Santelmann, H., Franklin, J., Busshoff, J., and Baethge, C. Test-retest reliability of schizoaffective disorder compared with schizophrenia, bipolar disorder, and unipolar depression—a systematic review and meta-analysis. Bipolar Disord., 17:753–768, 2015.

182. Santelmann, H., Franklin, J., Busshoff, J., and Baethge, C. Interrater reliability of schizoaffective disorder compared with schizophrenia, bipolar disorder, and unipolar depression—a systematic review and meta-analysis. Schizophr. Res., 176:357–363, 2016.

183. Saunders, K. E., and Hawton, K. Clinical assessment and crisis intervention for the suicidal bipolar disorder patient. Bipolar Disord., 15:575–583, 2013.

184. Schaffer, A., Isometsa, E. T., Tondo, L., Moreno, H., Turecki, G., Reis, C., Cassidy, F., Sinyor, M., Azorin, J. M., Kessing, L. V., Ha, K., Goldstein, T., Weizman, A., Beautrais, A., Chou, Y. H., Diazgranados, N., Levitt, A. J., Zarate, C. A., Jr., Rihmer, Z., and Yatham, L. N. International Society for Bipolar Disorders Task Force on Suicide: meta-analyses and meta-regression of correlates of suicide attempts and suicide deaths in bipolar disorder. Bipolar Disord., 17:1–16, 2015.

185. Severus, E., Taylor, M. J., Sauer, C., Pfennig, A., Ritter, P., Bauer, M., and Geddes, J. R. Lithium for prevention of mood episodes in bipolar disorders: systematic review and meta-analysis. Int. J. Bipolar Disord., 2:15, 2014.

186. Severus, W. E., Kleindienst, N., Seemuller, F., Frangou, S., Moller, H. J., and Greil, W. What is the optimal serum lithium level in the long-term treatment of bipolar disorder—a review? Bipolar Disord., 10:231–237, 2008.

187. Shear, M. K. Grief and mourning gone awry: pathway and course of complicated grief. Dialogues Clin. Neurosci., 14:119–128, 2012.

188. Shear, M. K. Clinical practice. Complicated grief. N. Engl. J. Med., 372:153–160, 2015.

189. Shear, M. K., Simon, N., Wall, M., Zisook, S., Neimeyer, R., Duan, N., Reynolds, C., Lebowitz, B., Sung, S., Ghesquiere, A., Gorscak, B., Clayton, P., Ito, M., Nakajima, S., Konishi, T., Melhem, N., Meert, K., Schiff, M., O'Connor, M. F.,

First, M., Sareen, J., Bolton, J., Skritskaya, N., Mancini, A. D., and Keshaviah, A. Complicated grief and related bereavement issues for DSM-5. Depress. Anxiety, 28:103–117, 2011.

190. Smoller, J. W., and Finn, C. T. Family, twin, and adoption studies of bipolar disorder. Am. J. Med. Genet. C. Semin. Med. Genet., 123:48–58, 2003.

191. Solomon, D. A., Leon, A. C., Coryell, W. H., Endicott, J., Li, C., Fiedorowicz, J. G., Boyken, L., and Keller, M. B. Longitudinal course of bipolar I disorder: duration of mood episodes. Arch. Gen. Psychiatry, 67:339–347, 2010.

192. Spielmans, G. I., Berman, M. I., Linardatos, E., Rosenlicht, N. Z., Perry, A., and Tsai, A. C. Adjunctive atypical antipsychotic treatment for major depressive disorder: a meta-analysis of depression, quality of life, and safety outcomes. PLOS Med., 10:e1001403, 2013.

193. Steinert, C., Hofmann, M., Kruse, J., and Leichsenring, F. The prospective long-term course of adult depression in general practice and the community. A systematic literature review. J. Affect. Disord., 152-154:65–75, 2014.

194. Stewart, A. E., Roecklein, K. A., Tanner, S., and Kimlin, M. G. Possible contributions of skin pigmentation and vitamin D in a polyfactorial model of seasonal affective disorder. Med. Hypotheses, 83:517–525, 2014.

195. Stohl, H., Kohm, A. D., and Dossett, E. A rock and a hard place: the selective serotonin reuptake inhibitor dilemmas in addressing perinatal mood and anxiety disorders. J. Neonatal Perinatal. Med., 9:1–5, 2016.

196. Tanaka, E. Toxicological interactions involving psychiatric drugs and alcohol: an update. J. Clin. Pharm. Ther., 28:81–95, 2003.

197. Tejedor, M. C., Diaz, A., Castillon, J. J., and Pericay, J. M. Attempted suicide: repetition and survival—findings of a follow-up study. Acta Psychiatr. Scand., 100:205–211, 1999.

198. Thronson, L. R., and Pagalilauan, G. L. Psychopharmacology. Med. Clin. North Am., 98:927–958, 2014.

199. Tondo, L., Baldessarini, R. J., and Floris, G. Long-term clinical effectiveness of lithium maintenance treatment in types I and II bipolar disorders. Br. J. Psychiatry, 178:S184–S190, 2001.

200. Tondo, L., Baldessarini, R. J., Hennen, J., Minnai, G. P., Salis, P., Scamonatti, L., Masia, M., Ghiani, C., and Mannu, P. Suicide attempts in major affective disorder patients with comorbid substance use disorders. J. Clin. Psychiatry, 60(Suppl 2):63–69, 1999.

201. Tondo, L., Vazquez, G. H., Baethge, C., Baronessa, C., Bolzani, L., Koukopoulos, A., Mazzarini, L., Murru, A., Pacchiarotti, I., Pinna, M., Salvatore, P., Sani, G., Selle, V., Spalletta, G., Girardi, P., Tohen, M., Vieta, E., and Baldessarini, R. J. Comparison of psychotic bipolar disorder, schizoaffective disorder, and schizophrenia: an international, multisite study. Acta Psychiatr. Scand., 133:34–43, 2016.

202. Tremblay, C. H., Grosskopf, S., and Yang, K. Brainstorm: occupational choice, bipolar illness and creativity. Econ. Hum. Biol., 8:233–241, 2010.

203. Undurraga, J., and Baldessarini, R. J. Randomized, placebo-controlled trials of antidepressants for acute major depression: thirty-year meta-analytic review. Neuropsychopharmacology, 37:851–864, 2012.

204. Vassos, E., Agerbo, E., Mors, O., and Pedersen, C. B. Urban–rural differences in incidence rates of psychiatric disorders in Denmark. Br. J. Psychiatry, 208:435–440, 2016.

205. Versiani, M., Cheniaux, E., and Landeira-Fernandez, J. Efficacy and safety of electroconvulsive therapy in the treatment of bipolar disorder: a systematic review. J. ECT, 27:153–164, 2011.

206. Villanueva, R. Neurobiology of major depressive disorder. Neural Plast., 2013:873278, 2013.

207. Vittengl, J. R., Jarrett, R. B., Weitz, E., Hollon, S. D., Twisk, J., Cristea, I., David, D., DeRubeis, R. J., Dimidjian, S., Dunlop, B. W., Faramarzi, M., Hegerl, U., Kennedy, S. H., Kheirkhah, F., Mergl, R., Miranda, J., Mohr, D. C., Rush, A. J., Segal, Z. V., Siddique, J., Simons, A. D., and Cuijpers, P. Divergent outcomes in cognitive-behavioral therapy and pharmacotherapy for adult depression. Am. J. Psychiatry, 173:481–490, 2016.

208. von Wolff A., Holzel, L. P., Westphal, A., Harter, M., and Kriston, L. Selective serotonin reuptake inhibitors and tricyclic antidepressants in the acute treatment of chronic depression and dysthymia: a systematic review and meta-analysis. J. Affect. Disord., 144:7–15, 2013.

209. Waraich, P., Goldner, E. M., Somers, J. M., and Hsu, L. Prevalence and incidence studies of mood disorders: a systematic review of the literature. Can. J. Psychiatry, 49:124–138, 2004.

210. Weissman, M. M., Bland, R. C., Canino, G. J., Faravelli, C., Greenwald, S., Hwu, H. G., Joyce, P. R., Karam, E. G., Lee, C. K., Lellouch, J., Lepine, J. P., Newman, S. C., Rubio-Stipec, M., Wells, J. E., Wickramaratne, P. J., Wittchen, H., and Yeh, E. K. Cross-national epidemiology of major depression and bipolar disorder. JAMA, 276:293–299, 1996.

211. Weissman, M. M., Bruce, M. L., Leaf, P. J., Florio, L. P., and Holzer, I. C. Affective disorders. In *Psychiatric Disorders in America: The Epidemiologic Catchment Area Study*, Robins, L. N., Regier, D. A. (eds.). New York: The Free Press, pp. 53–80, 1991.

212. Wesselhöft, R. T. Childhood depressive disorders. Dan. Med. J., 63:1–28, 2016.

213. Whiskey, E., and Taylor, D. A review of the adverse effects and safety of noradrenergic antidepressants. J. Psychopharmacol., 27:732–739, 2013.

214. Wichniak, A., Wierzbicka, A., and Jernajczyk, W. Sleep as a biomarker for depression. Int. Rev. Psychiatry, 25:632–645, 2013.

215. Wilcox, J. A., and Reid, D. P. The syndrome of catatonia. Behav. Sci. (Basel), 5:576–588, 2015.

216. Williams, K., and Anderson, I. Psychotherapy for depression—a review and practical guide. Prescriber, 25:10–16, 2014.

217. Wilson, J. E., Nian, H., and Heckers, S. The schizoaffective disorder diagnosis: a conundrum in the clinical setting. Eur. Arch. Psychiatry Clin. Neurosci., 264:29–34, 2014.

218. Winokur, G., Coryell, W., Keller, M., Endicott, J., and Akiskal, H. A prospective follow-up of patients with bipolar and primary unipolar affective disorder. Arch. Gen. Psychiatry, 50:457–465, 1993.

219. Winokur, G., Coryell, W., Keller, M., Endicott, J., and Leon, A. A family study of manic-depressive (bipolar I) disease. Is it a distinct illness separable from primary unipolar depression? Arch. Gen. Psychiatry, 52:367–373, 1995.

220. Winokur, G., and Pitts Jr, F. N. Affective disorder: VI. A family history study of prevalences, sex differences, and possible genetic factors. J. Psychiatr. Res., 3:113–123, 1965.

221. Xu, Y., Hackett, M., Carter, G., Loo, C., Galvez, V., Glozier, N., Glue, P., Lapidus, K., McGirr, A., Somogyi, A. A., Mitchell, P. B., and Rodgers, A. Effects of low-dose and very low-dose ketamine among patients with major depression: a systematic review and meta-analysis. Int. J. Neuropsychopharmacol., 19, 2016.

222. Yiend, J., Paykel, E., Merritt, R., Lester, K., Doll, H., and Burns, T. Long-term outcome of primary care depression. J. Affect. Disord., *118*:79–86, 2009.

223. Zhu, W., Ding, Z., Zhang, Y., Shi, J., Hashimoto, K., and Lu, L. Risks associated with misuse of ketamine as a rapid-acting antidepressant. Neurosci. Bull., *32*:557–564, 2016.

224. Zisook, S., Iglewicz, A., Avanzino, J., Maglione, J., Glorioso, D., Zetumer, S., Seay, K., Vahia, I., Young, I., Lebowitz, B., Pies, R., Reynolds, C., Simon, N., and Shear, M. K. Bereavement: course, consequences, and care. Curr. Psychiatry Rep., *16*:482, 2014.

CHAPTER 3

୶

Schizophrenic Disorders

Hallucinations and delusions are psychotic symptoms that reflect impaired contact with reality. These symptoms are widely considered to be hallmarks of mental disorder and thus are of great interest to psychiatrists. Psychotic symptoms may be seen in a wide variety of illnesses, including mood disorders, neurocognitive disorders, alcohol and drug use disorders, and a group of conditions that may be called the "schizophrenic disorders."

Schizophrenic disorders and mood disorders comprise the main psychotic disorders. In general, but not always, the schizophrenic disorders have a worse long-term prognosis compared with psychotic mood disorders, which tend to be more remitting (97).

Many investigators believe that schizophrenic disorders comprise a number of different conditions (11, 133, 164). Efforts to divide them into valid subgroups, however, have had limited success. Psychiatrists have historically grouped the schizophrenias into paranoid, catatonic, hebephrenic, and simple types, depending on whether the predominant symptoms are delusions, bizarre motor behavior, disturbances in affect and associations, or social withdrawal and inadequacy (15, 80). In practice, however, these diagnostic subtypes of schizophrenia have not been demonstrated to represent stable entities over time, and patients may fall into different subcategories at different points of the course of their illness (112).

The schizophrenic disorders have classically been divided into two main categories: one with a relatively poor prognosis, the other with a relatively good prognosis (97, 140). Terms historically applied to the poor-prognosis cases are chronic schizophrenia, process schizophrenia, nuclear schizophrenia, and nonremitting schizophrenia; the good-prognosis cases have been called schizophreniform disorder, acute schizophrenia, reactive schiz-ophrenia, schizoaffective disorder, and remitting schizophrenia (122).

Research has clarified that schizophrenic conditions have consider-able variability in outcome (56, 110, 116, 133). Consistent predictors of outcomes have been identified (116). Patients with more favorable prog-nosis are those whose previous general adjustment has been good, and their illness presents episodically with intervening periods of remission (56, 116, 135). Many patients show striking mood symptoms during the acute psy-chotic illness (79, 98, 113). They may seem perplexed and bewildered and may be mildly disoriented. Subsequent episodes may sometimes resemble mood disorders (113). Prominent mood disturbances during episodes of psychosis predict a more favorable course and outcome (97).

A cardinal feature of schizophrenia is the occurrence of delusions and hallucinations in a clear sensorium. Other noteworthy features are a blunted, shallow, or strikingly inappropriate affect; odd, sometimes bi-zarre, motor behavior; and disordered thinking in which goal directedness and normal associations between ideas are markedly distorted (loosening of associations and tangential thinking). Cognitive functioning is often im-paired, and many patients experience extensive loss of motivation, drive, and social functioning, referred to as "negative" symptoms.

HISTORICAL BACKGROUND

In now-classic studies, Emil Kraepelin (1856–1926), a German psychiatrist, built upon the work of his countrymen Kahlbaum (1828–1899) and Hecker (1843–1909), who described "catatonia" and "hebephrenia," respectively, to lay the groundwork for present views of schizophrenia (59, 80). Careful follow-up of hospitalized patients led Kraepelin to separate "manic depres-sive psychosis" from "dementia praecox." The latter term referred to what is now called "chronic schizophrenia." Even though Kraepelin believed de-mentia praecox to be a chronic disorder that frequently ended in marked deterioration of mental functions, he recognized that a small number of patients recovered completely. His "narrow" view of schizophrenia has been followed by most European psychiatrists, particularly those in the Scandinavian countries and Great Britain.

A broader approach to schizophrenia (and the name itself) was offered by Eugene Bleuler (1857–1939), a Swiss psychiatrist, who realized that he might be dealing with a group of disorders (15). His diagnostic criteria were not based on their ability to predict course and outcome, but on conformance to his hypothesis concerning the basic defect, namely, the "splitting" of psychic functions. By this he meant inconsistency, inappropriateness, and disorganization of affect, thought, and action, in the absence of obvious brain disease. Despite his less-strict approach to diagnosis and the variable course that his patients experienced, Bleuler believed that patients with schizophrenia never recovered completely, never returned to their premorbid state (*restituo ad integrum*). Because his "fundamental" symptoms included autistic thinking (defined by Bleuler as "divorce from reality"), blunted or inappropriate affect, ambivalence, and disturbed association of thought—all inherently difficult to define and specify—Bleuler's work set the stage for the very broad concepts of schizophrenia developed by psychoanalysts and adopted for years by many American psychiatrists.

Psychoanalysts viewed schizophrenia primarily as a manifestation of a "weak ego." Unable to cope with the problems of life and unable to use effectively the "defenses of the ego" to handle instinctual forces and anxiety, patients "regress" to a primitive level of functioning ("primary process") manifested by thought disorder, affective poverty, disorganization, and inability to conform to the demands of "reality" (20). In this psychoanalytic view of schizophrenia, all signs of weak ego (including a wide range of personality handicaps and abnormalities) or of "primary process" (such as hallucinations, delusions, poor reality-testing, tangential thinking, and ambivalence) are manifestations of the illness. It is not surprising, therefore, that the diagnosis was used in a wide range of clinical situations.

In the late 1930s, a number of European and American investigators began again to approach the problem of studying the schizophrenias for predicting course, response to treatment, and long-term outcomes. They recognized that proper evaluation of treatment requires knowledge of the natural history of the disorder in patients and their families, especially the factors associated with different clinical courses and outcomes. As a result, clinical and research approaches to the schizophrenic disorders have been based on extensive longitudinal follow-up studies, supplemented by family studies (122).

Differences between European and American psychiatrists in conceptualizing schizophrenic disorders were largely resolved after the introduction of systematic diagnostic criteria in *DSM-III*, in 1980. Most psychiatrists around the world came to accept the narrower approach to schizophrenia, referred to as "neo-Kraepelinian" (33). This consensus is largely based on empirical and systematic studies indicating that the narrower approach produces more consistent findings with regard to course, response to treatment, long-term outcome, and familial illness patterns.

EPIDEMIOLOGY

Chronic schizophrenia occurs in somewhat less than 1% of the population (27, 129, 134, 136), but because of its early onset, chronicity, and associated disability, it is one of the most important psychiatric illnesses. Historically, epidemiological studies have typically neither distinguished between good- and poor-prognosis forms of schizophrenia nor considered the possibility that some of the good-prognosis cases may represent other disorders. Available evidence suggests that the good-prognosis cases may be relatively common (125). The combined prevalence of both good- and poor-prognosis disorders is probably between 1% and 2%.

Schizophrenic disorders are found in all cultures. A number of studies have indicated that they are more prevalent among people from lower socioeconomic backgrounds (84). For some investigators, this has suggested that poverty, limited education, and associated handicaps predispose to schizophrenic illness. Studies have shown, however, that the association between schizophrenic illness and low socioeconomic status can be explained by "downward drift," a term that refers to the effect of an illness on the patient's socioeconomic status (14). If a disorder interferes with education and work performance, so that individuals are not able to complete advanced schooling or hold positions of responsibility, their socioeconomic status—characteristically defined by income, educational achievement, and job prestige—cannot be high.

Classic studies of schizophrenia in the United States and Europe have shown that the distribution of socioeconomic class among the fathers of children with the illness is not different from that in the general population, indicating that the lower socioeconomic status of patients with schizophrenic illness is at least partially the result of downward drift (84). Immigrants to European countries—especially ethnic minority groups and those from underdeveloped countries—have been found to have substantially higher rates of schizophrenia than in native-born groups (18, 154, 162). The intersection of low social status and schizophrenia in these immigrants cannot be entirely explained by selective downward social drift. Environmental stressors such as unemployment, social adversity, racial discrimination, and cultural hardships appear to have contributed to their risk for developing psychotic illness (131, 162).

In hundreds of studies, dating as far back as 1929, researchers have consistently identified an excess of births during the late winter and early spring months among individuals who develop schizophrenia in the Northern Hemisphere (12, 22, 110). Though most births in schizophrenia do not occur during these months and the effect size is small, the importance of these findings is that something associated with such births (e.g., increased exposure to perinatal influenza) may predispose to schizophrenic illness (22). This line of research is supported by a study documenting a seven-fold increase in risk for schizophrenia among children with maternal serological evidence of first-trimester exposure to influenza (107). Other research has demonstrated convincing evidence of increased rates of schizophrenia among individuals with prenatal exposure to maternal starvation during famines (22, 118, 137, 144).

Schizophrenia appears to have a slight male preponderance, with males having a 1.4-fold greater incidence of the disorder (1, 22). Males also seem to have poorer premorbid adjustment, more severe clinical manifestations, and a more chronic course (1, 86).

CLINICAL PICTURE

The main clinical features of schizophrenia include persistent hallucinations, delusions, disorganized speech and behavior, inappropriate or flattened emotional expression, and lack of motivation (8, 110). Patients with schizophrenia may be socially withdrawn, produce little spontaneous speech, and lack ability to initiate and sustain goal-directed activities. There is a decline in their work, interpersonal, and even self-care functioning. These patients may exhibit neurocognitive difficulties, especially in memory, attention, and executive functions.

Common delusions in schizophrenia are those of persecution and control in which patients believe others are spying on them, spreading false rumors about them, planning to harm them, trying to control their thoughts or actions, or reading their minds. For instance, a young woman complained bitterly that her brother was sending special mysterious messages to her by means of television in order to make her do things that would call attention to her and lead to trouble with the police. A young man was convinced that he was being followed and observed on the streets and in various buildings, but he concluded that this was being directed by his psychiatrist as a way to monitor his progress. Patients may express the belief that they are the victims of conspiracies by neighbors, the FBI, the Mafia, aliens, and so on. Delusions of depersonalization are also common. These may be feelings that bizarre bodily changes are taking place, sometimes as a result of the deliberate but obscure actions of others, for example: "My insides are rotting because they are poisoning my food. It's because they know I'm wise to them and have reported them to the police."

The most common hallucinations are auditory. They may involve solitary or multiple voices. The patient may or may not recognize the voices or talk back to them. The voices may seem to come from within the patient's body or from outside sources, such as radios or walls. The voices may criticize, ridicule, or threaten; often they urge the patient to do something she or he believes is wrong.

Visual hallucinations may not be as prevalent in schizophrenia as in bipolar disorder, but neither are they unusual (10). These hallucinations may vary from frightening, vague forms to images of dead or absent relatives to scenes of violence or hell. Olfactory hallucinations, which are infrequent, usually consist of unpleasant smells arising from the patient's own body. Tactile (haptic) hallucinations, also infrequent, may consist of feelings that one's genitals are being manipulated, that there are animals inside one's body, or that there is "grit" on one's skin that cannot be washed off.

Although the so-called typical flat schizophrenic affect is highly characteristic when it is severe, its diagnostic value is limited because it frequently is subtle, leading to disagreement about its presence. Even when clearly present, it is not easy to describe. Patients seem emotionally unresponsive, without warmth or empathy. They can talk about frightening or shocking thoughts without seeming to experience their usual emotional impact ("inappropriate" affect). It is often difficult to feel compassion and sympathy for the patient or to believe that he or she can empathize with others.

Recurrent posturing, grimacing, prolonged immobility, and "waxy flexibility" are dramatic examples of catatonic behavior. These may be independent symptoms or responses to auditory hallucinations.

The impaired goal-directedness of schizophrenic thought and speech may take various forms, all likely to occur in the same patient. These include blocking, in which the patient's thought and speech stop for periods of time only to begin again with an apparently different subject; tangential associations, in which connections between thoughts are difficult or impossible to follow; neologisms, in which the patient makes up new words; or "word salad," in which the patient's speech consists of words without any understandable sequence or meaning.

Delusions, hallucinations, bizarre and disorganized behavior, and formal thought disorder in schizophrenia have been collectively termed "positive" symptoms; blunted affect, social withdrawal, amotivation, apathy, anhedonia, and social and occupational deficits are considered "negative" symptoms (19, 40). The positive symptoms may fluctuate during the course of the illness and the negative symptoms tend to be more constant. The negative symptoms have consistently been shown to be associated with a poorer prognosis (40, 86). "Deficit" schizophrenia refers to the most severe form of the illness with enduring negative symptoms and cognitive problems (19). Positive- and negative-symptom groupings have not offered enduring utility for subtyping forms of schizophrenia. Recognition of the positive–negative symptom distinction has, however, stimulated clinicians to pay more attention to the full spectrum of clinical features of schizophrenia (40) and spurred the development of novel medications to target negative symptoms that were largely unresponsive to the earlier antipsychotic medications (121, 138).

From the time of Kraepelin's application of the name "dementia praecox" to the schizophrenias, the associated cognitive deficits have been recognized as a central feature of the illness. In the nineteenth century, however, the cognitive deficits were viewed merely as secondary to positive and negative symptoms that were considered the core psychopathology of schizophrenia. In the last two decades, the cognitive deficits have come to be appreciated as primary and central features of the illness and recognized as responsible for the socio-occupational decline seen in many of these patients (76). Schizophrenia research has identified impairments in higher neurocognitive abilities that map to prefrontal cortex circuitry abnormalities and frontotemporal structural brain changes (67, 76, 110). Specific deficits have been demonstrated in memory encoding and retrieval, sustained and selective attention and vigilance, perceptual and cognitive processing, response speed, visuospatial skills, and verbal fluency (16, 17, 76, 133). These cognitive abnormalities result in difficulties with neurobehavioral regulation and executive functions involving planning and pursuing the goal-directed activities that are essential to real-world functioning (76, 110).

Patients with schizophrenic disorders may display prominent alterations of mood, usually depression but sometimes euphoria, during the course of illness (79, 98, 113). Other affective symptoms—such as insomnia, anorexia, weight loss, alterations in interest and energy, impairment of mental concentration, guilt, and suicidal preoccupation—may also be present. In fact, many patients with schizophrenia experience episodes of depression that symptomatically resemble those seen in major depressive disorder (110, 112). Because the first-degree relatives of such patients do not appear to have an increased prevalence of mood disorders, their depression may be regarded as symptomatic of schizophrenia rather than the manifestation of a second illness.

BIOLOGICAL FINDINGS

Schizophrenia is now generally accepted to be a "brain-based" illness, but the exact etiology remains uncertain (11, 110). The likelihood that the schizophrenias represent a collection of syndromes representing the end state of different biological pathways only complicates the scientific search for the source of the illness (110, 164). Although neuropathology, neurochemistry, neuroimaging, and neurocognitive studies have demonstrated consistent brain abnormalities in schizophrenia, there are as yet no reliable biomarkers for schizophrenia and no diagnostic laboratory tests for the disorder (27, 54, 91, 110, 147).

Brain pathology in schizophrenia has been investigated through studies of postmortem brains and in brain imaging research. Postmortem brains of patients with schizophrenia have revealed subtle macroscopic and microscopic differences from nonschizophrenic brains, including reduced neuronal numbers and neuronal size (69). A computerized tomography (CT) study published in 1976 was the first imaging study to show enlarged ventricles in patients with schizophrenia compared to controls (11, 69). CT and other brain imaging techniques—magnetic resonance imaging (MRI), positron emission tomography (PET), single photon emission computed tomography (SPECT), functional magnetic resonance imaging (fMRI), diffusion tensor imaging (DTI), and magnetic resonance spectroscopy (MRS)—have opened new vistas into the investigation of brain structure and function in schizophrenia.

Consistently identified brain abnormalities in schizophrenia are low brain weight and decreased cortical volume. The most remarkable reductions of brain tissue are found in limbic and associated areas, including the temporal lobe, superior temporal gyrus, hippocampus, parahippocampal gyrus, anterior cingulate cortex, and amygdala (9, 53, 110). These abnormalities are more pronounced in gray matter than in white matter (110). A corresponding increased volume found in the lateral and third ventricles—on the order of 26%—has been one of the most consistent brain findings in schizophrenia (27, 61, 104, 127, 155).

A recognized methodological limitation of neuropathological and brain imaging studies is that first-episode and medication-naïve patients have generally not been included. Thus, some brain findings from these studies may represent artifacts of antipsychotic medication, illness chronicity, medical comorbidity, or even smoking (27, 127). Because recent research has demonstrated an evolving neuropathological picture over the course of the illness, especially progression of gray matter loss (72) and frontal cortex changes that reflect the course of symptoms and executive impairments

(58), it is evident that effects of age and duration of illness have not been adequately addressed in the patients studied (11). However, many of the brain abnormalities in schizophrenia have been demonstrated in young, first-episode, or never-medicated patients with the illness without association with age, illness chronicity, duration of antipsychotic treatment, length of previous hospitalization, or the use of electroconvulsive therapy. This suggests that these brain abnormalities are primary features of the illness rather than artifacts of associated characteristics of the individuals studied, and that they may be present early in the course of the illness (41, 64).

A long-standing assumption, dating back to Kraepelin (80) a century ago, is that schizophrenia is a neurodegenerative condition, based on observations of the progressive, deteriorating course of many of these patients (89, 153). More recently, however, the dominant view of schizophrenia is that it represents a neurodevelopmental condition (89). Strongly supporting this assumption is the finding that gliosis is not a consistent brain finding in schizophrenia (11), a finding that is more consistent with the neurodevelopmental hypothesis.

Considerable evidence has accumulated to implicate abnormalities in three main neurotransmitter systems—the dopaminergic, serotonergic, and glutamatergic systems—in schizophrenia (21, 27, 31). Historically, the main neurochemical theory has been the "dopamine hypothesis," which arose in the 1960s from animal experiments demonstrating that antipsychotic medications blocked dopamine receptors (87). The dopamine hypothesis postulates presynaptic dysfunction of the dopamine D_2 receptors, resulting in excessive synthesis and release of dopamine in the limbic striatum (62, 72). Elevated dopamine levels in the striatum have been identified in both postmortem and PET studies. This dopamine excess is considered the source of psychotic symptoms such as hallucinations and delusions (62, 110) and a main target of antipsychotic medications directed toward reduction of these symptoms (72). In the 1990s, the dopamine hypothesis was revised to suggest that the positive symptoms of schizophrenia result from hyperactive mesolimbic dopamine projections functioning to hyperstimulate striatal dopamine receptors of the D_2 subclass, and that the negative symptoms and cognitive impairments of schizophrenia result from hypoactive mesolimbic dopamine projections that hypostimulate prefrontal cortex dopamine receptors of the D_1 subclass (21, 87).

A "serotonin hypothesis" of schizophrenia assumes the disease is caused by chronic widespread serotonergic overdrive in the anterior cingulate cortex and the dorsolateral frontal lobe, disrupting the functioning of cortical neurons (42). Serotonin is central to neurobiological processes of emotional and mood regulation, and it is thought to be involved in negative symptoms as well as in depressive states that are observed in patients with schizophrenia (132). The evidence for a primary role of the serotonin system in schizophrenia is not as strong as the evidence implicating the dopamine system, and is largely derived from indirect drug challenge studies (132). A recent meta-analysis of postmortem studies, however, documented prefrontal elevations in activity of serotonin 5-hydroxytriptamine (5-HT) receptors of the 1A subtype and reductions in activity of 5-HT receptors of the 2A subtype in schizophrenia compared to activity in healthy controls (132). 5-HT1A stimulation has been shown to increase dopamine release, which may contribute to psychosis. 5-HT1A activity has been implicated in anxiety and has been implicated in mood states in schizophrenia. 5-HT2A stimulation may inhibit dopamine release in the frontal cortex; reduced activity has been identified in these receptors in schizophrenia, which may further contribute to psychosis (132).

The "glutamate hypothesis" of schizophrenia emerged from evidence that antagonists at the N-methyl-D-aspartate (NMDA) receptor, such as phencyclidine and ketamine, can induce the full range of psychotic symptoms (72, 110). Glutamate acts at the NMDA receptor and is the primary excitatory neurotransmitter in the brain (95). Glutamate is the precursor of gamma-aminobutyric acid (GABA), the brain's main inhibitory neurotransmitter. Compromise of glutamate function in schizophrenia thus diminishes the inhibitory effects of GABA, in turn promoting excessive dopamine activity in the mesolimbic pathway (72, 87, 141). Glutamate disturbances are thought to be especially associated with cognitive dysfunction in schizophrenia (110, 141).

Increasing evidence suggests dopamine as the final common pathway of various predisposing environmental and genetic contributors to the development of schizophrenia. Other neurotransmitters such as glutamate, GABA, serotonin, adenosine, and acetylcholine appear to act in concert with dopamine in this process (21, 87). Evidence of the contribution of these neurotransmitter systems to psychosis has stimulated research to develop and test pharmacological agents acting on various neurotransmitter receptors in efforts to improve pharmacotherapy for schizophrenia (94, 143).

A number of measurable neurophysiological abnormalities have been found to be associated with schizophrenia, through research methods including electroencephalography (EEG), magnetoencephalography (MEG), polysomnography (PSG), anti-saccade paradigms, event-related potential (ERP) recordings, and smooth-pursuit eye movement (SPEM) measurements

(147). The most remarkable neurophysiological abnormalities have been documented through 1) analysis of SPEMs (reflecting attentional and inhibitory deficits), 2) examination of ERP P50 component suppression of irrelevant stimuli (assessing early information-processing and sensory gating), 3) observation of fMRI activation in a "two-back" working-memory task (requiring recollection of the position of an image on a grid and matching it with an auditory stimulus), 4) oculomotor delayed-response testing of spatial working memory, 5) the continuous performance test (stimulus response mapping to measure vigilance), and 6) examination of neuromotor deviations (including coordination difficulties, involuntary movements, mirror movements, and deviations in muscle power and tone) (147). Even though neurophysiological abnormalities measured by these methods are demonstrated to be significantly associated with schizophrenia, they are not diagnostic because they are found in substantial proportions of people without schizophrenia (147).

Environmental variables have the potential to modify the genetic blueprints for brain development. Nongenetic influences on gene expression are referred to as "epigenetic." Based on available evidence, environmental factors that might contribute to epigenetic influences may include stressors in the fetal or postnatal environment, such as nutritional, infectious, and toxic exposures; childhood trauma and neglect; cannabis use; and various social adversities, such as poverty and discrimination (22, 110, 117, 118, 137, 144, 165). "Epigenetic factors" refers to a collection of nongenetic influences that modulate gene expression without changing the actual DNA sequences (137). These influences are thought to operate through biological mechanisms involving DNA cytosine methylation and histone modifications (4, 5, 137).

The age of greatest risk for schizophrenia being late adolescence to early adulthood has led investigators to consider brain development processes that may malfunction during this period. Profound changes in the brain occur during this time of development, in which high-order cognitive functions such as logical and abstract thinking and executive-planning capacities, especially in the prefrontal cortex, achieve maturation (165). During development, frequently used synaptic connections are strengthened and infrequently used connections are attenuated, and at adolescence the weak connections are removed by synaptic pruning of synapses, dendrites, and axons (110, 165). Gray matter of the prefrontal, parietal, and temporal cortex, as demonstrated in imagining studies, undergoes significant attrition through this critical period from late adolescence to early adulthood (165). If the frequently and infrequently used synapses cannot be differentiated, pruning becomes a random process, eliminating the important connections along with the less relevant ones (72). Disturbances of inhibitory neurons containing the calcium-binding protein parvalbumin have been implicated in initiation of abnormal synaptic pruning processes, and these inhibitory neurons may be damaged by oxidative stress (110, 165). Aberrant pruning compromises the integrity, stability, and fidelity of connectional architecture of excitatory glutamate synapses in the prefrontal cortex in particular that are responsible for reliable and predictable information processing (110, 165). These types of developmental synaptic plasticity abnormalities are hypothesized to be instrumental in the onset of schizophrenia (165).

Epigenetic modulations during brain development may initiate pathological processes leading to schizophrenia (4, 31). DNA methylation was one of the first epigenetic modifications to be recognized. DNA methylation prevents the binding of transcription factors with their specific DNA sequences, effectively silencing gene expression (4, 31). Abnormal DNA methylation renders glial cells dysfunctional, especially oligodendrocytes. Abnormalities in microglial functioning are considered important contributors to the pathogenesis of schizophrenia (31), likely related to their essential role in normal dendritic spine pruning and maintenance (110).

Synaptic pruning activities of microglia—the main immunocompetent cells in the developing brain (72)—involve immune inflammatory processes (110). Abnormal immune and inflammatory processes in brain development have been demonstrated to contribute risk for schizophrenia, involving multiple immune mediators, including cytokines (72, 110, 156). Maternal infections during pregnancy (reflected in an overrepresentation of births during late winter and spring in individuals who develop schizophrenia) (156) may increase risk for schizophrenia through immunological mechanisms. Other prenatal stressors increasing risk for schizophrenia include gestational and obstetric complications and famines during pregnancy (22, 118, 137, 144). Postnatal environmental stressors found to represent potential epigenetic contributors to risk for schizophrenia include urban residence, immigration, especially among minority groups, childhood trauma and neglect, and cannabis use (110, 117, 118, 165).

The biological studies of the brain in schizophrenia reviewed here collectively indicate that the disorder is unlikely to be explained by any lesion in a single structure. Rather, the disorder appears to involve widespread abnormalities in structures and connections throughout the brain supporting many different cognitive, emotional, and behavioral regulatory processes (41, 110, 165).

Although neurobiological studies, particularly imaging studies, have successfully demonstrated differences between groups of patients with schizophrenia from controls, many of these differences have been found to be nonspecific, overlapping substantially across other psychotic disorders, especially psychotic bipolar disorder, and even with many normal controls (113). These limitations have precluded clinical applications of biological measures for differential diagnosis (147, 164). Some researchers have observed, however, that longitudinal studies can detect biological differences in brain development trajectories between schizophrenia and bipolar illness that cross-sectional studies alone are inadequate to differentiate (58, 89).

Researchers have long sought to identify diagnosis-specific biomarkers (i.e., biological identifiers of an illness) and endophenotypes (which are quantifiable, reproducible, stable, heritable biological traits that are also abnormal in close relatives of individuals with the illness) for the psychotic disorders (112, 113, 147). Concerted efforts to differentiate psychotic disorders (schizophrenia, schizoaffective disorder, and bipolar psychosis) from one another on biological measures have failed (17, 113, 146). Thus, attempts to map biological data to clinical diagnoses in search of biological validation of the existing diagnostic categorization have not proven feasible. This situation has prompted researchers to try to reorganize diagnostic classification by mapping psychiatric disorders according to biological data in a new framework that is agnostic to existing diagnostic systems (112).

Using this approach, the Bipolar-Schizophrenia Network on Intermediate Phenotypes (B-SNIP) study grouped its results into purely biologically based entities referred to as "biotypes." The biotypes of psychotic syndromes that emerged do not conform to existing clinical diagnoses of schizophrenia or bipolar disorder, in essence transcending the currently established diagnostic categories (113). This new psychosis research trajectory represents a major departure from phenomenologically based syndromes in a search for purely neurobiological definitions of psychotic illness (113). Findings from these early exploratory studies will require replication, investigation of additional biomarkers, and examination of the findings in longitudinal studies. An accompanying means of detecting biologically defined disorders through clinical examination will be needed before such biologically based categories can be used in psychiatric practice (32).

This direction in research on psychotic disorders is not without controversy. Some researchers have concluded that the boundaries between psychotic disorders have not been established by brain morphology research, and that current progress in neurobiology is not yet compelling enough to justify a transition to a more biologically determined model of classification (34, 63). Unlike the rest of medicine, which has largely defined diseases on the basis of biological determinants, psychiatry needs further progress in the understanding of biological abnormalities and pathogenesis of psychosis to enable it to move beyond classification of these disorders based on phenomenology alone (32, 34, 113).

NATURAL HISTORY

As chronic schizophrenia typically begins insidiously, it is often hard to determine when the disorder started. In retrospect, many patients, if not most, evidence certain prepsychotic personality abnormalities: excessive shyness, social awkwardness, withdrawal from personal relationships, and inability to form close relationships—that is, schizoid personality features. A parent put it this way: "He was always afraid to make friends and felt that other people wouldn't like him. He couldn't be comfortable with girls, never knew what to say. I'd try to help him but it was very hard to change him. He'd cry and say it made him too uncomfortable to be with others." These traits may be present from early adolescence; often they are of concern to the patient's family for months or years before delusions or hallucinations become manifest.

In childhood and adolescence, long before the diagnostic symptoms of schizophrenia are evident, signs of neurodevelopmental problems may be evident among individuals who later develop schizophrenia. These prepsychotic abnormalities may be manifestations of the increased frequency of pregnancy and birth complications in the records of individuals who later developed schizophrenia (4, 22, 110). Prospective studies have provided considerable evidence that individuals at risk for schizophrenia may manifest early abnormalities. Compared to siblings and other controls, they exhibit more neuromotor developmental delays in infancy, delayed speech milestones, lower cognitive and motor performance, difficulties in reading and spelling, problems with sustaining attention, academic difficulties, poor premorbid adjustment and abnormal social interactions, and various traits identified in association with development of schizophrenia in childhood and early adolescence (55, 68, 101, 118, 159). In studies of videotapes made long before the onset of schizophrenia, raters blind to the diagnosis of schizophrenia in the children identified more negative emotional expressions, thought disorder, and negative symptoms in the children destined to develop schizophrenia than in their unaffected siblings (109, 160). Neurocognitive difficulties are thought to constitute core deficits that may manifest early in the course of the illness or even before the onset of symptoms (72, 110, 118, 156).

The peak period of onset of clinical problems that may be diagnosed as schizophrenia is in late adolescence and early adulthood (165). Delusions, hallucinations, and strange behavior usually become apparent in the late teens or 20s. At first, these aberrations may be brief and vague, leaving families uncertain of their significance. Gradually, the symptoms become more obvious and disturbing, usually leading to psychiatric consultation. Onset before age 12 is uncommon; the early childhood–onset type appears to represent the same disorder seen in adults, although with a more severe course (108, 119). Schizophrenia infrequently begins after age 40.

When a patient is seen for the first time, it may be difficult to predict what the course and prognosis will be. Good-prognosis cases generally begin more abruptly than poor-prognosis cases, without a history of long-standing personality abnormalities (71). Other factors associated with better outcomes include female gender, older age at onset of illness, educational attainment, employment history, better premorbid functioning, positive social support, and association of stressors with the onset of the illness. Factors associated with worse outcomes include insidious onset of illness, prominent negative symptoms, lack of insight, never-married status, and family history of schizophrenia (37, 71, 102, 152). Both greater duration of illness and duration of untreated psychosis have been associated with less favorable outcomes of illness (37, 71, 102, 114, 152, 157).

Schizophrenia has a variable and often fluctuating course. Today, most patients with schizophrenia live independently outside hospitals, although many require extensive support from relatives and from outpatient case management services (110). Even when not hospitalized, many people with this illness lead disturbed lives: They fail to form satisfactory personal relationships, are less likely to marry than their contemporaries, have poor job histories, and seldom achieve positions of responsibility. They may become neighborhood eccentrics or socially isolated residents in urban areas, doing irregular unskilled work or being supported by welfare. Those who lack insight into their illness and who have comorbid substance abuse are particularly vulnerable to homelessness. Schizophrenia is overrepresented in homeless populations by a factor of about 10, yet it is present only in a minority (about 10%) of homeless individuals (48).

Historically, the benchmark for determining schizophrenia outcomes has been achievement of remission—defined as substantial symptomatic improvement to levels no longer representing an active diagnosis (52, 152). The advent of modern antipsychotic medications has allowed up to one-half of patients to experience remission of psychotic symptoms. This advancement, however, has not uniformly translated to positive functional outcomes, because cognitive deficits remaining even after remission of psychotic symptoms are more contributory than psychotic symptoms to functional deficits and disability (52). Schizophrenia outcomes have recently been reconceptualized in terms of recovery—defined as re-establishment of functioning in domains of work, school, community, and home (52). Only one in seven patients have been found to achieve complete recovery as defined by normalization of social and vocational functioning and symptom remission lasting at least 2 years (52). The potential for recovery as an achievable goal for a substantial minority of patients (152), however, can provide a source of hope for patients undergoing treatment (52).

After the onset of schizophrenia, relapse is most common in the first 2–3 years, occurring in about one-third of patients in this time period (2, 102, 116). The lifetime risk for schizophrenic relapse after the first episode, however, has been estimated to be as high as 70%–80% (2, 44). More than one-half of patients have a chronic course of illness, and the majority of the remainder have an episodic-remitting course (58). Relapse is especially frequent in patients who discontinue their antipsychotic medication, and medication discontinuation is the biggest risk factor for relapse of schizophrenia (44). It has been hypothesized that relapse exerts neurotoxic effects on the brain through glutamatergic and dopaminergic transmitter systems (44, 116). Frequent relapses are associated with progressive functional deterioration, cognitive impairment, reduced treatment response, and worse clinical prognosis (116). A deteriorating course in symptom levels and executive functioning has been demonstrated to be associated with progressive changes in the frontal cortex and cognitive impairment (58). It is thus recommended that psychotic illness be identified early and adequate treatment be provided as soon as possible to prevent further deterioration that may result from continuing active illness.

Clinicians and investigators have long noted high rates of drug and alcohol use disorders among individuals with schizophrenia, demonstrated in recent research studies to occur in approximately one-half of all patients with schizophrenia (148). Self-medication of emotional distress may be a compelling explanation for the associated substance abuse, but there is considerable evidence that people with schizophrenia use substances for the same reasons and in the same manner as the general population, with additional contributions of impaired judgment and impulse control that psychosis may confer (6). Comorbid substance abuse makes the care of patients with psychotic illness much more difficult, as these patients have more positive symptoms, less treatment adherence, more frequent relapse requiring inpatient care, and more frequent homelessness and legal, medical, and social complications (35, 116, 124). Integrated treatment is the current standard of care for patients with comorbid schizophrenia and substance abuse (35).

Two historic developments have dramatically altered the general clinical course in the treatment of schizophrenia: the introduction of antipsychotics and the shift away from prolonged hospitalization. With antipsychotics, significant control of hallucinations, delusions, and bizarre behavior is possible for many patients. As a result, and also because of substantial reductions in hospital admissions and the duration of inpatient stays, patients spend far less time in psychiatric hospitals than was the case in earlier years. The advent of the newer second-generation antipsychotic medications has allowed many patients with previously incapacitating functional deficits based on amotivation and apathy to achieve new levels of occupational and social functioning. Clozapine in particular targets negative symptoms not substantially affected by traditional antipsychotics, leading to significant clinical improvement in many patients who have been refractory to other antipsychotic medications.

COMPLICATIONS

In no illness is it more difficult to distinguish between the typical clinical picture and the complications than in chronic schizophrenia. For example, difficulties in school or at work are common features of schizophrenia. Yet it is usually hard to tell whether these problems arise because of the patient's disordered thinking or loss of motivation, or whether they result from the reactions of teachers, fellow students and workers, or supervisors to the patient's abnormal behavior.

Suspicious, fearful, and deluded individuals may not perform well in school or at work because of preoccupation with abnormal thoughts; at the same time, withdrawn, preoccupied, and unresponsive students may draw criticism and other adverse responses from teachers and supervisors. These, in turn, will reinforce the individuals' pathological behaviors. The definition of the disorder encompasses its natural history and at the same time specifies the complications. These include impaired education, poor work history and job achievement, celibacy, and prolonged or repeated psychiatric hospitalization.

Because chronic schizophrenia typically begins early in life and is characterized by recurrent or persistent manifestations, patients' schooling and education suffer. Early school difficulties have been noted, but even among those who do well in elementary school, difficulties may arise in high school or college. Social withdrawal and loss of interest in studies may become evident. These changes, coupled with the need to leave school at the onset of more dramatic symptoms, may eventually lead to dropping out of school. If the illness peaks after the completion of formal education, the same clinical features may lead to marked reduction of effectiveness at work, demotions, being fired, frequent job changes, and financial dependency. People with schizophrenia are less likely than other people to be married (23).

Despite great reductions in chronic psychiatric hospitalization of patients with schizophrenia in recent decades, no other illness results in more time spent in psychiatric hospitals. Hospitalization is usually for repeated, relatively brief periods, but a few patients spend many years in hospitals.

A common misconception about schizophrenia is that people with this illness are likely to act on psychotic delusions and commit violent crimes such as murder. Available data suggest, however, that there is only a modestly greater risk of significant crimes committed by individuals with this illness than in general populations (103, 158). Risk for violent crime by individuals with schizophrenia is highly associated with substance abuse and increases with treatment discontinuation (158, 163). Individuals with schizophrenia are far more likely to be arrested for vagrancy, disturbing the peace, and other misdemeanors than for violent crimes and are only rarely involved in serious or violent felonies.

Approximately 1 out of 20 people with schizophrenia will eventually commit suicide (60, 110, 111, 115, 157). The most vulnerable time is near the beginning of illness onset, often following discharge from an inpatient hospital stay (115, 157). Suicide risk in schizophrenia is related to psychotic symptoms such as paranoia and command hallucinations, depressive symptoms and hopelessness, agitation and motor restlessness, and awareness of effects of the illness on cognitive functioning (57, 157). Additionally, previous suicide attempts, recent loss, poor treatment adherence, and substance abuse have been identified as suicide risk factors in schizophrenia (157). Social support, positive coping skills, life satisfaction, and engagement in treatment appear to be protective against suicide risk in schizophrenia (99, 157).

Patients with schizophrenia have remarkable rates of morbidity and mortality from all causes, resulting in a reduced life expectancy by 20 years compared to the general population (88, 110). Lifestyle factors such as smoking, excessive alcohol and drug use, unhealthy diet, and lack of exercise likely contribute to medical complications in these patients (105). Underutilization of prevention and treatment for medical illness may also contribute, as well as the known adverse metabolic side effects of antipsychotic medications (110).

FAMILY AND GENETIC STUDIES

A family history of psychosis appears to be the strongest risk factor for schizophrenia. There is a 10-fold elevated risk of schizophrenia in the close relatives of patients with schizophrenia (73). The prevalence of schizophrenia increases with closeness of relationship to a family member with schizophrenia: 2%–4% with a second-degree relative and 10%–15% with a first-degree relative (129, 137, 145). The specific lifetime risk for developing schizophrenia is 9% for individuals with an affected sibling, 13% for individuals with one affected parent, and 46% for individuals with two affected parents (55, 137). Schizophrenia risk is highly heritable, as reflected in 80%–85% of the variance in risk that is explained by genetic effects (26, 27, 129, 136). Despite this high heritability, the vast majority (about 60%–80%) of people with schizophrenia have no known first- or second-degree relatives with schizophrenia (145).

A series of twin studies conducted over a 70-year period provides overwhelming evidence of higher concordance rates (prevalence of the disorder in relatives of affected individuals) for schizophrenia among monozygotic twins (40%–50%) (27) than among dizygotic twins (around 10%–15%) (26, 136) of the same sex. (See results of these studies listed in Table 3.1.) However, dizygotic twins have only a slightly higher prevalence of schizophrenia than in their ordinary siblings of the same sex when one member of the pair is affected (137).

Studies of the offspring of twins have shed additional light on hereditary disposition to schizophrenia. A study of monozygotic twins discordant for schizophrenia found no different rates of schizophrenia in the children of unaffected and affected twins (17% each) (46, 50). In contrast, a study of dizygotic twin pairs discordant for schizophrenia found higher rates of schizophrenia among offspring of affected (17%) compared to unaffected (2%) twins (50). These findings suggest that at least some schizophrenic illnesses have a hereditary predisposition, and that a schizophrenic genotype or diathesis may not be expressed unless it is accompanied by critical nonfamilial, environmental factors.

Adoption studies provide more specific evidence to untangle genetic from environmental factors (26). Most of these studies were carried out in the last century (26). These studies have found that children separated early in life from parents with schizophrenia and raised by unrelated adoptive parents are far more likely to have schizophrenia as adults than are adopted-away offspring of parents without the disorder (26). A more recent and much larger study using a Swedish population registry has further substantiated the results of these earlier studies (90). Conversely, studies of biological relatives of adopted-away offspring with schizophrenia have

TABLE 3.1 SCHIZOPHRENIA CONCORDANCE RATES IN MONOZYGOTIC (MZ) AND DIZYGOTIC (DZ) TWINS

Investigator(s), Year (Country) (Ref. No.)	MZ Twins		DZ Twins (Same Sex)	
	Full Criteria Met for Schizophrenia (%)	Including Uncertain/ Spectrum Cases (%)	Full Criteria Met for Schizophrenia (%)	Including Uncertain/ Spectrum Cases (%)
Luxenberger, 1928 (Germany) (92)	50	71	0	0
Rosanoff et al., 1934 (USA) (123)	44	61	9	13
Essen-Möller, 1941 (Sweden) (45)	14	71	8	17
Kallmann, 1941 (USA) (74)		69		17
Slater and Shields, 1953 (UK) (139)		65		14
Inouye, 1963 (Japan) (65)		60		18
Tienari, 1963 (Finland) (150)	6	31	5	5
Kringlen, 1964 (Norway) (81)	25		16	
Kringlen, 1966 (Norway) (82)	28	38	6	14
Gottesman and Shields, 1966 (UK) (51)	42	54	9	18
Kringlen, 1968 (Norway) (83)	25	38	4	10
Fischer et al., 1969 (Denmark) (47)	24	40	10	19
Allen et al., 1972 (USA) (7)		27		5
Tienari, 1975 (Finland) (149)				
pairwise method	15		7	
proband method	33		14	
Kendler and Robinette, 1983 (USA) (77)		31		7
Onstad et al., 1991 (Norway) (106)				
pairwise method	33		1	
proband method	48		4	

TABLE 3.1 CONTINUED

Investigator(s), Year (Country) (Ref. No.)	MZ Twins		DZ Twins (Same Sex)	
	Full Criteria Met for Schizophrenia (%)	Including Uncertain/ Spectrum Cases (%)	Full Criteria Met for Schizophrenia (%)	Including Uncertain/ Spectrum Cases (%)
Tsujita et al., 1992 (151)		50		14
Kläning, 1996 (Denmark) (78)	44		11	
Cannon et al., 1998 (Finland) (24)		46		9
Franzek and Beckmann, 1998 (Germany) (49)				
pairwise method	67	46	17	17
proband method	79	61	17	24
Cardno et al., 1999 (England) (25)	39		5	

found several-fold higher rates of schizophrenia than in biological relatives of adopted-away offspring without the disorder (26).

Family studies have investigated the concept of a familial schizophrenia spectrum, which dates to observations by Kraepelin and Bleuler that many family members of patients with schizophrenia who do not have schizophrenia appear to have long-standing, schizophrenia-like characteristics (36). Studies have shown a familial and even a genetic relationship between schizophrenia and schizotypal personality, thus supporting the validity of a familial schizophrenia-spectrum concept (36). Schizotypal personality, described in *DSM-5*, includes social withdrawal, reduced cognitive capacity, emotional dysregulation, and attenuated psychotic features, but does not include delusions or hallucinations (161). Predisposition to schizophrenia spectrum disorders has been demonstrated through twin and family studies with heritability estimated around 30%–50% (36).

Increasing evidence has accumulated to indicate a partial overlap in family susceptibility for schizophrenia and bipolar disorder (13, 93, 96, 112). Schizophrenia appears to occur more frequently than expected by chance in families of individuals with bipolar disorder, and bipolar disorder appears to occur more frequently than expected by chance in families of individuals with schizophrenia (34). Additionally, twin studies have demonstrated a shared genetic liability for psychosis in schizophrenia, schizoaffective disorder, and bipolar disorder (34). The heritability between schizophrenia and bipolar disorder documented in family studies is substantial, on the order of 60%, somewhat lower than the within-disorder heritability rates of 80%–85% for schizophrenia and for bipolar disorder (26). The apparent shared genetic liability between schizophrenia and bipolar disorder identified in family studies, however, has not been demonstrated in genetic studies and is not considered sufficient to warrant a change in the nosological conceptualization of these separately conceptualized disorders (34).

Unlike genetic research on other medical disorders, studies of schizophrenia have failed to provide a coherent genetic map of this illness; a high proportion of the risk for schizophrenia remains genetically unassigned (110, 136). Research findings to date suggest that no single gene or gene locus will likely account for the disorder in a substantial proportion of cases, and that genetic liability for schizophrenia is likely polygenic, involving many genes, each contributing a small risk, and interacting with each other and with environmental risk factors (136). Genetic risk for schizophrenia is likely to be highly pleiotropic, with one gene or allele affecting multiple apparently unrelated phenotypic traits not corresponding to existing definitions of disease (110). Thus, it appears there no simple solutions will emerge with regard to the genetics of schizophrenia.

To date, more than 100 distinct genes have been found to be associated with schizophrenia risk (110, 136). Recent research has revealed that common variants with small effects (single-nucleotide polymorphisms) contribute up to 32% of the risk for schizophrenia in a polygenic model (129, 145). Rare variants with large effects known as copy number variants that represent deletions or duplications of large regions of the genome further contribute to genetic risk of schizophrenia, especially sporadic cases, in a heterogeneity model (145).

It has long been suspected that there must be important environmental factors in the etiology of schizophrenia. Such consideration has been prompted both by the failure to find complete concordance in monozygotic twins and by research demonstrating environmental risk factors for schizophrenia, such as maternal starvation in famines and maternal influenza infection during fetal development (22, 118, 137, 144). Because the environments of twins are most similar during gestation and infancy and then tend to diverge over time, resulting in the largest differences by the time of adulthood, this suggests that the environmental influences in liability to schizophrenia most likely occur early in life (142).

DIFFERENTIAL DIAGNOSIS

A small number of patients presenting with depression will, at follow-up, be found to be suffering from chronic schizophrenia (128). This is much more likely to be the case when the depression is accompanied by striking delusions or hallucinations. Although many good-prognosis cases of schizophrenia are likely manifestations of mood disorders, the question of differential diagnosis is often one of diagnostic convention or style. Certain delusions (those of poverty, sinfulness, disease) are common in depression, and others (those of overconfidence and unusual powers) in mania. Delusions of control, persecution, and depersonalization are more likely to present as part of illness eventually to be declared as schizophrenia.

Obsessive-compulsive disorder, early in its course, occasionally is difficult to distinguish from schizophrenia (166), especially if the obsessions are bizarre or if the patient lacks insight into the abnormal nature of the obsessional thoughts and impulses. The risk of schizophrenia is small after the first year or two of obsessive-compulsive illness and when the obsessions are classical.

A clinical picture resembling schizophrenia has been described in association with complex partial seizure disorder (43). This clinical picture may be indistinguishable from typical schizophrenia in individual cases, but the absence of a higher prevalence of schizophrenia in close relatives suggests that it is a separate entity (28). Other features of the clinical presentation, such as soft or hard neurological signs, history of seizures, olfactory and somatosensory hallucinations, absence episodes, automatisms, EEG focal abnormalities, especially on the left side, and MRI evidence of temporal-limbic lesions, are suggestive of complex partial seizure disorder.

Patients with systemic medical illnesses affecting the brain, such as lupus erythematosus, may develop psychiatric symptoms that vary over time from those of depression to those of a neurocognitive disorder, with a schizophrenic picture in between. Psychotic features, especially hallucinations and delusions, often with paranoid and persecutory themes, are common in many neurocognitive disorders, such as those based in delirium, dementia, or another medical condition (8). Visual hallucinations are more common in neurocognitive disorders than in psychotic mood disorders and schizophrenia (8). The differential diagnosis between primary psychotic illness and neurocognitive disorders is particularly important in older patients, because serious medical conditions may masquerade as psychotic illness (120). Even when striking delusions and hallucinations are present, persistent disorientation and memory impairment point to a neurocognitive disorder. If disorientation and memory impairment are transient and less striking than the delusions, hallucinations, and bizarre behavior, a diagnosis of a psychotic disorder is more likely. Disorganized speech and behavior that are commonly seen in primary psychotic disorders are not characteristic of the psychosis occurring as part of neurocognitive disorders (8). Ultimately, the diagnosis of a primary psychotic disorder is made by elimination of secondary medical causes of psychosis, based on careful history and physical examination, collateral history, and appropriate laboratory evaluation (120).

A classic psychotic syndrome originating in very heavy alcohol use is delirium tremens, which was differentiated from alcohol-induced psychotic disorders in 1847 by Marcel (70). In 1913, Kraepelin further delineated Wernicke's encephalopathy, Korsakoff psychosis, and alcohol-induced dementia from alcohol-induced psychotic disorders (70). Alcohol-induced psychotic disorders have also been referred to as "alcoholic hallucinosis," referring to a syndrome of striking hallucinations (typically auditory) or delusions (typically persecutory or derogatory) with clear consciousness and without formal thought disorder, occurring within 1 month of alcohol intoxication or withdrawal (8). The outcome of alcoholic-induced psychotic disorder is variable, with most symptoms usually subsiding within a few weeks; however, resolution of hallucinations can take up to 6 months (70). Some cases of alcohol-induced psychotic disorder can persist and become chronic, resembling schizophrenia.

Psychotomimetic drugs such as lysergic acid diethylamide (LSD) and phencyclidine (PCP) can cause acute psychotic states that may be clinically indistinguishable from naturally occurring schizophrenia on initial assessment, especially in acute care settings such as the emergency department (29, 30). Psychotomimetic drugs are responsible for a substantial percentage of cases of acute psychosis seen in emergency departments or in patients admitted to psychiatric inpatient units. Untangling the contributors to psychosis may be difficult, especially in acute care settings, because it typically requires information from collateral sources and longitudinal observation of the course of the disorder in association with substance use (124). These drug-induced psychotic states usually subside within 10–14 days after discontinuation of drug use. In a few chronic cases, the situation is similar to that seen in alcohol-induced psychotic disorders, in which it is uncertain which came first—the substance abuse or the psychosis. Patients with preexisting schizophrenia may also suffer acute intensification of psychosis as the result of using psychotomimetic drugs.

NMDA antagonist hallucinogens (e.g., PCP, ketamine, dextromethorphan) tend to produce positive, negative, and cognitive symptoms of psychotic syndromes. Presentation with positive symptoms alone is more suggestive of stimulants (e.g., methamphetamine, cocaine) and serotonergic hallucinogens (e.g., LSD) (124).

CLINICAL MANAGEMENT

Antipsychotic medication is the keystone of effective schizophrenia treatment. A policy of early discharge from psychiatric hospitals was made possible in part by the advent of antipsychotic medications, beginning with the discovery of chlorpromazine in the 1950s (110). The first-generation antipsychotic medications, also including haloperidol and thioridazine, dramatically helped reduce positive symptoms of schizophrenia such as delusions, hallucinations, and bizarre behavior, but they were not particularly effective for negative symptoms such as amotivation and emotional and social withdrawal. These antipsychotic medications exert their therapeutic effects through dopamine receptor D_2 blockade (110). They are classified in relation to their potency, with the prescribed doses being inversely proportional to potency. The high-potency medications are most likely to cause extrapyramidal side effects, such as rigidity, dystonic reactions, akathisia, and tremor. The low-potency medications are associated with more sedation and autonomic side effects (126). Anticholinergic effects of some of these medications, as well as anticholinergic medications used to remedy extrapyramidal side effects, may further contribute to cognitive problems in schizophrenia.

The advent of newer second-generation antipsychotic medications, beginning with clozapine in the 1990s, further improved treatment of schizophrenia, and for the first time targeted negative symptoms as well as being equally effective for positive symptoms. These medications (e.g., risperidone, olanzapine, and quetiapine) all act at serotonin as well as dopamine D_2 receptors, and as a result are less likely to produce extrapyramidal side effects (85). Unwelcome side effects may occur with these agents, such as sedation, hypotension, seizures, weight gain, and hyperglycemia and other features of metabolic syndrome (85). Therefore, regular monitoring of vital signs and laboratory metabolic indicators is indicated.

Patients vary considerably in their metabolism of antipsychotic medications; therefore, individualization of dosage is indicated. Larger doses are usually needed during acute exacerbations but may be reduced as the patient's symptoms abate. Because there are no biomarkers or pharmacological tests to guide the choice of antipsychotic agent, the selection of medication is typically based on the side-effect profile (85). Antipsychotic medication is generally titrated up to a therapeutic dose to assess treatment effects. Most antipsychotic effects occur within the first week, with marginal improvements thereafter (85). After 4 to 6 weeks without adequate treatment response, it is recommended to switch to another antipsychotic agent with a different receptor-binding profile. Treatment is generally continued for at least 1 year for first episodes and at least 5 years for patients with multiple episodes of illness (85).

Clozapine is particularly effective for refractory illness and for suicidal ideation, with a 50%–60% response in patients who are refractive to all other antipsychotics (85). A specific safety concern for treatment with clozapine is agranulocytosis, which is uncommon (<1% of patients treated and increases with dosage level) but can be medically catastrophic, and even fatal in 1 of 10,000 treated patients. Optimally safe prescription of this antipsychotic drug therefore requires close monitoring of white blood cell counts (85) in addition to the standard laboratory monitoring of metabolic status recommended for other antipsychotic agents.

Antipsychotic polypharmacy, defined as the use of two or more antipsychotic agents simultaneously, is generally discouraged. There is no evidence, outside of specific justifications for this practice in unusual circumstances, to suggest that more than one antipsychotic agent is more effective than a single antipsychotic, yet this practice often occurs. Antipsychotic polypharmacy is also further associated with potential for excessive dosing, adverse drug–drug interactions, and dosing complexity that further compromises patient adherence to medication schedules (85).

High-dose antipsychotic treatment above standard recommended dosing levels has not been demonstrated to increase effectiveness in general. High dosages are associated with adverse effects (which are dose related), especially when combinations of antipsychotics are used, and are thus recommended only for extraordinary circumstances and with careful monitoring for metabolic effects and especially electrocardiographic changes such as QT_c prolongation (85).

Treatment of all chronic diseases is compromised by treatment nonadherence. This problem is greater for schizophrenia, however, than for most other chronic diseases, observed in 75% of patients with schizophrenia over a 2-year period after discharge from psychiatric hospitalization (85). Treatment nonadherence can result from intolerable side effects, lack of insight into illness that frequently accompanies schizophrenia, continued psychotic symptoms, and poor therapeutic alliance (85). Long-acting depot formulations of some antipsychotic medications have helped the problem of unsatisfactory treatment adherence (85).

Although antipsychotic drugs remain the mainstay of schizophrenia treatment, this pharmacotherapy is far more effective when it can be delivered as part of a comprehensive treatment plan that includes extensive psychological and social support. This requires a multidisciplinary approach by a coordinated team of healthcare professionals and agencies delivering an assortment of vocational and educational services and rehabilitation in the community care setting (110). Ideally, care for patients with schizophrenia also provides support to families, who often end up being responsible for major aspects of the day-to-day care for their loved ones with schizophrenia.

The first 2 or 3 years after the first onset of illness in schizophrenia are thought to be a period in which the illness is most modifiable and interventions may be most effective at reducing progression of the illness and its negative consequences (38, 39, 66, 100). In particular, greater duration of untreated psychosis has been found to be strongly predictive of clinical outcomes of schizophrenia, especially negative symptoms, quality of life, and functional capacity (3). These findings have prompted the development of specialist early intervention services providing intensive services for patients in their first psychotic episode and for the first 2 or 3 years (38, 39, 66, 100). These services have been demonstrated to have beneficial effects on outcome in the first few years (75), but their long-term effect remains uncertain (130).

REFERENCES

1. Abel, K. M., Drake, R., and Goldstein, J. M. Sex differences in schizophrenia. Int. Rev. Psychiatry, 22:417–428, 2010.
2. Addington, D. E., Patten, S. B., McKenzie, E., and Addington, J. Relationship between relapse and hospitalization in first-episode psychosis. Psychiatr. Serv., 64:796–799, 2013.
3. Addington, J., Heinssen, R. K., Robinson, D. G., Schooler, N. R., Marcy, P., Brunette, M. F., Correll, C. U., Estroff, S., Mueser, K. T., Penn, D., Robinson, J. A., Rosenheck, R. A., Azrin, S. T., Goldstein, A. B., Severe, J., and Kane, J. M. Duration of untreated psychosis in community treatment settings in the United States. Psychiatr. Serv., 66:753–756, 2015.
4. Akbarian, S. Epigenetics of schizophrenia. Curr. Top. Behav. Neurosci., 4:611–628, 2010.
5. Akbarian, S. Epigenetic mechanisms in schizophrenia. Dialogues Clin. Neurosci., 16:405–417, 2014.
6. Akerele, E. O., and Levin, F. R. Substance abuse among patients with schizophrenia. J. Psychiatr. Pract., 8:70–80, 2002.
7. Allen, M. G., Cohen, S., and Pollin, W. Schizophrenia in veteran twins: a diagnostic review. Am. J. Psychiatry, 128:939–945, 1972.
8. American Psychiatric Association. *Diagnostic and Statistical Manual for Mental Disorders,* 5th edition. Washington, DC: Author, 2013.

9. Arnold, S. J., Ivleva, E. I., Gopal, T. A., Reddy, A. P., Jeon-Slaughter, H., Sacco, C. B., Francis, A. N., Tandon, N., Bidesi, A. S., Witte, B., Poudyal, G., Pearlson, G. D., Sweeney, J. A., Clementz, B. A., Keshavan, M. S., and Tamminga, C. A. Hippocampal volume is reduced in schizophrenia and schizoaffective disorder but not in psychotic bipolar I disorder demonstrated by both manual tracing and automated parcellation (FreeSurfer). Schizophr. Bull., *41*:233–249, 2015.

10. Baethge, C., Baldessarini, R. J., Freudenthal, K., Streeruwitz, A., Bauer, M., and Bschor, T. Hallucinations in bipolar disorder: characteristics and comparison to unipolar depression and schizophrenia. Bipolar Disord., 7:136–145, 2005.

11. Bakhshi, K., and Chance, S. A. The neuropathology of schizophrenia: a selective review of past studies and emerging themes in brain structure and cytoarchitecture. Neuroscience, *303*:82–102, 2015.

12. Bembenek, A. [Seasonality of birth in schizophrenia patients. Literature review]. Psychiatr. Pol., *39*:259–270, 2005.

13. Berrettini, W. Evidence for shared susceptibility in bipolar disorder and schizophrenia. Am. J. Med. Genet. C. Semin. Med. Genet., *123*:59–64, 2003.

14. Bhatia, T., Chakraborty, S., Thomas, P., Naik, A., Mazumdar, S., Nimgaonkar, V. L., and Deshpande, S. N. Is familiality associated with downward occupation drift in schizophrenia? Psychiatry Investig., 5:168–174, 2008.

15. Bleuler, E. *Dementia Praecox or the Group of Schizophrenias*, Zinkin, J. (trans.). New York: International Universities Press, 1950.

16. Bora, E. Differences in cognitive impairment between schizophrenia and bipolar disorder: considering the role of heterogeneity. Psychiatry Clin. Neurosci., 70:424–433, 2016.

17. Bortolato, B., Miskowiak, K. W., Kohler, C. A., Vieta, E., and Carvalho, A. F. Cognitive dysfunction in bipolar disorder and schizophrenia: a systematic review of meta-analyses. Neuropsychiatr. Dis. Treat., *11*:3111–3125, 2015.

18. Bourque, F., van der Ven, E., Fusar-Poli, P., and Malla, A. Immigration, social environment and onset of psychotic disorders. Curr. Pharm. Des., *18*:518–526, 2012.

19. Boutros, N. N., Mucci, A., Diwadkar, V., and Tandon, R. Negative symptoms in schizophrenia. Clin. Schizophr. Relat. Psychoses, 8:28–35B, 2014.

20. Brenner, D. *Elementary Textbook of Psychoanalysis*. New York: International Universities Press, 1955.

21. Brisch, R., Saniotis, A., Wolf, R., Bielau, H., Bernstein, H. G., Steiner, J., Bogerts, B., Braun, K., Jankowski, Z., Kumaratilake, J., Henneberg, M., and Gos, T. The role of dopamine in schizophrenia from a neurobiological and evolutionary perspective: old fashioned, but still in vogue. Front. Psychiatry, 5:47, 2014.

22. Brown, A. S. The environment and susceptibility to schizophrenia. Prog. Neurobiol., *93*:23–58, 2011.

23. Burns, T. Evolution of outcome measures in schizophrenia. Br. J. Psychiatry Suppl., *50*:s1–s6, 2007.

24. Cannon, T. D., Kaprio, J., Lonnqvist, J., Huttunen, M., and Koskenvuo, M. The genetic epidemiology of schizophrenia in a Finnish twin cohort. A population-based modeling study. Arch. Gen. Psychiatry, *55*:67–74, 1998.

25. Cardno, A. G., Marshall, E. J., Coid, B., Macdonald, A. M., Ribchester, T. R., Davies, N. J., Venturi, P., Jones, L. A., Lewis, S. W., Sham, P. C., Gottesman, I. I., Farmer, A. E., McGuffin, P., Reveley, A. M., and Murray, R. M. Heritability estimates for psychotic disorders: the Maudsley twin psychosis series. Arch. Gen. Psychiatry, *56*:162–168, 1999.

26. Cardno, A. G., and Owen, M. J. Genetic relationships between schizophrenia, bipolar disorder, and schizoaffective disorder. Schizophr. Bull., 40:504–515, 2014.

27. Cariaga-Martinez, A., Saiz-Ruiz, J., and Alelu-Paz, R. From linkage studies to epigenetics: what we know and what we need to know in the neurobiology of schizophrenia. Front. Neurosci., 10:202, 2016.

28. Cascella, N. G., Schretlen, D. J., and Sawa, A. Schizophrenia and epilepsy: is there a shared susceptibility? Neurosci. Res., 63:227–235, 2009.

29. Caton, C. L., Drake, R. E., Hasin, D. S., Dominguez, B., Shrout, P. E., Samet, S., and Schanzer, B. Differences between early-phase primary psychotic disorders with concurrent substance use and substance-induced psychoses. Arch. Gen. Psychiatry, 62:137–145, 2005.

30. Caton, C. L., Samet, S., and Hasin, D. S. When acute-stage psychosis and substance use co-occur: differentiating substance-induced and primary psychotic disorders. J. Psychiatr. Pract., 6:256–266, 2000.

31. Chen, X. S., Huang, N., Michael, N., and Xiao, L. Advancements in the underlying pathogenesis of schizophrenia: implications of DNA methylation in glial cells. Front. Cell. Neurosci., 9:451, 2015.

32. Clementz, B. A., Sweeney, J. A., Hamm, J. P., Ivleva, E. I., Ethridge, L. E., Pearlson, G. D., Keshavan, M. S., and Tamminga, C. A. Identification of distinct psychosis biotypes using brain-based biomarkers. Am. J. Psychiatry, 173:373–384, 2016.

33. Compton, W. M., and Guze, S. B. The neo-Kraepelinian revolution in psychiatric diagnosis. Eur. Arch. Psychiatry Clin. Neurosci., 245:196–201, 1995.

34. Cosgrove, V. E., and Suppes, T. Informing DSM-5: biological boundaries between bipolar I disorder, schizoaffective disorder, and schizophrenia. BMC Med., 11:127, 2013.

36. De Witte, N. A., Crunelle, C. L., Sabbe, B., Moggi, F., and Dom, G. Treatment for outpatients with comorbid schizophrenia and substance use disorders: a review. Eur. Addict. Res., 20:105–114, 2014.

35. Debbane, M., Eliez, S., Badoud, D., Conus, P., Fluckiger, R., and Schultze-Lutter, F. Developing psychosis and its risk states through the lens of schizotypy. Schizophr. Bull., 41(Suppl 2):S396–S407, 2015.

37. Diaz-Caneja, C. M., Pina-Camacho, L., Rodriguez-Quiroga, A., Fraguas, D., Parellada, M., and Arango, C. Predictors of outcome in early-onset psychosis: a systematic review. NPJ Schizophr., 1:14005, 2015.

38. Dixon, L. B., Goldman, H. H., Bennett, M. E., Wang, Y., McNamara, K. A., Mendon, S. J., Goldstein, A. B., Choi, C. W., Lee, R. J., Lieberman, J. A., and Essock, S. M. Implementing coordinated specialty care for early psychosis: the RAISE connection program. Psychiatr. Serv., 66:691–698, 2015.

39. Dixon, L. B., and Stroup, T. S. Medications for first-episode psychosis: making a good start. Am. J. Psychiatry, 172:209–211, 2015.

40. Dollfus, S., and Lyne, J. Negative symptoms: history of the concept and their position in diagnosis of schizophrenia. Schizophr. Res., 186:1–7, 2017.

41. Drevets, W. C., Botteron, K., and Barch, D. M. Neuroimaging in psychiatry. In *Adult Psychiatry*, second edition, Rubin, E. H., Zorumski, C. F. (eds.). Malden, MA: Blackwell, pp. 45–75, 2005.

42. Eggers, A. E. A serotonin hypothesis of schizophrenia. Med. Hypotheses, 80:791–794, 2013.

43. Elliott, B., Joyce, E., and Shorvon, S. Delusions, illusions and hallucinations in epilepsy: 2. Complex phenomena and psychosis. Epilepsy Res., 85:172–186, 2009.

44. Emsley, R., Chiliza, B., Asmal, L., and Harvey, B. H. The nature of relapse in schizophrenia. BMC Psychiatry, 13:50, 2013.
45. Essen-Möller, E. *Psychiatrische Untersuchungen an einer Serie von Zwillingen.* Copenhagen: Ejnar Munksgaard, 1941.
46. Fischer, M. Psychoses in the offspring of schizophrenic monozygotic twins and their normal co-twins. Br. J. Psychiatry, 118:43–52, 1971.
47. Fischer, M., Harvald, B., and Hauge, M. A Danish twin study of schizophrenia. Br. J. Psychiatry, 115:981–990, 1969.
48. Foster, A., Gable, J., and Buckley, J. Homelessness in schizophrenia. Psychiatr. Clin. North Am., 35:717–734, 2012.
49. Franzek, E., and Beckmann, H. Different genetic background of schizophrenia spectrum psychoses: a twin study. Am. J. Psychiatry, 155:76–83, 1998.
50. Gottesman, I. I., and Bertelsen, A. Confirming unexpressed genotypes for schizophrenia. Risks in the offspring of Fischer's Danish identical and fraternal discordant twins. Arch. Gen. Psychiatry, 46:867–872, 1989.
51. Gottesman, I. I., and Shields, J. Contributions of twin studies to perspectives in schizophrenia. Vol. 3. In *Progress in Experimental Personality Research*, Maher, B. A. (ed.). New York: Academic Press, pp. 1–84, 1966.
52. Green, M. F. Impact of cognitive and social cognitive impairment on functional outcomes in patients with schizophrenia. J. Clin. Psychiatry, 77(*Suppl* 2):8–11, 2016.
53. Haijma, S. V., Van, H. N., Cahn, W., Koolschijn, P. C., Hulshoff Pol, H. E., and Kahn, R. S. Brain volumes in schizophrenia: a meta-analysis in over 18 000 subjects. Schizophr. Bull., 39:1129–1138, 2013.
54. Hallak, J. E., de Paula, A. L., Chaves, C., Bressan, R. A., and Machado-de-Sousa, J. P. An overview on the search for schizophrenia biomarkers. CNS Neurol. Disord. Drug Targets, 14:996–1000, 2015.
55. Hameed, M. A., and Lewis, A. J. Offspring of parents with schizophrenia: a systematic review of developmental features across childhood. Harv. Rev. Psychiatry, 24:104–117, 2016.
56. Harrow, M., Jobe, T. H., and Faull, R. N. Do all schizophrenia patients need antipsychotic treatment continuously throughout their lifetime? A 20-year longitudinal study. Psychol. Med., 42:2145–2155, 2012.
57. Hawton, K., Sutton, L., Haw, C., Sinclair, J., and Deeks, J. J. Schizophrenia and suicide: systematic review of risk factors. Br. J. Psychiatry, 187:9–20, 2005.
58. Heilbronner, U., Samara, M., Leucht, S., Falkai, P., and Schulze, T. G. The longitudinal course of schizophrenia across the lifespan: clinical, cognitive, and neurobiological aspects. Harv. Rev. Psychiatry, 24:118–128, 2016.
59. Hoff, P. The Kraepelinian tradition. Dialogues Clin. Neurosci., 17:31–41, 2015.
60. Hor, K., and Taylor, M. Suicide and schizophrenia: a systematic review of rates and risk factors. J. Psychopharmacol., 24:81–90, 2010.
61. Horga, G., Bernacer, J., Dusi, N., Entis, J., Chu, K., Hazlett, E. A., Haznedar, M. M., Kemether, E., Byne, W., and Buchsbaum, M. S. Correlations between ventricular enlargement and gray and white matter volumes of cortex, thalamus, striatum, and internal capsule in schizophrenia. Eur. Arch. Psychiatry Clin. Neurosci., 261:467–476, 2011.
62. Howes, O. D., and Murray, R. M. Schizophrenia: an integrated sociodevelopmental-cognitive model. Lancet, 383:1677–1687, 2014.
63. Hyman, S. E. Diagnosing the DSM: diagnostic classification needs fundamental reform. Cerebrum, 2011:6, 2011.

64. Ichimaya, T., Okubo, Y., Suhara, T., and Sudo, Y. Reduced volume of the cerebellar vermis in neuroleptic-naive schizophrenia. Biol. Psychiatry, 49:20–27, 2001.

65. Inouye, E. Similarity and dissimilarity of schizophrenia in twins. In *Proceedings of the 3rd World Congress on Psychiatry.* Toronto: University of Toronto Press, 1963.

66. Insel, T. R. RAISE-ing our expectations for first-episode psychosis. Am. J. Psychiatry, 173:311–312, 2016.

67. Isaac, C., and Januel, D. Neural correlates of cognitive improvements following cognitive remediation in schizophrenia: a systematic review of randomized trials. Socioaffect. Neurosci. Psychol., 6:30054, 2016.

68. Isohanni, M., Murray, G. K., Jokelainen, J., Croudace, T., and Jones, P. B. The persistence of developmental markers in childhood and adolescence and risk for schizophrenic psychoses in adult life. A 34-year follow-up of the Northern Finland 1966 birth cohort. Schizophr. Res., 71:213–225, 2004.

69. Johnstone, E. C., Crow, T. J., Frith, C. D., Husband, J., and Kreel, L. Cerebral ventricular size and cognitive impairment in chronic schizophrenia. Lancet, 2:924–926, 1976.

70. Jordaan, G. P., and Emsley, R. Alcohol-induced psychotic disorder: a review. Metab. Brain Dis., 29:231–243, 2014.

71. Juola, P., Miettunen, J., Veijola, J., Isohanni, M., and Jaaskelainen, E. Predictors of short- and long-term clinical outcome in schizophrenic psychosis—the Northern Finland 1966 Birth Cohort study. Eur. Psychiatry, 28:263–268, 2013.

72. Kahn, R. S., and Sommer, I. E. The neurobiology and treatment of first-episode schizophrenia. Mol. Psychiatry, 20:84–97, 2015.

73. Kakela, J., Panula, J., Oinas, E., Hirvonen, N., Jaaskelainen, E., and Miettunen, J. Family history of psychosis and social, occupational and global outcome in schizophrenia: a meta-analysis. Acta Psychiatr. Scand., 130:269–278, 2014.

74. Kallmann, F. J. The genetic theory of schizophrenia. An analysis of 691 twin index families. Am. J. Psychiatry, 103:309–322, 1941.

75. Kane, J. M., Robinson, D. G., Schooler, N. R., Mueser, K. T., Penn, D. L., Rosenheck, R. A., Addington, J., Brunette, M. F., Correll, C. U., Estroff, S. E., Marcy, P., Robinson, J., Meyer-Kalos, P. S., Gottlieb, J. D., Glynn, S. M., Lynde, D. W., Pipes, R., Kurian, B. T., Miller, A. L., Azrin, S. T., Goldstein, A. B., Severe, J. B., Lin, H., Sint, K. J., John, M., and Heinssen, R. K. Comprehensive versus usual community care for first-episode psychosis: 2-year outcomes from the NIMH RAISE Early Treatment Program. Am. J. Psychiatry, 173:362–372, 2016.

76. Kar, S. K., and Jain, M. Current understandings about cognition and the neurobiological correlates in schizophrenia. J. Neurosci. Rural Pract., 7:412–418, 2016.

77. Kendler, K. S., and Robinette, C. D. Schizophrenia in the National Academy of Sciences–National Research Council Twin Registry: a 16-year update. Am. J. Psychiatry, 140:1551–1563, 1983.

78. Kläning, U. Schizophrenia in twins: incidence and risk factors. Unpublished doctoral dissertation, University of Aarhus, Denmark, 1996.

79. Kotov, R., Leong, S. H., Mojtabai, R., Erlanger, A. C., Fochtmann, L. J., Constantino, E., Carlson, G. A., and Bromet, E. J. Boundaries of schizoaffective disorder: revisiting Kraepelin. JAMA Psychiatry, 70:1276–1286, 2013.

80. Kraepelin, E. *Dementia Praecox and Paraphrenia,* Barclay, R. M. and Robertson, G. M. (trans.). Edinburgh: E. & S. Livingstone, 1919.

81. Kringlen, E. Schizophrenia in male monozygotic twins. Acta Psychiatr. Scand., 40(*Suppl*):1–76, 1964.

82. Kringlen, E. Schizophrenia in twins. An epidemiological-clinical study. Psychiatry, 29:172–184, 1966.

83. Kringlen, E. *Heredity and Environment in the Functional Psychoses: An Epidemiological-Clinical Twin Study, Vol. I and II (Case Histories)*. London: William Heinemann, 1968.

84. Kwok, W. Is there evidence that social class at birth increases risk of psychosis? A systematic review. Int. J. Soc. Psychiatry, 60:801–808, 2014.

85. Lally, J., and Maccabe, J. H. Antipsychotic medication in schizophrenia: a review. Br. Med. Bull., 114:169–179, 2015.

86. Lang, F. U., Kosters, M., Lang, S., Becker, T., and Jager, M. Psychopathological long-term outcome of schizophrenia—a review. Acta Psychiatr. Scand., 127:173–182, 2013.

87. Lau, C. I., Wang, H. C., Hsu, J. L., and Liu, M. E. Does the dopamine hypothesis explain schizophrenia? Rev. Neurosci., 24:389–400, 2013.

88. Laursen, T. M., Nordentoft, M., and Mortensen, P. B. Excess early mortality in schizophrenia. Annu. Rev. Clin. Psychol., 10:425–448, 2014.

89. Liberg, B., Rahm, C., Panayiotou, A., and Pantelis, C. Brain change trajectories that differentiate the major psychoses. Eur. J. Clin. Invest., 46:658–674, 2016.

90. Lichtenstein, P., Yip, B. H., Bjork, C., Pawitan, Y., Cannon, T. D., Sullivan, P. F., and Hultman, C. M. Common genetic determinants of schizophrenia and bipolar disorder in Swedish families: a population-based study. Lancet, 373:234–239, 2009.

91. Linden, D. E. The challenges and promise of neuroimaging in psychiatry. Neuron, 73:8–22, 2012.

92. Luxenburger, H. Bericht uber psychiatrischen Serieuntersuchungen an Zwillingen. Z. Ges. Neurol. Psychiatrie, 176:297–326, 1928.

93. Maier, W., Hofgen, B., Zobel, A., and Rietschel, M. Genetic models of schizophrenia and bipolar disorder: overlapping inheritance or discrete genotypes? Eur. Arch. Psychiatry Clin. Neurosci., 255:159–166, 2005.

94. Miyamoto, S., Miyake, N., Jarskog, L. F., Fleischhacker, W. W., and Lieberman, J. A. Pharmacological treatment of schizophrenia: a critical review of the pharmacology and clinical effects of current and future therapeutic agents. Mol. Psychiatry, 17:1206–1227, 2012.

95. Moghaddam, B., and Javitt, D. From revolution to evolution: the glutamate hypothesis of schizophrenia and its implication for treatment. Neuropsychopharmacology, 37:4–15, 2012.

96. Moller, H. J. Bipolar disorder and schizophrenia: distinct illnesses or a continuum? J. Clin. Psychiatry, 64(Suppl 6):23–27, 2003.

97. Moller, H. J., Bottlender, R., Gross, A., Hoff, P., Wittmann, J., Wegner, U., and Strauss, A. The Kraepelinian dichotomy: preliminary results of a 15-year follow-up study on functional psychoses: focus on negative symptoms. Schizophr. Res., 56:87–94, 2002.

98. Moller, H. J., Bottlender, R., Wegner, U., Wittmann, J., and Strauss, A. Long-term course of schizophrenic, affective and schizoaffective psychosis: focus on negative symptoms and their impact on global indicators of outcome. Acta Psychiatr. Scand. Suppl., 407:54–57, 2000.

99. Montross, L. P., Zisook, S., and Kasckow, J. Suicide among patients with schizophrenia: a consideration of risk and protective factors. Ann. Clin. Psychiatry, 17:173–182, 2005.

100. Mueser, K. T., Penn, D. L., Addington, J., Brunette, M. F., Gingerich, S., Glynn, S. M., Lynde, D. W., Gottlieb, J. D., Meyer-Kalos, P., McGurk, S. R., Cather, C.,

Saade, S., Robinson, D. G., Schooler, N. R., Rosenheck, R. A., and Kane, J. M. The NAVIGATE program for first-episode psychosis: rationale, overview, and description of psychosocial components. Psychiatr. Serv., 66:680–690, 2015.

101. Murray, G. K., Jones, P. B., Moilanen, K., Veijola, J., Miettunen, J., Cannon, T. D., and Isohanni, M. Infant motor development and adult cognitive functions in schizophrenia. Schizophr. Res., 81:65–74, 2006.

102. Murru, A., and Carpiniello, B. Duration of untreated illness as a key to early intervention in schizophrenia: a review. Neurosci. Lett., 669:59–67, 2018.

103. Nordstrom, A., Kullgren, G., and Dahlgren, L. Schizophrenia and violent crime: the experience of parents. Int. J. Law Psychiatry, 29:57–67, 2006.

104. Olabi, B., Ellison-Wright, I., McIntosh, A. M., Wood, S. J., Bullmore, E., and Lawrie, S. M. Are there progressive brain changes in schizophrenia? A meta-analysis of structural magnetic resonance imaging studies. Biol. Psychiatry, 70:88–96, 2011.

105. Olfson, M., Gerhard, T., Huang, C., Crystal, S., and Stroup, T. S. Premature mortality among adults with schizophrenia in the United States. JAMA Psychiatry, 72:1172–1181, 2015.

106. Onstad, S., Skre, I., Torgersen, S., and Kringlen, E. Twin concordance for DSM-III-R schizophrenia. Acta Psychiatr. Scand., 83:395–401, 1991.

107. Opler, M. G., and Susser, E. S. Fetal environment and schizophrenia. Environ. Health Perspect., 113:1239–1242, 2005.

108. Ordóñez, A. E., Sastry, N. V., and Gogtay, N. Functional and clinical insights from neuroimaging studies in childhood-onset schizophrenia. CNS Spectr., 20:442–450, 2015.

109. Ott, S. L., Allen, J., and Erlenmeyer-Kimling, L. The New York High-Risk Project: observations on the rating of early manifestations of schizophrenia. Am. J. Med. Genet., 105:25–27, 2001.

110. Owen, M. J., Sawa, A., and Mortensen, P. B. Schizophrenia. Lancet, 388:86–97, 2016.

111. Palmer, B. A., Pankratz, V. S., and Bostwick, J. M. The lifetime risk of suicide in schizophrenia: a reexamination. Arch. Gen. Psychiatry, 62:247–253, 2005.

112. Pearlson, G. D. Etiologic, phenomenologic, and endophenotypic overlap of schizophrenia and bipolar disorder. Annu. Rev. Clin. Psychol., 11:251–281, 2015.

113. Pearlson, G. D., Clementz, B. A., Sweeney, J. A., Keshavan, M. S., and Tamminga, C. A. Does biology transcend the symptom-based boundaries of psychosis? Psychiatr. Clin. North Am., 39:165–174, 2016.

114. Penttila, M., Jaaskelainen, E., Hirvonen, N., Isohanni, M., and Miettunen, J. Duration of untreated psychosis as predictor of long-term outcome in schizophrenia: systematic review and meta-analysis. Br. J. Psychiatry, 205:88–94, 2014.

115. Popovic, D., Benabarre, A., Crespo, J. M., Goikolea, J. M., Gonzalez-Pinto, A., Gutierrez-Rojas, L., Montes, J. M., and Vieta, E. Risk factors for suicide in schizophrenia: systematic review and clinical recommendations. Acta Psychiatr. Scand., 130:418–426, 2014.

116. Porcelli, S., Bianchini, O., De, G. G., Aguglia, E., Crea, L., and Serretti, A. Clinical factors related to schizophrenia relapse. Int. J. Psychiatry Clin. Pract., 20:54–69, 2016.

117. Radhakrishnan, R., Wilkinson, S. T., and D'Souza, D. C. Gone to pot—a review of the association between cannabis and psychosis. Front. Psychiatry, 5:54, 2014.

118. Rapoport, J. L., Giedd, J. N., and Gogtay, N. Neurodevelopmental model of schizophrenia: update 2012. Mol. Psychiatry, 17:1228–1238, 2012.
119. Rapoport, J. L., and Gogtay, N. Childhood onset schizophrenia: support for a progressive neurodevelopmental disorder. Int. J. Dev. Neurosci., 29:251–258, 2011.
120. Reinhardt, M. M., and Cohen, C. I. Late-life psychosis: diagnosis and treatment. Curr. Psychiatry Rep., 17:1, 2015.
121. Remington, G., Foussias, G., Fervaha, G., Agid, O., Takeuchi, H., Lee, J., and Hahn, M. Treating negative symptoms in schizophrenia: an update. Curr. Treat. Options Psychiatry, 3:133–150, 2016.
122. Robins, E., and Guze, S. B. Establishment of diagnostic validity in psychiatric illness: its application to schizophrenia. Am. J. Psychiatry, 126:983–987, 1970.
123. Rosanoff, A. J., Handy, I. M., Plesset, I. R., and Brush, S. The etiology of so-called schizophrenic psychoses. With special reference to their occurrence in twins. Am. J. Psychiatry, 81:247–286, 1934.
124. Ross, S., and Peselow, E. Co-occurring psychotic and addictive disorders: neurobiology and diagnosis. Clin. Neuropharmacol., 35:235–243, 2012.
125. Ruggeri, M., Lasalvia, A., Tansella, M., Bonetto, C., Abate, M., Thornicroft, G., Allevi, L., and Ognibene, P. Heterogeneity of outcomes in schizophrenia. 3-year follow-up of treated prevalent cases. Br. J. Psychiatry, 184:48–57, 2004.
126. Sampford, J. R., Sampson, S., Li, B. G., Zhao, S., Xia, J., and Furtado, V. A. Fluphenazine (oral) versus atypical antipsychotics for schizophrenia. Cochrane Database Syst. Rev., 7:CD010832, 2016.
127. Sayo, A., Jennings, R. G., and Van Horn, J. D. Study factors influencing ventricular enlargement in schizophrenia: a 20 year follow-up meta-analysis. Neuroimage, 59:154–167, 2012.
128. Schulz, P. E., and Arora, G. Depression. Continuum (Minneap. Minn.), 21:756–771, 2015.
129. Schwab, S. G., and Wildenauer, D. B. Genetics of psychiatric disorders in the GWAS era: an update on schizophrenia. Eur. Arch. Psychiatry Clin. Neurosci., 263(Suppl 2):S147–S154, 2013.
130. Secher, R. G., Hjorthoj, C. R., Austin, S. F., Thorup, A., Jeppesen, P., Mors, O., and Nordentoft, M. Ten-year follow-up of the OPUS specialized early intervention trial for patients with a first episode of psychosis. Schizophr. Bull., 41:617–626, 2015.
131. Selten, J. P., Cantor-Graae, E., and Kahn, R. S. Migration and schizophrenia. Curr. Opin. Psychiatry, 20:111–115, 2007.
132. Selvaraj, S., Arnone, D., Cappai, A., and Howes, O. Alterations in the serotonin system in schizophrenia: a systematic review and meta-analysis of postmortem and molecular imaging studies. Neurosci. Biobehav. Rev., 45:233–245, 2014.
133. Shmukler, A. B., Gurovich, I. Y., Agius, M., and Zaytseva, Y. Long-term trajectories of cognitive deficits in schizophrenia: a critical overview. Eur. Psychiatry, 30:1002–1010, 2015.
134. Simeone, J. C., Ward, A. J., Rotella, P., Collins, J., and Windisch, R. An evaluation of variation in published estimates of schizophrenia prevalence from 1990 horizontal line 2013: a systematic literature review. BMC Psychiatry, 15:193, 2015.
135. Simonsen, E., Friis, S., Haahr, U., Johannessen, J. O., Larsen, T. K., Melle, I., Opjordsmoen, S., Rund, B. R., Vaglum, P., and McGlashan, T. Clinical epidemiologic first-episode psychosis: 1-year outcome and predictors. Acta Psychiatr. Scand., 116:54–61, 2007.
136. Singh, S., Kumar, A., Agarwal, S., Phadke, S. R., and Jaiswal, Y. Genetic insight of schizophrenia: past and future perspectives. Gene, 535:97–100, 2014.

137. Singh, S. M., and O'Reilly, R. (Epi)genomics and neurodevelopment in schizophrenia: monozygotic twins discordant for schizophrenia augment the search for disease-related (epi)genomic alterations. Genome, *52*:8–19, 2009.

138. Siskind, D., McCartney, L., Goldschlager, R., and Kisely, S. Clozapine v. first- and second-generation antipsychotics in treatment-refractory schizophrenia: systematic review and meta-analysis. Br. J. Psychiatry, *209*:385–392, 2016.

139. Slater, E., and Shields, J. *Psychotic and Neurotic Illnesses in Twins.* London: Her Majesty's Stationery Office, 1953.

140. Slopen, N. B., and Corrigan, P. W. Recovery in schizophrenia: reality or mere slogan. Curr. Psychiatr. Rep., 7:316–320, 2005.

141. Snyder, G. L., Vanover, K. E., Zhu, H., Miller, D. B., O'Callaghan, J. P., Tomesch, J., Li, P., Zhang, Q., Krishnan, V., Hendrick, J. P., Nestler, E. J., Davis, R. E., Wennogle, L. P., and Mates, S. Functional profile of a novel modulator of serotonin, dopamine, and glutamate neurotransmission. Psychopharmacology (Berl)., *232*:605–621, 2015.

142. Sullivan, P. F., Kendler, K. S., and Neale, M. C. Schizophrenia as a complex trait: evidence from a meta-analysis of twin studies. Arch. Gen. Psychiatry, *60*:1187–1192, 2003.

143. Sumiyoshi, T., Kunugi, H., and Nakagome, K. Serotonin and dopamine receptors in motivational and cognitive disturbances of schizophrenia. Front. Neurosci., 8:395, 2014.

144. Susser, E., and Keyes, K. M. Prenatal nutritional deficiency and psychosis: where do we go from here? JAMA Psychiatry, 74:349–350, 2017.

145. Svrakic, D. M., Zorumski, C. F., Svrakic, N. M., Zwir, I., and Cloninger, C. R. Risk architecture of schizophrenia: the role of epigenetics. Curr. Opin. Psychiatry, 26:188–195, 2013.

146. Tamminga, C. A., Pearlson, G., Keshavan, M., Sweeney, J., Clementz, B., and Thaker, G. Bipolar and schizophrenia network for intermediate phenotypes: outcomes across the psychosis continuum. Schizophr. Bull., *40(Suppl 2)*:S131–S137, 2014.

147. Thibaut, F., Boutros, N. N., Jarema, M., Oranje, B., Hasan, A., Daskalakis, Z. J., Wichniak, A., Schmitt, A., Riederer, P., and Falkai, P. Consensus paper of the WFSBP Task Force on Biological Markers: criteria for biomarkers and endophenotypes of schizophrenia part I: neurophysiology. World J. Biol. Psychiatry, *16*:280–290, 2015.

148. Thoma, P., and Daum, I. Comorbid substance use disorder in schizophrenia: a selective overview of neurobiological and cognitive underpinnings. Psychiatry Clin. Neurosci., *67*:367–383, 2013.

149. Tienari, E. Schizophrenia in Finnish male twins. In *Studies of Schizophrenia. British Journal of Psychiatry, Special Publication No. 10*, Lader, M. H. (ed.), pp. 29–35, 1975.

150. Tienari, P. Psychiatric illnesses in identical twins. Acta Psychiatr. Scand., *39*:1–195, 1963.

151. Tsujita, T., Okazaki, Y., Fujimaru, K., Minami, Y., Mutoh, Y., Maeda, H., Fukazawa, T., Yamashita, H., and Nakane, Y. *Twin Concordance Rate of DSM-III-R Schizophrenia in a New Japanese Sample.* Abstracts of the Seventh International Congress on Twin Studies, Tokyo, Japan, 1992.

152. Valencia, M., Fresan, A., Barak, Y., Juarez, F., Escamilla, R., and Saracco, R. Predicting functional remission in patients with schizophrenia: a cross-sectional study of symptomatic remission, psychosocial remission, functioning, and clinical outcome. Neuropsychiatr. Dis. Treat., *11*:2339–2348, 2015.

153. van den Heuvel, M. P., and Fornito, A. Brain networks in schizophrenia. Neuropsychol. Rev., *24*:32–48, 2014.
154. van der Ven, E., Veling, W., Tortelli, A., Tarricone, I., Berardi, D., Bourque, F., and Selten, J. P. Evidence of an excessive gender gap in the risk of psychotic disorder among North African immigrants in Europe: a systematic review and meta-analysis. Soc. Psychiatry Psychiatr. Epidemiol., *51*:1603–1613, 2016.
155. van Erp, T. G., Hibar, D. P., Rasmussen, J. M., Glahn, D. C., Pearlson, G. D., Andreassen, O. A., Agartz, I., Westlye, L. T., Haukvik, U. K., Dale, A. M., Melle, I., Hartberg, C. B., Gruber, O., Kraemer, B., Zilles, D., Donohoe, G., Kelly, S., McDonald, C., Morris, D. W., Cannon, D. M., Corvin, A., Machielsen, M. W., Koenders, L., de Haan, L., Veltman, D. J., Satterthwaite, T. D., Wolf, D. H., Gur, R. C., Gur, R. E., Potkin, S. G., Mathalon, D. H., Mueller, B. A., Preda, A., Macciardi, F., Ehrlich, S., Walton, E., Hass, J., Calhoun, V. D., Bockholt, H. J., Sponheim, S. R., Shoemaker, J. M., van Haren, N. E., Hulshoff Pol, H. E., Ophoff, R. A., Kahn, R. S., Roiz-Santianez, R., Crespo-Facorro, B., Wang, L., Alpert, K. I., Jonsson, E. G., Dimitrova, R., Bois, C., Whalley, H. C., McIntosh, A. M., Lawrie, S. M., Hashimoto, R., Thompson, P. M., and Turner, J. A. Subcortical brain volume abnormalities in 2028 individuals with schizophrenia and 2540 healthy controls via the ENIGMA consortium. Mol. Psychiatry, *21*:547–553, 2016.
156. Venkatasubramanian, G., and Debnath, M. Neuroimmunological aberrations and cerebral asymmetry abnormalities in schizophrenia: select perspectives on pathogenesis. Clin. Psychopharmacol. Neurosci., *12*:8–18, 2014.
157. Ventriglio, A., Gentile, A., Bonfitto, I., Stella, E., Mari, M., Steardo, L., and Bellomo, A. Suicide in the early stage of schizophrenia. Front. Psychiatry, 7:116, 2016.
158. Volavka, J. Violence in schizophrenia and bipolar disorder. Psychiatr. Danub., *25*:24–33, 2013.
159. Vourdas, A., Pipe, R., Corrigall, R., and Frangou, S. Increased developmental deviance and premorbid dysfunction in early onset schizophrenia. Schizophr. Res., *62*:13–22, 2003.
160. Walker, E. F., Grimes, K. E., Davis, D. M., and Smith, A. J. Childhood precursors of schizophrenia: facial expressions of emotion. Am. J. Psychiatry, *150*:1654–1660, 1993.
161. Walter, E. E., Fernandez, F., Snelling, M., and Barkus, E. Genetic consideration of schizotypal traits: a review. Front. Psychol., 7:1769, 2016.
162. Werbeloff, N., Levine, S. Z., and Rabinowitz, J. Elaboration on the association between immigration and schizophrenia: a population-based national study disaggregating annual trends, country of origin and sex over 15 years. Soc. Psychiatry Psychiatr. Epidemiol., 47:303–311, 2012.
163. Witt, K., van, D. R., and Fazel, S. Risk factors for violence in psychosis: systematic review and meta-regression analysis of 110 studies. PLoS One, 8:e55942, 2013.
164. Wong, A. H., and Van Tol, H. H. Schizophrenia: from phenomenology to neurobiology. Neurosci. Biobehav. Rev., *27*:269–306, 2003.
165. Woo, T. U. Neurobiology of schizophrenia onset. Curr. Top. Behav. Neurosci., *16*:267–295, 2014.
166. Zink, M. Comorbid obsessive-compulsive symptoms in schizophrenia: insight into pathomechanisms facilitates treatment. Adv. Med., *2014*:317980, 2014.

CHAPTER 4

oѵɔ

Panic and Phobic Disorders

In current diagnostic nomenclature, panic disorder and agoraphobia are two distinct disorders that are diagnosed independently of one another (3, 100). In previous versions of the criteria, these diagnoses were linked (e.g., panic disorder with or without agoraphobia and agoraphobia without panic disorder). This chapter will cover both panic and phobic disorders.

Panic disorder is a chronic illness characterized by recurrent, acute panic attacks. Panic attacks are discrete episodes of anxiety or fearfulness with definite onset, rapid increase, and spontaneous termination. During attacks patients may have overwhelming feelings of impending doom. The attacks are accompanied by symptoms associated with the autonomic nervous system: palpitations, tachycardia, rapid or shallow breathing, dizziness, and tremor. Between attacks, patients may be relatively asymptomatic though some experience fatigue, headache, and symptoms of anxiety attacks that persist. A panic attack is a symptom rather than a disorder, and panic attacks can be part of the course of any psychiatric illness. When panic attacks occur together, independent of other significant psychiatric symptoms, the diagnosis of panic disorder is made.

Panic is distinguished from ordinary fear by the lack of an appropriate stimulus precipitating the emotions. Sometimes, however, patients experience panic attacks in response to a fear-provoking situation, such as facing an angry employer or giving a public speech. In these cases the clinician must decide whether the anxiety is grossly out of proportion to the fear-provoking stimulus, as well as make a diagnosis based on the complete history. Most patients with panic disorder report some panic attacks without any fear-provoking stimulus, but on other occasions they overreact to situations that would produce some degree of apprehension in individuals without the disorder.

Phobic disorder is a chronic condition dominated by one or more phobias. A phobia is an intense, recurrent, unreasonable fear of a specific object, activity, or situation that results in a compelling desire to avoid the dreaded object, activity, or situation. DSM-5 subdivides phobias into specific phobias (e.g., fear of animals), social anxiety disorder that consists of social phobias (e.g., fear of public speaking), and agoraphobia (3). Agoraphobia is characterized by multiple phobias involving a fear of being in places where help might not be available in the event of an anxiety attack.

HISTORICAL BACKGROUND

> My cheek is cold and white, alas!
> O lift me from the grass!
> I die! I faint! I fall!
> . . .
> My cheek is cold and white, alas!
> My heart beats loud and fast.
>
> Percy Bysshe Shelley
> *The Indian Serenade* (p. 370) (102)

It has been suggested that Shelley was having a panic attack when he wrote these lines (20). If so, he probably would have called it something else. In the nineteenth century, "anxiety reactions" referring to fainting—which was fashionable among women of that era—were called "vapors." Modern patients with panic disorder also sometimes faint—probably from hyperventilating. In Victorian times the prototype of a refined young woman was "a swooner, pale and trembling, who responded to unpleasant or unusual social situations by taking to the floor in a graceful and delicious maneuver, in no way resembling the crash of the epileptic" (p. 1401) (20). A Jane Austen heroine found one social situation "too pathetic for the feelings of Sophie and myself. We fainted alternately on a sofa" (p. 1401) (20). Overly tight corsets may have been responsible for some of the fainting. A nineteenth-century physician, Dr. John Brown, cured fainting by "cutting the stay laces, which ran before the knife and cracked like a bow string" (p. 1401) (20).

One of the first medical terms to describe anxiety disorders was "neurasthenia," defined by an American physician, G. M. Beard, in 1869 (9). Neurasthenia broadly included patients with hysteria, obsessional illness, and anxiety disorders, as well as hypochondria and swooning (15). The term "anxiety neurosis" was first used by Freud in 1895. It was not until 1980 that the concept of neurosis was dropped from American Psychiatric Association general nomenclature, and the term "panic disorder" replaced the older term "anxiety neurosis" as the disorder's official name (1). Panic disorder was later subdivided into two types, with and without agoraphobia (2), but ultimately panic disorder and agoraphobia were separated into two distinct disorders (3).

The term "phobia" originates from the name of a Greek god, Phobos, whose likeness was painted on masks and shields for the purpose of frightening the enemy (58). The word *phobia* first appeared in medical terminology in Rome 2,000 years ago, when hydrophobia was used to describe a symptom of rabies. Hippocrates also described cases of phobic fears.

During the nineteenth century, *phobia* appeared increasingly in descriptions of morbid fears, beginning with syphilophobia, defined in a medical dictionary published in 1848 as "a morbid dread of syphilis giving rise to fancied symptoms of the disease" (p. 93) (55). Later authorities compiled long lists of phobias, naming each in Greek or Latin terms after the object or situation feared. Thus, as Nemiah pointed out, "the patient who was spared the pangs of taphaphobia (fear of being buried alive) or ailurophobia (fear of cats) might yet fall prey to belonophobia (fear of needles), siderodromophobia (fear of railways), or triskaidekaphobia (fear of thirteen at table), and pantaphobia was the diagnostic fate of that unfortunate soul who feared them all" (p. 895) (69).

The term "phobia" was not applied in a psychiatric sense until the nineteenth century. In 1871, Westphal described three men who feared public places and labeled the condition "agoraphobia," *agora* derived from the Greek word for "place of assembly or marketplace" (98). Westphal recommended companionship, alcohol, or the use of a cane to treat the condition. Numerous theories were advanced to explain phobias, including poor upbringing (52).

Phobias and panic attacks have long been known to occur in a variety of psychiatric conditions. Controversy has continued since the late nineteenth century over the relationship of phobias and panic to other psychiatric disorders, such as obsessional and mood disorders, substance abuse, and personality disorders (5, 36, 42, 58, 85, 105).

EPIDEMIOLOGY

Panic and phobic disorders are among the most common psychiatric syndromes (19, 78). As many as 2%–4% of the adult population may have panic disorder at some time in their lifetimes (6, 25, 43, 44, 79), and women have at least twice the prevalence of men (6, 25, 41, 62). Panic disorder appears to be more common in whites than in African Americans and Hispanics (26). The previous linkage of panic disorder and agoraphobia in the diagnostic criteria was not without basis, because one-third to one-half of general-population panic disorder cases are associated with agoraphobia, and this proportion is greater, 80% or more, in clinical samples (6, 13, 26, 42).

Panic disorder has inconsistently been found to be associated with low educational level and socioeconomic status (25, 26). The disorder has been found to be associated with self-reported childhood abuse history, but the association was modest, much of it explained by other childhood and family factors (18, 33).

Many people with panic disorder experience a mild form and, like those with phobic disorders, do not seek medical care for their symptoms (6, 19). Many others consult family practitioners or internists rather than psychiatrists. Patients with panic disorder who see psychiatrists may represent a small group with a high prevalence of comorbid mood disorder (6).

Two population studies using structured diagnostic interviews have provided lifetime prevalence rates of phobic disorders. In the 1980s, the Epidemiologic Catchment Area (ECA) study (80) examined more than 19,000 representative members of the US population with the National Institutes of Mental Health (NIMH) Diagnostic Interview Schedule. In the 1990s, the National Comorbidity Survey (NCS) study interviewed more than 8,000 representative US population members with the World Health Organization (WHO) Composite International Diagnostic Interview (CIDI) (43). These systematic studies found higher lifetime prevalence of phobic disorders than in previous studies, 14% in the ECA study and 22% in the NCS. Specific diagnosis rates in the NCS were 13% for social phobia, 11% for specific phobia, and 5% for agoraphobia. Despite the higher overall prevalence of phobic disorders in these studies, the findings challenged prevailing notions of the ubiquitous nature of specific phobias, such as fear of snakes and heights, especially in childhood and among women.

The reported prevalence of phobic disorders varies according to the sample surveyed, the interview employed, and the choice of diagnostic criteria (6, 31, 62). A possible explanation for the higher prevalence of phobias in these population studies than in earlier studies is that respondents were shown lists of feared objects and situations, unlike many previous studies that may have depended on people to remember phobic fears more spontaneously. Because inconsistency in methods between studies is a common problem in psychiatric epidemiology, findings often must be considered only tentative. Use of different diagnostic criteria and instruments of measure across epidemiological studies has undoubtedly contributed to disparities in prevalence rates reported for phobic disorders. In clinical samples, discrepancy in prevalence data for phobias may also be attributed to two other reasons. First, some physicians may include what others consider normal fears in their statistics. Second, many people are embarrassed about their phobias and tend to be secretive about them. It is not unusual in psychiatric practice to see patients for years before they describe, almost in passing, a phobia that has bothered them for a long time.

In both the ECA and NCS studies, the prevalence of phobic disorders in the 12 months preceding the interview was lower than the lifetime prevalence by about half, suggesting that phobic disorders are either episodic or temporary. This finding contradicts previous clinical observations and studies characterizing phobias as chronic conditions. Because few individuals with phobias ever receive treatment for them, most of the difference between lifetime and 12-month rates cannot be attributed to medications or psychotherapy.

Both the ECA study and the NCS found phobias to be more prevalent among women than men. The ECA study found that phobias are more prevalent among African Americans than whites and Hispanics (25, 38). People with phobic disorders are less likely to be employed and their socioeconomic status is lower compared to other people. They are also less likely to be married (38, 40, 99).

CLINICAL PICTURE

Panic attacks are the hallmark of panic disorder. The attacks usually begin suddenly, sometimes in a public place or at a social gathering, or even at home. There is a sense of foreboding, fear, and apprehension; a sense that one has suddenly become seriously ill; and a feeling that one's life may be threatened by such illness. Some patients, especially those with agoraphobia, describe a disturbing sense of their body changing or becoming distorted (depersonalization) (91). These feelings are hard to define and appear to be an unpleasant, scary sense of being unreal, strange, and disembodied, cut off from one's surroundings. Feelings of alien change may extend to the surrounding world (derealization). Symptoms of labored breathing, smothering, palpitation, blurred vision, tremulousness, and weakness usually accompany the apprehension and foreboding. Patients examined during such an attack manifest signs of distress: tachycardia, sweating, tachypnea, tremor, hyperactive deep tendon reflexes, and dilated pupils.

Panic disorder is defined in *DSM-5* (3) as a syndrome of recurrent, unexpected panic attacks, which are episodes of intense fear or discomfort that begin abruptly and intensify rapidly, accompanied by several symptoms that may include trembling, palpitations, sweating, shortness of breath, dizziness, chest pain, and abdominal distress. These are accompanied by sustained worry about further attacks or maladaptive behavioral changes to avoid attacks.

Panic attacks vary in frequency among patients. Some experience them on a daily basis; others have them only once or twice a year. Other symptoms may occur between attacks. Table 4.1 lists these symptoms and their frequency as reported in a classic study of this disorder (16). The symptoms can occur in practically any pattern.

Cardiorespiratory symptoms are the most frequent chief complaints that panic disorder patients report to physicians: "I have heart spells," "I think I'll smother," or "There is no way for me to get enough air." The chief complaint is occasionally psychological, but more often the chief complaint reveals that the patient considers the disorder medical, and perhaps very serious, as illustrated in the following case report.

A 51-year-old electrical engineer was brought to an emergency room by ambulance, complaining of severe left anterior chest pain. His breathing was labored and he complained of numbness and tingling in his lips and fingers. His pulse rate was 110. He was perspiring heavily and visibly frightened. However, the electrocardiogram was normal, and blood enzymes were within normal limits. He was observed over the next several hours and then discharged asymptomatic.

The history revealed that the patient had first experienced severe chest pain at the age of 21 while watching a movie. He had experienced many subsequent episodes of chest pain accompanied by dyspnea and anxiety and had been taken to an emergency room on at least 10 previous occasions. Although the examinations were always normal, he had undergone a variety of cardiovascular procedures, including cardiac catheterization. He had never been seen by a psychiatrist and at no time had been told that he very likely suffered from a common psychiatric disorder characterized by panic attacks.

Symptoms may become associated with specific situations that patients will try to avoid. For example, they may choose aisle seats in theaters,

TABLE 4.1 SYMPTOMS OF PANIC DISORDER

Symptoms	60 Patients (%)	102 Controls* (%)
Palpitation	97	9
Tires easily	93	19
Breathlessness	90	13
Nervousness	88	27
Chest pain	85	10
Sighing	79	16
Dizziness	78	16
Faintness	70	12
Apprehensiveness	61	3
Headache	58	26
Paresthesias	58	7
Weakness	56	3
Trembling	54	17
Breathing unsatisfactory	53	4
Insomnia	53	4
Unhappiness	50	2
Shakiness	47	16
Fatigued all the time	45	6
Sweating	42	33
Fear of death	42	2
Smothering	40	3
Syncope	37	11
Nervous chill	24	0
Urinary frequency	18	2
Vomiting and diarrhea	14	0
Anorexia	12	3
Paralysis	0	0
Blindness	0	0

*Healthy controls consisted of 50 men and 11 women from a large industrial plant and 41 healthy postpartum women from the Boston Lying-In Hospital.
Adapted from Cohen and White (16).

preferably close to exits, so that if an attack occurs, they will not be confined. Or patients may avoid social situations in which an attack would be both frightening and embarrassing.

Phobias can be distinguished from "normal" fears by their intensity, duration, irrationality, and the disablement resulting from avoidance of the feared situation. *DSM-5* divides phobic disorders into three types: specific phobia, social phobia, and agoraphobia.

A *specific phobia* is an isolated fear of a single object or situation, leading to avoidance of the object or situation. The fear is irrational and excessive but not always disabling because the object or situation can sometimes be easily avoided (e.g., snakes, if you are a city dweller). Impairment may be considerable if the phobic object is common and cannot be avoided, such as a fear of elevators for someone who must use elevators at work.

Specific phobias almost always involve a single isolated phobia. People with specific phobias typically are no more (or less) anxious than anyone else until exposed to the phobic object or situation. Then they become overwhelmingly uncomfortable and fearful, sometimes having panic attack symptoms (palpitations, sweating, dizziness, difficulty breathing). People with phobias also fear the possibility of confronting the phobic stimulus. Called "anticipatory anxiety," this leads to avoidance of situations in which the stimulus might be present.

Some common specific phobias are fear of animals, heights, closed spaces, wind, storms, lightning, loud noises, driving a car, flying in airplanes, riding in subways, hypodermic needles, and blood. Less common ones include fear of running water and of going to the hairdresser. There is even the case of the tennis player who wore gloves because he was afraid of fuzz, and tennis balls are fuzzy. Phobias can develop toward almost any object or situation.

Animal phobias are perhaps the most common specific phobias, or at least the most commonly studied. They occur often in childhood and are usually transient. Among adults, more women than men are subject to animal phobias. The phobia usually involves only one kind of animal but may lead to frequent distress with mild social disablement if the animals are domestic, such as dogs or cats (32).

Fear of heights is another common phobia. The fear may be totally unrealistic. The person may be close enough to the ground so that a fall would not cause injury. Some people with phobias will not walk down a flight of stairs if they see the open stairwell. Some will not look out a window from the second floor or above, particularly if the window goes from floor to ceiling. Others will not cross a bridge on foot, though they may go by car.

Social phobia is another form of isolated phobia that generally leads to only mild forms of impairment. It involves fears of eating in public, public speaking, receiving criticism from superiors, urinating in the presence of others, practicing musical instruments because the neighbors will hear mistakes, and swimming or undressing in front of others because of shame at one's appearance. Social phobia often involves two or more phobias. The individual with social phobia fears embarrassment, humiliation, or rejection if the fearful behavior is noticed by others. Social phobia does not generally lead to total avoidance of the situations, but occasionally, severe handicap may result, as illustrated next.

The young wife of a business executive refused to entertain associates of her husband with a dinner party or attend dinner parties in restaurants or someone else's home. Her husband made excuses for her but felt his career was being damaged by their lack of social life. At first her explanation for refusing to join in dinner parties was that it was a waste of time or too much trouble. Later she confessed, tearfully and with much embarrassment, that she was afraid of being unable to eat if strangers were watching. Questioned by her concerned husband, she said she was afraid that once food was in her mouth she would be unable to swallow it and then find herself in the embarrassing situation of not knowing where to dispose of the food. She was also afraid that she would gag on the food and possibly vomit. She could eat in front of her husband with no difficulty until she told him about the phobia and then became concerned that he was watching her eat and expecting her to gag or vomit. From then on she ate alone in the kitchen. The marriage survived, but barely (32).

Unlike specific and social phobias, *agoraphobia* has a complex clinical picture involving the combination of a wide range of phobic fears, including the following:

1. *Public transportation*: Trains, buses, subways, airplanes. When crowded, these vehicles may be intolerable to people with agoraphobia. Waiting in line is almost as bad, whether for a bus or a movie.
2. *Other confining places*: Tunnels, bridges, elevators, the hairdresser or barber's chair, and the dentist's chair. These fears belong to the category of claustrophobia, but most people with claustrophobia have only a single phobia and do not actually have agoraphobia. Paradoxically, people with agoraphobia may also be fearful of open spaces, such as empty parking lots.
3. *Being home alone*: Some people with agoraphobia require constant companionship, to the despair of friends, neighbors, and family.
4. *Being away from home* or another "safe" place where help cannot be readily obtained if needed: The agoraphobia sufferer is sometimes comforted just knowing there is a police officer or a doctor somewhere nearby.

When confronted with these types of situations, people with these phobias worry that they will be trapped in a terrible situation. No one would be available to help in the event that they would become incapacitated (e.g., by falling) or be embarrassed (e.g., with incontinence) or overcome by panic symptoms.

Klein and associates observed that most agoraphobia patients describe a history of panic attacks preceding the onset of phobias, and anticipatory anxiety about another panic attack leads to phobic avoidance of places where panic attacks might occur (47). Thus, a bridge phobia may not involve a fear of bridges per se, but may develop from a fear of experiencing panic on a bridge. Phobias about buses, trains, or airplanes may arise from concern that a panic attack might occur in a vehicle from which escape is impossible or embarrassing. Although *DSM-III-R* adopted Klein's conceptualization of agoraphobia within the context of panic disorder, these two disorders were again separated in *DSM-5*.

BIOLOGICAL FINDINGS

Over the last two centuries, many theories of the origin of anxiety syndromes and anxiety disorders have evolved, from constitutional weakness of the nervous system to social and psychological factors to more recent biological hypotheses. Although the cause of panic disorder remains unknown, discovery of physiological abnormalities associated with panic disorder and advances in understanding of the neural circuitry of anxiety states have led to the elaboration of plausible theoretical models of anxiety disorders.

Physiological findings are well documented in anxiety disorders. People with panic disorder have greater cardiac and respiratory reactivity during fear exposure compared to healthy controls (64, 65). In people with panic or phobic disorders, breathing carbon dioxide may induce respiratory alkalosis and exaggerated elevations in brain lactate, eliciting panic attacks as well (60, 83, 89, 95). Elevated levels of lactate or carbon dioxide signal an inborn survival mechanism to warn the body of impending suffocation or danger. It is speculated that in panic disorder, this "suffocation alarm" feedback system may be dysregulated (64, 89).

The neurobiology of anxiety disorders remains poorly understood at this time (19). However, it is generally accepted that abnormalities in the limbic system and the hypothalamic-pituitary-adrenal (HPA) axis functioning underlie the neuropathology of anxiety disorders (19). Much attention has been focused on the locus ceruleus, a nucleus that represents a major part of the noradrenergic system. The locus ceruleus serves as a relay center for the body's alarm system and projects to the limbic system and cortex. Dysregulated activation of the locus ceruleus generates inappropriate subjective fear responses, precipitating inefficient cardiorespiratory compensatory mechanisms (21). Drugs that increase the firing rate of locus ceruleus neurons increase anxiety levels, and drugs that block the firing of these neurons have opposite effects (21). Several medications used to relieve anxiety and prevent spontaneous panic attacks also reduce panic and anxiety symptoms: beta blockers such as propranolol, benzodiazepines such as alprazolam, tricyclic antidepressants such as amitriptyline, and serotonin-selective reuptake inhibitor (SSRI) antidepressants such as paroxetine, sertraline, fluvoxamine, and citalopram (70).

No neurobiological markers have been identified for the diagnosis of anxiety disorders (19). Findings from research on brain fear-response circuitry and neurobiological investigation of patients with anxiety disorders have led to the identification of abnormalities in brain structure and functioning that may be involved in the psychopathology of anxiety disorders (60). Imaging studies have demonstrated brain changes in panic disorder, including increased activity in the amygdala, hippocampus, thalamus, midbrain, caudal pons, medulla, and cerebellum (60). Lactate-induced anxiety attacks in patients with panic disorder have been found to be associated with increased blood flow to the right orbitofrontal and left occipital cortex and decreased blood flow to the amygdala and hippocampus (28). Neurotransmitter abnormalities implicated in anxiety disorders include dysregulation of the serotonin neurotransmitter system and inhibition of gamma-amino-butyric acid (GABA) or increased excitatory transmission by glutamate (60).

NATURAL HISTORY

Panic disorder most often begins in the third decade of life, and most cases begin between the ages of 18 and 35 (6, 26, 35, 44). A study of 38 families with transgenerational occurrence of the disorder found the mean age of onset to be younger in subsequent generations (age 23 in younger generations compared to 37 in the older generation) (8). Panic disorder may begin acutely with a discrete anxiety attack, but it also may begin insidiously with feelings of tenseness, nervousness, fatigue, or dizziness for years before the first anxiety attack. Some patients may remember the exact time and circumstances of the first attack, such as a stressful experience (e.g., while making a speech in class).

Many patients with panic disorder attribute their symptoms to medical problems and present to medical or emergency care settings with their symptoms (6, 29). The initial medical contacts of panic disorder patients are not always helpful. Patients commonly present with complaints of cardiorespiratory symptoms, fearing heart disease. Physicians unacquainted with the natural history of panic disorder may reinforce these patients' fears by referring them to a specialist and warning them to limit exertion.

Somatic symptoms reported by patients with panic disorder are not confined to the cardiorespiratory system. Some patients present with symptoms of irritable bowel syndrome (29, 54). These patients usually consult a gastroenterologist. Among their most common presenting symptoms are abdominal cramping, diarrhea, constipation, nausea, belching, flatus, and sometimes dysphagia without objective findings of structural bowel disease. Panic disorder is not the only psychiatric disorder associated with such complaints, however, as major depressive disorder and somatoform disorders may also present similarly (66, 72). Patients with panic disorder also have many other somatic symptoms, including musculoskeletal symptoms, dizziness, headaches, chest pain, and palpitations (22, 63, 90). Many of these patients receive diagnoses of disorders without identified pathology (termed "functional" disorders), such as fibromyalgia, chronic fatigue syndrome, and migraine as well as irritable bowel syndrome (14, 29, 39, 54, 88).

The course of panic disorder is variable (103). Symptoms may be chronic, but more commonly they wax and wane in an irregular pattern that may or may not be associated with events and circumstances interpreted by the patient as stressful (19). Despite their symptoms, most patients with panic disorder live productively without social impairment. Longitudinal studies have found that more than half of patients recover, but relapse is common (76). Remission is less likely after 2 years of continuous illness (103).

The median age of onset for agoraphobia is 20 years (6). The first anxiety attack often occurs against a background of worry and unhappiness: job dissatisfaction, domestic crisis, serious medical illness, a death in the family. Nevertheless, people with agoraphobia do not associate the first anxiety attack with a specific stress that would justify panic. Isaac Marks quotes a patient as saying (p. 86) (57):

> I was standing at the bus stop wondering what to cook for dinner when suddenly I felt panicky and sweaty, my knees felt like jelly, and I had to hold on to the lamppost and I was afraid I would die. I got on the bus and was terribly nervous, but just managed to totter home. Since then I haven't liked to go out on the street and have never been on a bus again.

One-half to three-quarters of patients with mild or moderate agoraphobia will recover or substantially improve within 5–10 years after the illness began. The severely disabled housebound patient may remain that way indefinitely. Some cases are short-lived, but nobody knows how many. If the symptoms of agoraphobia persist for a year, they are almost certain to last much longer (57).

Specific and social phobias have an earlier onset than agoraphobia, with a median age of onset of 7 years for specific phobias and 13 years for social phobias (6). Unlike specific phobias and agoraphobia, which affect many more women than men, social phobias affect the sexes more equally (19, 99). Most social phobias develop over several months, beginning without any apparent precipitating event, and stabilize after a period of years with a gradual diminution of severity in middle life.

Specific phobias beginning in childhood and early adolescence tend to improve and eventually disappear, approximately half of them disappearing within 5 years (10). Phobias beginning after adolescence persist longer and gradually worsen in about one-third of patients. Specific phobias that persist into adulthood usually do not remit (3). The longitudinal course of social phobia is more chronic: only about one-third of patients achieve remission within a decade, and one-third of those who remit will subsequently relapse (76).

Some predictors of outcomes of anxiety disorders have been identified. In panic disorder, comorbidity with major depressive disorder reduces the recovery rates by about half and approximately doubles the likelihood of relapse (13). Personality disorder, observed in more than one-third of one sample of patients with social phobia and in one-fifth of a sample of patients with panic disorder, was found to be associated with a more chronic 1- to 5-year follow-up course in social phobia but not in panic disorder (61). In panic disorder (76, 78) and social phobia (99), patients with an earlier age of onset of the disorder have been found to have a more severe and persistent course of the illness. Men and women fare about equally well (or poorly) in outcomes of panic and phobic disorders (103).

COMPLICATIONS

The most common complication of panic disorder is major depressive disorder, which presents as a comorbid disorder in half or more of cases (51). There is a predilection for the initial onset of the anxiety disorder to precede the first appearance of depression (51).

The frequent comorbidity of major depression with panic disorder has generated speculation that panic disorder may be a variant or an epiphenomenon of major depressive disorder (23). Both conditions are relieved by antidepressant medications (60). Additionally, depressive and anxiety disorders overlap in relatives of patients with depression and anxiety disorders (76). Arguments against the illnesses being identical are as follows: 1) panic disorder has an earlier age of onset than major depressive disorder; 2) these disorders demonstrate diagnostic consistency in longitudinal studies (76); 3) panic attacks can usually be precipitated in people with a history of spontaneous panic attacks by carbon dioxide inhalation, and this rarely happens in patients with depression only (89, 95); and 4) failure of suppression in the dexamethasone suppression test occurs in about half of patients with depression but is rare in individuals with spontaneous panic attacks (96).

Major depressive disorder is also a common comorbidity in patients with social phobia. Social phobia is associated with psychiatric comorbidity in 50%–80% of cases, and panic disorder and substance use disorders are also commonly comorbid with social phobia (42, 99). Specific phobias have far lower rates of associated psychiatric comorbidities (45).

Evidence from epidemiological research has documented an overabundance of alcohol problems among people with panic or phobic disorders, and, conversely, an increased prevalence of panic and phobic disorders among individuals with alcohol use disorders (4, 17, 19, 42, 92, 99). The odds of having an alcohol use disorder are approximately doubled or tripled among people with an anxiety disorder (50, 87). There are three possible causal interpretations of these associations: 1) anxiety symptoms might lead to problems with alcohol, potentially through a hypothesized process of "self-medication" of anxiety symptoms with alcohol; 2) anxiety might result from neurological changes induced by alcohol use or withdrawal (as many people with alcohol use disorders are observed to have panic attacks, particularly when hung over); or 3) there may be no direct causal relationship but rather an indirect connection between alcohol and anxiety problems through associations with other causal factors, such as common genetic vulnerabilities (17, 19).

Drug abuse may also arise as a complication of panic disorder, the occasional result of overzealous prescription of habit-forming medication by well-meaning physicians. The odds of having a drug use disorder are approximately doubled for people with an anxiety disorder (50).

Anxiety disorders have historically been reported to be associated with reduced longevity, but studies in the past decade have challenged this finding (19, 82). Methodological problems in research studies, including use of self-report symptom measures rather than structured diagnostic interviews assessing full diagnostic criteria, brief length of follow-up, and lack of control for comorbid depressive disorders, appear to have contributed to morbidity findings (82). Most of the excess mortality in anxiety disorders has been found to result from comorbidity with depressive illness (19).

It was long assumed that anxiety disorders do not increase risk for suicide, logically following observations that a major fear among patients with anxiety disorders is the fear of dying (93). A study published in 1989 found an increased risk of suicide in panic disorder (97), and other studies subsequently reported associations of suicidality with panic disorder (93) and social anxiety disorder (4). A concern with suicidality studies, however, was that more general risk factors for suicide attempts, such as female sex, substance use disorder, and comorbid major depressive disorder, are also associated with anxiety disorders, confounding suicidality in these other conditions with comorbid anxiety disorders (93).

Anxiety disorders are associated with varying degrees of functional impairment and disability (4, 19, 100). Many individuals with anxiety disorders are able to function and experience a satisfactory quality of life. In isolated phobias, the disability tends to be mild and is limited to responses to the phobic object or situation. At the other end of the disability spectrum, patients with agoraphobia may become completely housebound and unable to work, which occurs in approximately one-third of these patients (3). Patients with agoraphobia often recruit other people to do their shopping and take their children to school. The anxiety disorders associated with the highest levels of functional impairment and disability are panic disorder and agoraphobia. Patients meeting criteria for both of these disorders have even greater impairment and disability (100). Levels of functional disability in social phobia lie somewhere between those of panic disorder and specific phobias (19).

Sexual maladjustments, such as premature ejaculation, anorgasmia, and sexual aversion, are known complications of panic and phobic disorders (104). Oddly, the sexual difficulties often antedate the anxiety symptoms.

FAMILY AND GENETIC STUDIES

Panic disorder is a strikingly familial condition (60, 83, 100). First-degree relatives of individuals with panic disorder have a seven times higher likelihood of developing panic disorder compared to the general population (60, 83). Twin studies find a much higher concordance of panic disorder among monozygotic twins than in dizygotic twins, with a heritability estimate of 30%–50% (60, 83, 100). These findings support a genetic predisposition to panic disorder.

Agoraphobia has been found to have an even higher heritability, on the order of 60% (83, 100). Relatives of probands with agoraphobia have an increased risk of both agoraphobia and panic disorder, about 30% each (100). Agoraphobia without comorbid panic disorder, however, does not appear to be familial. Agoraphobia in general, however, is associated with familial transmission of panic disorder (100).

Twin studies have found the various anxiety disorders to have shared familial associations (83, 89). For example, first-degree relatives of patients with panic disorder not only have an increased likelihood of panic disorder but also of phobic disorders (60, 100).

Specific phobias have the least demonstrated heritability of the phobic disorders, estimated at 20%–40% (94). Social phobia is intermediate between agoraphobia and specific phobias in genetic heritability (60).

Panic disorder and major depressive disorder appear to overlap in family transmission (83), which might suggest a common diathesis (83). However, patients with primary major depression alone have been found to have increased rates of major depressive disorder but not panic disorder among their relatives; conversely, patients with primary panic disorder and secondary depression have increased rates of panic disorder but not major depressive disorder among family members (23). These findings contradict notions that panic disorder and major depressive disorder may represent an epiphenomenon or a complication of one another, or that comorbid major depressive disorder and panic disorder may constitute a distinct syndrome transmitted in families.

Patients with panic disorder and agoraphobia have higher rates of alcohol use disorders among their first-degree family members compared to first-degree family members of controls (34, 84). These findings suggest a familial association between panic disorder and alcohol use disorders.

Research on the genetics of anxiety disorders has lagged behind genetic research on other psychiatric disorders (87). Large-scale genome-wide association studies have only begun to identify common variant associations (87). No robust genetic findings have emerged for anxiety disorders to date (83).

DIFFERENTIAL DIAGNOSIS

The diagnosis of panic disorder requires the exclusion of medical conditions that give rise to similar symptoms. Medical illnesses that produce symptoms resembling those of panic disorder include cardiac arrhythmias (especially paroxysmal atrial tachycardia), angina, chronic obstructive pulmonary disease, asthma, hyperthyroidism, and pheochromocytoma (3, 24, 56). Symptoms such as palpitations and chest pain occurring as part of panic disorder are not easily differentiated from manifestations of a primary cardiac disorder (24).

Many individuals with panic disorder seek treatment first in the emergency department or other medical setting (27, 49). Unfortunately, clinicians not familiar with panic disorder as a specific diagnostic entity may mistakenly attribute the symptoms to a physical condition. Among patients presenting to emergency rooms with chest pain, 94% of panic disorder may go unrecognized in this setting (49).

Individuals reporting a history of chest pain have four times the prevalence of panic disorder as other people (37). The presence of panic disorder, however, does not rule out cardiac disease: 21% of panic disorder patients admitted to a coronary care unit had medical findings, including myocardial infarction (85). Of acute coronary care inpatients with negative cardiac workups, more than half were found to have panic disorder (85). Five variables have been identified in association with panic disorder diagnosed among patients presenting to a hospital emergency department with chest pain: 1) absence of coronary artery disease, 2) atypical quality of chest pain, 3) female sex, 4) younger age, and 5) report of high levels of anxiety (37).

Panic and gastrointestinal symptoms commonly co-occur (68, 86). As many as one-third or more of patients with irritable bowel syndrome have been identified to have somatization disorder (68, 72), a disorder characterized by complaints of multiple medically unexplained symptoms, both physical and psychological, across multiple organ systems. Somatization disorder may thus account for the apparent association of panic disorder with irritable bowel syndrome (71).

How far to pursue a physical explanation for symptoms that may represent panic disorder depends on clinical judgment, but considerable resources are often invested in tests and consultations. The healthcare costs for panic disorder patients with medical illness have been calculated to be approximately twice the costs for patients with medical illness alone (53). There is evidence that identifying and addressing the panic disorder with appropriate treatment significantly improves outcomes, and also presumably reduces medical care costs (53).

Panic attacks can occur as part of any psychiatric illness. Panic attacks commonly occur in patients with major depressive disorder, obsessional illness, phobic disorder, somatization disorder, and alcoholism. Similarly, phobic symptoms are not confined to phobic disorders and may accompany many other psychiatric disorders.

The mistake probably made most often in the evaluation of anxiety symptoms is that of overlooking major depressive disorder. Among other factors, a family history of mood disorder should alert one to the possibility that a patient with an anxiety symptom may have major depressive disorder with anxious features rather than an anxiety disorder. Also, panic symptoms beginning for the first time after the age of 40 are commonly part of a depressive syndrome rather than a manifestation of panic disorder. Among patients with well-documented histories of phobic disorder or panic disorder, the development of major depressive episodes with the full range of mood symptoms is common, and these episodes may be indistinguishable from major depressive disorder except for the prior history of significant phobic or panic symptoms. Conversely, major depressive episodes not uncommonly present with panic attacks or phobic qualities, such as fearfulness of social situations or disease as part of the episode, potentially distracting the clinician from appreciating the major depressive disorder.

Most somatization disorder patients acknowledge significant anxiety. Somatization disorder involves a broad range of medical complaints with frequent hospitalizations and operations not typical of panic and phobic disorders. Panic and phobic disorder patients do not undergo hospitalization and surgery more frequently than other individuals. The main differentiating feature is that panic and phobic disorders are not characterized by dramatic and medically unexplained complaints in nearly *every* area of the review of symptoms, as is the case in somatization disorder. Further, sexual and menstrual complaints and conversion symptoms (unexplained neurological complaints), common in somatization disorder, are not frequently encountered among patients with panic or phobic disorders.

Panic disorder, phobic disorder, and obsessive-compulsive disorder may be difficult to distinguish from one another. All three conditions begin early in life and have a chronic but sometimes fluctuating course, and they often co-occur within single patients. The distinction between phobic and panic disorder depends on whether phobias dominate the clinical picture. The most conspicuous feature of panic disorder is anxiety attacks unrelated to external situations in which the subjective experience of fear is accompanied by cardiorespiratory symptoms. Phobias and panic attacks also frequently occur as part of obsessive-compulsive disorder. Obsessive-compulsive disorder involves distinctive obsessional symptoms and checking and compulsive rituals such as counting that are not a part of phobic or panic disorders. Although ruminations and compulsions may occur in mild or incomplete forms among patients with panic disorder, they are not characteristically severe.

Panic disorder can be mistaken for posttraumatic stress disorder. Panic disorder is not among the conditions most likely to be precipitated by exposure to a traumatic event (73). In one series (67), patients who had experienced a life-threatening accident subsequently experienced a long period (6 months to 3 years) of free-floating anxiety, muscular tension, irritability, impaired concentration, repetitive nightmares of the accident, and social withdrawal. None of the patients, however, had cardiorespiratory or other autonomic symptoms, the hallmark of typical panic disorder.

Excessive worriers sometimes receive a diagnosis of generalized anxiety disorder. Despite the term, generalized anxiety disorder often involves anxiety about specific events such as work or school disturbance. The person is restless, easily tired, irritable, and may have trouble concentrating as well as sleep difficulty. Fears (which are usually chronic) in generalized anxiety disorder are distinguishable from phobia by their shifting focus and absence of avoidance behavior. Although generalized anxiety disorder has been found to afflict about 6% of the population at some time during their lives (44), the validity and reliability of the diagnosis remain questionable.

Panic attacks occasionally occur in patients with schizophrenia, especially during exacerbations of psychosis. When phobic-like symptoms occur in schizophrenia, they are usually bizarre and unaccompanied by insight.

CLINICAL MANAGEMENT

Psychiatric referral is rarely necessary for panic disorder if the patient's physician has diagnosed the disorder correctly, understands its natural history, and is willing to discuss the disorder with the patient. Telling the patient that there is nothing wrong physically is usually not enough. Some patients resent the implication that their symptoms might be "psychological." Others continue to believe that they have a serious illness. The physician should agree that something is wrong and should describe the syndrome in lay terms. Many patients are relieved by such an explanation and thereby become receptive to further reassurance.

As noted earlier, some patients with gastrointestinal or musculoskeletal complaints meet the criteria for panic disorder. In these cases, once sufficient medical evaluation has been completed, treatment should focus primarily on the basic underlying disorder—the panic disorder—so that the presenting physical complaints are viewed in this context and treated as conservatively as possible. In medical settings, clinicians should conduct a complete psychiatric evaluation to determine whether the patient has an anxiety disorder or whether the anxiety symptoms are a manifestation of another psychiatric disorder, such as major depressive disorder or somatization disorder.

In the 1960s, Klein and colleagues in New York (46) and Marks and colleagues in England (56) found that antidepressants prevented panic attacks (74). The New York group focused on the tricyclic antidepressant (TCA) imipramine and the British group on monoamine oxidase inhibitors (MAOIs). Both types of drugs apparently had similar efficacy in preventing panic attacks, although there was some disagreement about the relief persisting after the drugs were discontinued and also about the role of supportive or behavioral therapy in augmenting the effects of the drugs.

The more newly developed SSRIs (e.g., fluoxetine, paroxetine) are equally effective, better tolerated, and safer than TCAs and MAOIs for the treatment of anxiety disorders (21, 48). There is some evidence that serotonin-norepinephrine reuptake inhibitor (SNRI) (e.g., venlafaxine) antidepressants and other "newer generation" antidepressants (e.g., mirtazapine) may be beneficial for patients not responding to SSRI treatment (48) and may have more favorable side-effect profiles (21, 48). Pharmacotherapy with SSRIs and SNRIs has become standard treatment for panic disorder and agoraphobia (21, 48). The main side effects of the newer antidepressant medications include gastrointestinal symptoms, headache, and sedation, particularly early in treatment, as well as sexual dysfunction and increased anxiety. These side effects, however, can be managed by medication choice, careful advancement of dosage, and attention to the patient (7). Increased anxiety that may occur in the early weeks of treatment with antidepressant medications can be managed by temporary addition of a benzodiazepine during the initial phase of treatment (7).

Benzodiazepines have been found to be as effective as antidepressants in the treatment of anxiety disorders (7, 48, 75, 77). There is some indication that benzodiazepines are even more effective than antidepressants at relieving the somatic symptoms of anxiety disorders, but less effective at relieving the psychological symptoms (21). The onset of action is faster for benzodiazepines than for antidepressants, with effectiveness even on the first dose (48, 77). Adverse effects of benzodiazepines include drowsiness, ataxia, and cognitive and motor impairment (77). Benzodiazepines are better tolerated than antidepressants and may thus have lower likelihood of treatment dropout (7). Potential for abuse and dependence and problems of tolerance limit the utility of benzodiazepines as first-line agents and make them a better short-term than long-term solution (7, 21, 48, 77). Unlike antidepressants, benzodiazepines are not helpful for the co-morbid major depression that commonly accompanies panic disorder (7).

There has been much speculation about the action of antidepressant and benzodiazepine drugs in reducing anxiety and preventing panic attacks. Recent studies have indicated that antidepressants appear to prevent panic attacks by decreasing brain norepinephrine turnover and activating serotonin systems (7), and that benzodiazepines exert their anxiolytic effects through potentiating effects of the inhibitory neurotransmitter GABA (48).

Anticonvulsant medications may also reduce anxiety symptoms through reduction of limbic excitability, mediated through GABA receptors (30). Although some of these agents represent potentially promising treatments (21, 48, 77), research on these agents for treatment of anxiety disorders has been at best equivocal, thus these agents are not considered first-line treatments (7, 30).

Before the current emphasis on pharmacotherapy, the most popular approach to the treatment of specific and social phobias involved behavioral techniques based on learning theory, such as "systematic desensitization," introduced by Wolpe (101). This method consists of training patients to relax and then gradually exposing them to increasingly intensive versions of the phobic stimulus, which theoretically cancels the sensation of fear if the stimulus is not overwhelming. Exposure-based therapies used today have roots in classic desensitization paradigms. These therapies have historically invoked stimuli generated by the patient's imagination, but in recent applications, virtual reality technology provides real-seeming but imaginary scenes of phobic situations germane to patients' fears.

The main psychological treatments for panic and phobic disorders in current use involve cognitive-behavioral and cognitive therapies, exposure therapy, and response-prevention therapies (12). Elements fundamental to cognitive-behavioral therapy are exposure, reduction of safety-seeking behaviors, attention focus modification, and cognitive restructuring (59). The main drawback to psychotherapies for panic and phobic disorders is the time commitment and effort required of the patient (11). Prolonged and expensive forms of psychotherapy are rarely indicated.

A review of psychotherapeutic interventions for social phobia found cognitive and behavioral interventions superior to wait-list controls and supportive therapy (81). Comparison studies of cognitive-behavioral therapy and pharmacotherapy, however, have failed to demonstrate any consistent advantage of combining psychotherapy and pharmacotherapy over either intervention alone for phobic and panic disorders (12).

Regardless of the theoretical orientation of the treating clinician, it is generally agreed that at some point the patient must confront the feared situation. Most treatments—medications, psychotherapy, and behavior modification techniques—are designed to reduce panic and anxiety to the extent that the patient can tolerate exposure to his or her anxieties.

REFERENCES

1. American Psychiatric Association. *Diagnostic and Statistical Manual of Mental Disorders*, 3rd edition. Washington, DC: Author, 1980.
2. American Psychiatric Association. *Diagnostic and Statistical Manual of Mental Disorders*, 3rd revised edition. Washington, DC: Author, 1987.
3. American Psychiatric Association. *Diagnostic and Statistical Manual for Mental Disorders*, 5th edition. Washington, DC: Author, 2013.
4. Asher, M., Asnaani, A., and Aderka, I. M. Gender differences in social anxiety disorder: a review. Clin. Psychol. Rev., *56*:1–12, 2017.
5. Baillie, A. J., and Rapee, R. M. Panic attacks as risk markers for mental disorders. Soc. Psychiatry Psychiatr. Epidemiol., *40*:240–244, 2005.
6. Bandelow, B., and Michaelis, S. Epidemiology of anxiety disorders in the 21st century. Dialogues Clin. Neurosci., *17*:327–335, 2015.
7. Batelaan, N. M., van Balkom, A. J., and Stein, D. J. Evidence-based pharmacotherapy of panic disorder: an update. Int. J. Neuropsychopharmacol., *15*:403–415, 2012.
8. Battaglia, M., Bertella, S., Bajo, S., Binaghi, F., and Bellodi, L. Anticipation of age at onset in panic disorder. Am. J. Psychiatry, *155*:590–595, 1998.
9. Beard, G. M. Neurasthenia or nervous exhaustion. Boston Med. Surg. J., *3*:217, 1869.
10. Beesdo, K., Knappe, S., and Pine, D. S. Anxiety and anxiety disorders in children and adolescents: developmental issues and implications for DSM-V. Psychiatr. Clin. North Am., *32*:483–524, 2009.
11. Bennett, J. A., Moioffer, M., Stanton, S. P., Dwight, M., and Keck, P. E., Jr. A risk-benefit assessment of pharmacological treatments for panic disorder. Drug Safety, *18*:419–430, 1998.
12. Black, D. W. Efficacy of combined pharmacotherapy and psychotherapy versus monotherapy in the treatment of anxiety disorders. CNS Spectr., *11*:29–33, 2006.
13. Bruce, S. E., Yonkers, K. A., Otto, M. W., Eisen, J. L., Weisberg, R. B., Pagano, M., Shea, M. T., and Keller, M. B. Influence of psychiatric comorbidity on recovery and recurrence in generalized anxiety disorder, social phobia, and panic disorder: a 12-year prospective study. Am. J. Psychiatry, *162*:1179–1187, 2005.
14. Buskila, D., and Cohen, H. Comorbidity of fibromyalgia and psychiatric disorders. Curr. Pain Headache Rep., *11*:333–338, 2007.
15. Chatel, J. C., and Peele, R. A centennial review of neurasthenia. Am. J. Psychiatry, *126*:1404–1413, 1970.
16. Cohen, M., and White, P. Life situations, emotions, and neurocirculatory asthenia (anxiety neurosis, neurasthenia, effort syndrome). Res. Publ. Assoc. Res. Nerv. Ment. Dis., *29*:832–869, 1949.
17. Cosci, F., Schruers, K. R., Abrams, K., and Griez, E. J. Alcohol use disorders and panic disorder: a review of the evidence of a direct relationship. J. Clin. Psychiatry, *68*:874–880, 2007.
18. Cougle, J. R., Timpano, K. R., Sachs-Ericsson, N., Keough, M. E., and Riccardi, C. J. Examining the unique relationships between anxiety disorders and childhood

physical and sexual abuse in the National Comorbidity Survey–Replication. Psychiatry Res., 177:150–155, 2010.

19. Craske, M. G., Stein, M. B., Eley, T. C., Milad, M. R., Holmes, A., Rapee, R. M., and Wittchen, H. U. Anxiety disorders. Nat. Rev. Dis. Primers, 3:17024, 2017.

20. Dalessio, D. J. Hyperventilation: the vapors, effort syndrome, neurasthenia. JAMA, 239:1401–1402, 1978.

21. Dell'Osso, B., Buoli, M., Baldwin, D. S., and Altamura, A. C. Serotonin norepinephrine reuptake inhibitors (SNRIs) in anxiety disorders: a comprehensive review of their clinical efficacy. Hum. Psychopharmacol., 25:17–29, 2010.

22. Dieterich, M., Staab, J. P., and Brandt, T. Functional (psychogenic) dizziness. Handb. Clin. Neurol., 139:447–468, 2016.

23. Dindo, L., and Coryell, W. Comorbid major depression and panic disorder: significance of temporal sequencing to familial transmission. J. Affect. Dis., 82:119–123, 2004.

24. Domschke, K., Stevens, S., Pfleiderer, B., and Gerlach, A. L. Interoceptive sensitivity in anxiety and anxiety disorders: an overview and integration of neurobiological findings. Clin. Psychol. Rev., 30:1–11, 2010.

25. Eaton, W. W., Dryman, A., and Weissman, M. M. Panic and phobia. In *Psychiatric Disorders in America: The Epidemiologic Catchment Area Study*, Robins, L. N., Regier, D. A. (eds.). New York: The Free Press, pp. 155–179, 1991.

26. Eaton, W. W., Kessler, R. C., Wittchen, H. U., and Magee, W. J. Panic and panic disorder in the United States. Am. J. Psychiatry, 151:413–420, 1994.

27. Eken, C., Oktay, C., Bacanli, A., Gulen, B., Koparan, C., Ugras, S. S., and Cete, Y. Anxiety and depressive disorders in patients presenting with chest pain to the emergency department: a comparison between cardiac and non-cardiac origin. J. Emerg. Med., 39:144–150, 2010.

28. Engel, K., Bandelow, B., Gruber, O., and Wedekind, D. Neuroimaging in anxiety disorders. J. Neural Transm. (Vienna), 116:703–716, 2009.

29. Fadgyas-Stanculete, M., Buga, A. M., Popa-Wagner, A., and Dumitrascu, D. L. The relationship between irritable bowel syndrome and psychiatric disorders: from molecular changes to clinical manifestations. J. Mol. Psychiatry, 2:4, 2014.

30. Freire, R. C., Hallak, J. E., Crippa, J. A., and Nardi, A. E. New treatment options for panic disorder: clinical trials from 2000 to 2010. Expert Opin. Pharmacother., 12:1419–1428, 2011.

31. Furmark, T. Social phobia: overview of community surveys. Acta Psychiatr. Scand., 105:84–93, 2002.

32. Goodwin, D. W. *Phobia: The Facts*. London: Oxford University Press, 1983.

33. Goodwin, R. D., Fergusson, D. M., and Horwood, L. J. Childhood abuse and familial violence and the risk of panic attacks and panic disorder in young adulthood. Psychol. Med., 35:881–890, 2005.

34. Goodwin, R. D., Lipsitz, J. D., Chapman, T. F., Mannuzza, S., Klein, D. F., and Fyer, A. J. Alcohol use disorders in relatives of patients with panic disorder. Compr. Psychiatry, 47:88–90, 2006.

35. Helzer, J. E., Burnam, A., and McEvoy, L. T. Alcohol abuse and dependence. In *Psychiatric Disorders in America: The Epidemiologic Catchment Area Study*, Robins, L. N., Regier, D. A. (eds.). New York: The Free Press, pp. 81–115, 1991.

36. Horn, P. J., and Wuyek, L. A. Anxiety disorders as a risk factor for subsequent depression. Int. J. Psychiatry Clin. Pract., 14:244–247, 2010.

37. Huffman, J. C., and Pollack, M. H. Predicting panic disorder among patients with chest pain: an analysis of the literature. Psychosomatics, 44:222–236, 2003.

38. Hybels, C. F., Blazer, D. G., and Kaplan, B. H. Social and personal resources and the prevalence of phobic disorder in a community population. Psychol. Med., 30:705–716, 2000.

39. Janssens, K. A., Zijlema, W. L., Joustra, M. L., and Rosmalen, J. G. Mood and anxiety disorders in chronic fatigue syndrome, fibromyalgia, and irritable bowel syndrome: results from the LifeLines Cohort Study. Psychosom. Med., 77:449–457, 2015.

40. Kawakami, N., Abdulghani, E. A., Alonso, J., Bromet, E. J., Bruffaerts, R., Caldas-de-Almeida, J. M., Chiu, W. T., de Girolamo, G., de Graaf, R., Fayyad, J., Ferry, F., Florescu, S., Gureje, O., Hu, C., Lakoma, M. D., Leblanc, W., Lee, S., Levinson, D., Malhotra, S., Matschinger, H., Medina-Mora, M. E., Nakamura, Y., Oakley Browne, M. A., Okoliyski, M., Posada-Villa, J., Sampson, N. A., Viana, M. C., and Kessler, R. C. Early-life mental disorders and adult household income in the World Mental Health Surveys. Biol. Psychiatry, 72:228–237, 2012.

41. Kessler, R. C. The impairments caused by social phobia in the general population: implications for intervention. Acta Psychiatr. Scand. Suppl., 417:19–27, 2003.

42. Kessler, R. C., Chiu, W. T., Demler, O., Merikangas, K. R., and Walters, E. E. Prevalence, severity, and comorbidity of 12-month DSM-IV disorders in the National Comorbidity Survey Replication. Arch. Gen. Psychiatry, 62:617–627, 2005.

43. Kessler, R. C., McGonagle, K. A., Zhao, S., Nelson, C. B., Hughes, M., Eshleman, S., Wittchen, H. U., and Kendler, K. S. Lifetime and 12-month prevalence of DSM-III-R psychiatric disorders in the United States. Results from the National Comorbidity Survey. Arch. Gen. Psychiatry, 51:8–19, 1994.

44. Kessler, R. C., Petukhova, M., Sampson, N. A., Zaslavsky, A. M., and Wittchen, H.-U. Twelve-month and lifetime prevalence and lifetime morbid risk of anxiety and mood disorders in the United States. Int. J. Methods Psychiatr. Res., 21:169–184, 2012.

45. King-Kallimanis, B., Gum, A. M., and Kohn, R. Comorbidity of depressive and anxiety disorders for older Americans in the National Comorbidity Survey-Replication. Am. J. Geriatr. Psychiatry, 17:782–792, 2009.

46. Klein, D. F. Importance of psychiatric diagnosis in prediction of clinical drug effects. Arch. Gen. Psychiatry, 16:118–126, 1967.

47. Klein, D. F., Zitrin, C. M., Woerner, M. G., and Ross, D. C. Treatment of phobias. II. Behavior therapy and supportive psychotherapy: are there any specific ingredients? Arch. Gen. Psychiatry, 40:139–145, 1983.

48. Koen, N., and Stein, D. J. Pharmacotherapy of anxiety disorders: a critical review. Dialogues Clin. Neurosci., 13:423–437, 2011.

49. Kontos, M. C., Diercks, D. B., and Kirk, J. D. Emergency department and office-based evaluation of patients with chest pain. Mayo Clin. Proc., 85:284–299, 2010.

50. Lai, H. M., Cleary, M., Sitharthan, T., and Hunt, G. E. Prevalence of comorbid substance use, anxiety and mood disorders in epidemiological surveys, 1990-2014: a systematic review and meta-analysis. Drug Alcohol Depend., 154:1–13, 2015.

51. Lamers, F., van Oppen, P., Comijs, H. C., Smit, J. H., Spinhoven, P., van Balkom, A. J., Nolen, W. A., Zitman, F. G., Beekman, A. T., and Penninx, B. W. Comorbidity patterns of anxiety and depressive disorders in a large cohort study: the Netherlands Study of Depression and Anxiety (NESDA). J. Clin. Psychiatry, 72:341–348, 2011.

52. Lang, P. J. Fear reduction and fear behavior. "Problems in treating a construct". Chicago: 3rd Conference on Research in Psychotherapy, June, 1966.

53. Livermore, N., Sharpe, L., and McKenzie, D. Prevention of panic attacks and panic disorder in COPD. Eur. Respir. J., 35:557–563, 2010.

54. Lydiard, R. B. Increased prevalence of functional gastrointestinal disorders in panic disorder: clinical and theoretical implications. CNS Spectr., *10*:899–908, 2005.
55. Macalpine, I. Syphilophobia; a psychiatric study. Br. J. Vener. Dis., *33*:92–99, 1957.
56. Marks, I., and Lader, M. Anxiety states (anxiety neurosis): a review. J. Nerv. Ment. Dis., *156*:3–18, 1973.
57. Marks, I. M. *Fears and Phobias*. New York: Academic Press, 1969.
58. Marks, I. M. The classification of phobic disorders. Br. J. Psychiatry, *116*:377–386, 1970.
59. Marom, S., and Hermesh, H. Cognitive behavior therapy (CBT) in anxiety disorders. Isr. J. Psychiatry Relat. Sci., *40*:135–144, 2003.
60. Martin, E. I., Ressler, K. J., Binder, E., and Nemeroff, C. B. The neurobiology of anxiety disorders: brain imaging, genetics, and psychoneuroendocrinology. Clin. Lab. Med., *30*:865–891, 2010.
61. Massion, A. O., Dyck, I. R., Shea, M. T., Phillips, K. A., Warshaw, M. G., and Keller, M. B. Personality disorders and time to remission in generalized anxiety disorder, social phobia, and panic disorder. Arch. Gen. Psychiatry, *59*:434–440, 2002.
62. McLean, C. P., Asnaani, A., Litz, B. T., and Hofmann, S. G. Gender differences in anxiety disorders: prevalence, course of illness, comorbidity and burden of illness. J. Psychiatr. Res., *45*:1027–1035, 2011.
63. Metzler, D. H., Mahoney, D., and Freedy, J. R. Anxiety disorders in primary care. Prim. Care, *43*:245–261, 2016.
64. Meuret, A. E., Rosenfield, D., Hofmann, S. G., Suvak, M. K., and Roth, W. T. Changes in respiration mediate changes in fear of bodily sensations in panic disorder. J. Psychiatr. Res., *43*:634–641, 2009.
65. Meuret, A. E., Seidel, A., Rosenfield, B., Hofmann, S. G., and Rosenfield, D. Does fear reactivity during exposure predict panic symptom reduction? J. Consult. Clin. Psychol., *80*:773–785, 2012.
66. Miller, A., North, C. S., Clouse, R. E., Alpers, D. H., and Wetzel, R. D. Irritable bowel syndrome, psychiatric illness, personality, and abuse: is somatization disorder the missing link? Ann. Clin. Psychiatry, *13*:25–30, 2001.
67. Modlin, H. C. Postaccident anxiety syndrome: psychosocial aspects. Am. J. Psychiatry, *123*:1008–1012, 2003.
68. Mykletun, A., Jacka, F., Williams, L., Pasco, J., Henry, M., Nicholson, G. C., Kotowicz, M. A., and Berk, M. Prevalence of mood and anxiety disorder in self reported irritable bowel syndrome (IBS). An epidemiological population based study of women. BMC Gastroenterol., *10*:88, 2010.
69. Nemiah, J. C. Phobic disorders (phobic neuroses). In *Comprehensive Textbook of Psychiatry*, fourth edition, Kaplan, H. I., Sadock, B. J. (eds.). Baltimore: Williams and Wilkins, 1985.
70. Ninan, P. T., and Dunlop, B. W. Neurobiology and etiology of panic disorder. J. Clin. Psychiatry, *66(Suppl 4)*:3–7, 2005.
71. North, C. S. The classification of hysteria and related disorders: historical and phenomenological considerations. Behav. Sci. (Basel), *5*:496–517, 2015.
72. North, C. S., Downs, D., Clouse, R. E., Alrakawi, A., Dokucu, M. E., Cox, J., Spitznagel, E. L., and Alpers, D. H. The presentation of irritable bowel syndrome in the context of somatization disorder. Clin. Gastroenterol. Hepatol., *2*:787–795, 2004.
73. North, C. S., and Pfefferbaum, B. Mental health response to community disasters: a systematic review. JAMA, *310*:507–518, 2013.

74. Noyes, R., Jr., and Perry, P. Maintenance treatment with antidepressants in panic disorder. J. Clin. Psychiatry, *51(Suppl A)*:24–30, 1990.

75. Offidani, E., Guidi, J., Tomba, E., and Fava, G. A. Efficacy and tolerability of benzodiazepines versus antidepressants in anxiety disorders: a systematic review and meta-analysis. Psychother. Psychosom., *82*:355–362, 2013.

76. Penninx, B. W., Nolen, W. A., Lamers, F., Zitman, F. G., Smit, J. H., Spinhoven, P., Cuijpers, P., de Jong, P. J., van Marwijk, H. W., van der Meer, K., Verhaak, P., Laurant, M. G., de Graaf, R., Hoogendijk, W. J., van der Wee, N., Ormel, J., van Dyck, R., and Beekman, A. T. Two-year course of depressive and anxiety disorders: results from the Netherlands Study of Depression and Anxiety (NESDA). J. Affect. Disord., *133*:76–85, 2011.

77. Perna, G., Alciati, A., Riva, A., Micieli, W., and Caldirola, D. Long-term pharmacological treatments of anxiety disorders: an updated systematic review. Curr. Psychiatry Rep., *18*:23, 2016.

78. Ramsawh, H. J., Weisberg, R. B., Dyck, I., Stout, R., and Keller, M. B. Age of onset, clinical characteristics, and 15-year course of anxiety disorders in a prospective, longitudinal, observational study. J. Affect. Disord., *132*:260–264, 2011.

79. Robins, L. N., Helzer, J. E., Weissman, M. M., Orvaschel, H., Gruenberg, E., Burke, J. D., and Regier, D. A. Lifetime prevalence of specific psychiatric disorders in three sites. Arch. Gen. Psychiatry, *41*:949–958, 1984.

80. Robins, L. N., Locke, B. Z., and Regier, D. A. An overview of psychiatric disorders in America. In *Psychiatric Disorders in America: The Epidemiologic Catchment Area Study*, Robins, L. N., Regier, D. A. (eds.). New York: The Free Press, pp. 328–386, 1991.

81. Rowa, K., and Antony, M. M. Psychological treatments for social phobia. Can. J. Psychiatry, *50*:308–316, 2005.

82. Saeed, M. S., Ikram, M. A., Hofman, A., and Tiemeier, H. Anxiety does not predict mortality. A population-based study. World Psychiatry, *14*:103–104, 2015.

83. Schumacher, J., Kristensen, A. S., Wendland, J. R., Nothen, M. M., Mors, O., and McMahon, F. J. The genetics of panic disorder. J. Med. Genet., *48*:361–368, 2011.

84. Shih, R. A., Belmonte, P. L., and Zandi, P. P. A review of the evidence from family, twin and adoption studies for a genetic contribution to adult psychiatric disorders. Int. Rev. Psychiatry, *16*:260–283, 2004.

85. Simon, N. M., and Fischmann, D. The implications of medical and psychiatric comorbidity with panic disorder. J. Clin. Psychiatry, *66(Suppl 4)*:8–15, 2005.

86. Singh, P., Agnihotri, A., Pathak, M. K., Shirazi, A., Tiwari, R. P., Sreenivas, V., Sagar, R., and Makharia, G. K. Psychiatric, somatic and other functional gastrointestinal disorders in patients with irritable bowel syndrome at a tertiary care center. J. Neurogastroenterol. Motil., *18*:324–331, 2012.

87. Smith, J. P., and Randall, C. L. Anxiety and alcohol use disorders: comorbidity and treatment considerations. Alcohol Res., *34*:414–431, 2012.

88. Smitherman, T. A., Kolivas, E. D., and Bailey, J. R. Panic disorder and migraine: comorbidity, mechanisms, and clinical implications. Headache, *53*:23–45, 2013.

89. Smoller, J. W. The genetics of stress-related disorders: PTSD, depression, and anxiety disorders. Neuropsychopharmacology, *41*:297–319, 2016.

90. Soares-Filho, G. L., Arias-Carrion, O., Santulli, G., Silva, A. C., Machado, S., Valenca, A. M., and Nardi, A. E. Chest pain, panic disorder and coronary artery disease: a systematic review. CNS Neurol. Disord. Drug Targets, *13*:992–1001, 2014.

91. Stein, D. J. Agoraphobia and panic disorder: options for ICD-11. World Psychiatry, *11*:89–93, 2012.

92. Stinson, F. S., Dawson, D. A., Patricia, C. S., Smith, S., Goldstein, R. B., June, R. W., and Grant, B. F. The epidemiology of DSM-IV specific phobia in the USA: results from the National Epidemiologic Survey on Alcohol and Related Conditions. Psychol. Med., 37:1047–1059, 2007.

93. Thibodeau, M. A., Welch, P. G., Sareen, J., and Asmundson, G. J. Anxiety disorders are independently associated with suicide ideation and attempts: propensity score matching in two epidemiological samples. Depress. Anxiety, 30:947–954, 2013.

94. Van Houtem, C. M., Laine, M. L., Boomsma, D. I., Ligthart, L., van Wijk, A. J., and de Jongh, A. A review and meta-analysis of the heritability of specific phobia subtypes and corresponding fears. J. Anxiety Disord., 27:379–388, 2013.

95. Vickers, K., Jafarpour, S., Mofidi, A., Rafat, B., and Woznica, A. The 35% carbon dioxide test in stress and panic research: overview of effects and integration of findings. Clin. Psychol. Rev., 32:153–164, 2012.

96. Vreeburg, S. A., Zitman, F. G., van, P. J., DeRijk, R. H., Verhagen, J. C., van, D. R., Hoogendijk, W. J., Smit, J. H., and Penninx, B. W. Salivary cortisol levels in persons with and without different anxiety disorders. Psychosom. Med., 72:340–347, 2010.

97. Weissman, M. M., Klerman, G. L., Markowitz, J. S., and Ouellette, R. Suicidal ideation and suicide attempts in panic disorder and attacks. N. Engl. J. Med., 321:1209–1214, 1989.

98. Westphal, C. Agoraphobie: eine neuropathische Erscheinuung. Arch. Psychiatr. Nervenkr., 3:138–221, 1871.

99. Wittchen, H. U., and Fehm, L. Epidemiology and natural course of social fears and social phobia. Acta Psychiatr. Scand. Suppl., 417:4–18, 2003.

100. Wittchen, H. U., Gloster, A. T., Beesdo-Baum, K., Fava, G. A., and Craske, M. G. Agoraphobia: a review of the diagnostic classificatory position and criteria. Depress. Anxiety, 27:113–133, 2010.

101. Wolpe, J. *Psychotherapy by Reciprocal Inhibition*. Stanford, CA: Stanford University Press, 1958.

102. Woodberry, P. E. ed. *The Complete Poetical Works of Shelley*. Boston: Houghton, Mifflin, 1901.

103. Yonkers, K. A., Bruce, S. E., Dyck, I. R., and Keller, M. B. Chronicity, relapse, and illness—course of panic disorder, social phobia, and generalized anxiety disorder: findings in men and women from 8 years of follow-up. Depress. Anxiety, 17:173–179, 2003.

104. Zemishlany, Z., and Weizman, A. The impact of mental illness on sexual dysfunction. Adv. Psychosom. Med., 29:89–106, 2008.

105. Zimmerman, M., and Mattia, J. I. Axis I diagnostic comorbidity and borderline personality disorder. Compr. Psychiatry, 40:245–252, 1999.

CHAPTER 5

✦

Posttraumatic Stress Disorder

Posttraumatic stress disorder (PTSD) is a disorder that can emerge after exposure to an extreme traumatic stressor involving actual or threatened death or serious injury. It should not be assumed that the inclusion of PTSD in this text necessarily signifies established validity of this disorder. Recent comprehensive reviews of PTSD addressing its diagnostic validity have found that, although considerable progress has been accomplished toward this end, further research is needed (143, 166). Validation of diagnostic criteria for PTSD, in a process outlined several years ago by Robins and Guze (189), has still not documented several elements: that the symptoms correlate more with each other than with other disorders, that the disorder is distinguishable from other disorders (especially anxiety and depressive disorders), and that the disorder runs in families (143, 166, 190, 193, 210). The criteria tested in the *DSM-5* field trials (184), however, were demonstrated to have good interrater reliability (kappa = .69). Even though PTSD has not been demonstrated to represent a unified construct such as that established for other validated psychiatric disorders identified in this text, the empirically based references in this chapter testify to the developing knowledge base for PTSD.

PTSD is an unusual diagnosis among psychiatric disorders, owing to the conditional nature of this diagnosis that requires exposure to a traumatic event for consideration of this diagnosis. Individuals who have not been exposed to a traumatic event cannot meet criteria for PTSD. This unusual feature of the definition of PTSD has created difficulties in the application of this diagnosis in both clinical and research settings.

To qualify as "traumatic," a stressful event must pose a *threat to life or limb*. DSM-5 (9) carefully stipulates that the threat to life or limb must be immediate and result from accidental or unnatural causes. Therefore, a diagnosis of cancer that may increase risk for death months or years in the future and sudden, unexpected deaths resulting from natural causes such as a heart attack or a stroke do not qualify as trauma for consideration of a diagnosis of PTSD. Normal childbirth does not qualify. Exceptional medical incidents that would qualify under the definition of trauma, according to *DSM-5* criteria, include anaphylactic shock, waking during surgery, and life-threatening hemorrhage in one's child. Incidents such as stepping on an improvised explosive device in a combat zone, narrowly escaping death in a tornado, exposure to direct nuclear fallout of an atomic bomb, being shot or stabbed, and injury in a severe motor vehicle crash are classic qualifying types of trauma in Criterion A for the diagnosis of PTSD.

Stressful events not posing a threat to life or limb, such as being fired or being confronted with divorce proceedings, would not qualify as traumatic merely on the basis of associated emotional distress, if tangible physical danger is not involved (9). In short, even though all traumatic events can be classified under a larger category of stressful events, not all stressful events can be classified as traumatic.

The occurrence of a traumatic event is not sufficient for consideration of a diagnosis of PTSD (9). The individual must also have a qualifying exposure to the traumatic event. If a traumatic event occurs in Oregon, for example, people who were in Florida at the time would not be directly exposed to it. To count toward the diagnosis, the traumatic event must be experienced through a qualifying exposure; it may be experienced directly, personally witnessed, or experienced indirectly through the exposure of a loved one to a traumatic event. Examples of directly experienced traumatic events are exposure to the physical dangers of military combat, being physically attacked or sexually assaulted, being injured in a bad traffic accident, or being endangered in a disaster such as a tornado or a plane crash. Examples of witnessed events are seeing people injured or killed in a bad traffic accident, seeing someone murdered, or unexpectedly discovering a dead body. Witnessed exposures limited to electronic media (such as seeing live media coverage of strangers who were victims in the September 11, 2001 attacks) do not qualify. Indirect exposure to trauma through the direct experience of loved ones could occur with learning of the violent or accidental death or life-threatening experience of a close family member, such as an assault, homicide, suicide, or a lethal accident. *DSM-5* added a fourth type of qualifying exposure involving repeated or extreme exposure to aversive details of trauma, such as through work-related exposures of first responders and forensic workers. Only repeated or extreme work-related exposures count as exposures through electronic media.

Criterion A (the "trauma criterion") (9) is the entry point for consideration of diagnostic candidacy for PTSD (166). This criterion has not been addressed appropriately in claims of PTSD in litigation and applications for disability compensation (131, 208). For example, a woman complained in a lawsuit against her employer that she developed PTSD because she was not promoted on her job in as timely a manner as she desired. Another woman filed a lawsuit against her beauty shop claiming PTSD on the basis of damage to her hair by her beautician. It can be argued that these experiences do not rank with qualifying traumas such as amputation of one's hand in a chain saw accident or witnessing a co-worker being crushed to death by heavy equipment. Although it has been observed that stress-related symptoms commonly occur outside the context of exposure to traumatic events as defined here, it is the origination of the symptoms in association with a qualifying exposure to a defined traumatic event that differentiates PTSD from other kinds of stress-related complaints, symptoms, or syndromes (33, 166). It is not the subjective psychological distress following a stressful experience that determines whether the incident is classified as a traumatic exposure, but rather the objective characteristics of the event itself as representing a threat to life or limb. Separation of the objective characteristics of the incident from the subjective response of individuals exposed to it is critical to conceptualization of PTSD.

Diagnosis of PTSD requires new or worsening symptoms following trauma exposure, which continue for more than 1 month, in four categories: intrusive re-experience (requiring at least one of five symptoms), avoidance (requiring at least one of two symptoms), negative cognitions and mood (requiring at least two of seven symptoms), and hyperarousal (requiring at least two of six symptoms) (9). Intrusive re-experience (Criterion B) includes flashbacks, nightmares, and recurrent vivid images related to the event. Avoidance symptoms (Criterion C) may occur in response to internal reminders such as memories, thoughts, or feelings or external reminders such as locations related to the event. Negative alterations in cognitions and mood associated with the traumatic event (Criterion D) include psychogenic amnesia, numbing of emotions, negative cognitions, and negative emotions. Hyperarousal symptoms (Criterion E) include exaggerated startle response, disturbed concentration and sleep, irritability and anger outbursts, and reckless and self-destructive behaviors. Additionally, the symptoms must cause clinically significant distress or functional impairment and not be due to the physiological effects of alcohol, other drugs, or a medical condition.

HISTORICAL BACKGROUND

Emotional responses to catastrophic events were recorded as long as 4,000 years ago in cuneiform records of the destruction of the city of Ur (2000 B.C.) (115):

> In its places, where the festivities of the land took place, the people lay in heaps.
> At night a bitter lament having been raised unto me,
> I, although, for that night tremble,
> Fled not before that night's violence.
> The storm's cyclone like destruction—verily its terror has filled me full.
> Because of its [affliction] in my nightly sleeping place,
> In my nightly sleeping place verily there is no peace for me. (Verses 95–99 and 217)

Homer's *Iliad* described military soldiers' reactions to the horrors of war. These reactions were grief, guilt over fallen comrades, feeling dead, and berserk rage attacks (204), not unlike the descriptions of posttraumatic reactions among combat soldiers, especially among Vietnam veterans depicted in popular feature films.

A witness to the 1666 Great Fire of London described recurrent sleep disturbances and intrusive images associated with the experience (54):

> How strange that to this very day I cannot sleep at night without great fear of being overcome by fire. And last night I lay awake until almost 2 o'clock in the morning because I could not stop thinking about the fire.

Medical literature on psychiatric trauma syndromes can be traced to 1867 when John Erichsen described railroad spine syndrome in connection with collisions occurring with use of the newfangled steam-powered train in England (65, 221). Symptoms of railroad spine syndrome were sleep disturbance, distressing dreams, anxiety, irritability, memory and concentration problems, and multiple somatic symptoms. Erichsen considered the syndrome organically based, involving physical damage to the spinal cord (p. 77) (63):

> [I] direct your attention to a class of cases in which the injury inflicted upon the back is either very slight in degree, or in which the blow, if more severe, has fallen upon some other part of the body than the spine, and in which, consequently, its influence upon the cord has been of a less direct and often of a less instantaneous character. Nothing is more common than that the

symptoms of spinal mischief do not develop for several days after heavy falls on the back.

Page (173), however, disagreed, arguing in favor of extreme fear as the cause. Around the same time, however, Putnam (181) considered railroad spine syndrome to represent a form of hysterical neurosis. Railway spine evolved into a pejorative term that included "obscure affections of the brain and spinal cord" (207) and "real or imaginary affections of the spine" (80). It may be no accident that personal insurance was introduced around the same time as railway transportation. Railway accidents were among the first tragedies for which people could sue for damages (118).

American Civil War soldiers emerging from battlefields developed a syndrome consisting of exertional chest pain, rapid feeble pulse, shortness of breath, sleep disturbance with unpleasant dreams and jerking during sleep, headaches, dizziness, and gastrointestinal symptoms, chiefly diarrhea (82). Da Costa (53) formally named this constellation of complaints "irritable heart syndrome," reflecting his belief that overreaction and excessive excitement caused irritability of the heart. The syndrome has also been referred to as "Da Costa syndrome" and "effort syndrome." The possibility of emotional origins to these combat-related symptoms was not entertained, perhaps in part because conditions considered "hysterical" had not been observed to occur regularly in men (215). In the late nineteenth century, however, Briquet and Charcot (137) described several male cases of hysteria. Charcot proposed that neurological damage precipitated by traumatic events led to hysteria (62). Babinski and Froment (14) disagreed, however, invoking the process of suggestion as producing the symptoms rather than neurological damage from traumatic events.

Observing alleged sexual trauma in early childhood as a recurring feature of hysteria, Freud elaborated a traumatic theory of hysterical neurosis (69). Just 2 years later, however, he abandoned this position (70) in favor of a view that the reported traumatic events represented fantasies (70). Contemporaneously, Janet concluded that the shocking events alleged as etiological in hysteria might actually be imaginary (101). He proposed instead that dissociative processes are central to the psychopathology of hysteria and traumatic neurosis (224). (Dissociation is a theoretical process involving postulated disruption in the integrative functions of consciousness, memory, identity, or perception of the environment. Classical dissociative presentations include dissociative amnesia; fugue; depersonalization, which is a sensation of change or unreality of oneself; and derealization, which is a perception of change or unreality of one's environment or world.) Although it has been hypothesized that dissociative disorders are caused by the experience of unbearable trauma (209), empirical support is lacking, and dissociative disorders are not among those typically observed in studies of disaster survivors and combat veterans.

World War I saw the emergence of "soldier's heart," a posttraumatic syndrome with many associated nervous symptoms, leading to 80,000 discharges from the US Army (52). Finding no cardiac abnormalities in these cases, MacKenzie concluded that they were psychiatrically based (124). Myers applied the term "shell shock" to combat-related psychological syndromes (141). As described by Mott, shell shock constituted a variety of hysterical symptoms (paralysis, contractions, and disordered gait), neurasthenia symptoms (lassitude, fatigue, headaches, and terrifying dreams), exaggerated startle reflex, chronic jerking mannerisms, and spasms of the head and neck stimulated by noise (140).

At the end of World War I, skepticism was growing over the concept of shell shock, and suspicions of malingering arose (20, 98). By the beginning of World War II, the syndrome of shell shock had given way to the concept of war neurosis, implying psychogenic origins (108, 127).

Although reference to "trauma" had previously been reserved for physical, as opposed to psychological, experiences, in World War II and the Korean War, extreme psychological stress first came under the broad umbrella of emotional "trauma" (108). Studies of World War II prisoners of war and survivors of the horrors of Nazi concentration camps revealed ensuing problems of irritability and anger, restlessness and tension, chronic fears, depression, paranoia, decreased interest, poor concentration, social isolation, and changes in personality (19, 26, 229). The Vietnam War galvanized attention to posttraumatic psychiatric syndromes, which further increased in the 1980s and 1990s (118).

Posttraumatic syndromes have long been described in civilian victims of disasters and in industrial and occupational medicine. Following the 1871 passage of damage claims laws in Germany and in the midst of subsequent economic crisis in Germany, concerns arose about illness faked for compensation (91). In this context, a new term, "compensation neurosis," was introduced (65). American compensation laws passed in 1911 heralded a sharp increase in cases of industrial neurosis (57). Significant economic repercussions soon followed, fostering vigilance for "unscrupulous malingerers" faking injuries to obtain compensation (139). Persistent concerns about motivation for compensation complicated the evaluation of claims of Holocaust survivors and Vietnam veterans (72, 208).

The first community-based study of disasters is attributed to Stierlin (214), who in 1911 found sleep disturbance and nightmares in 25% of survivors of the Messina earthquake. Stierlin described two associated psychological syndromes. The first, considered to represent a psychotic or hysterical state, termed "fright psychosis," involved features of clouded consciousness, amnesia, disorientation, fearful affect, and hallucinations persisting 3 days. A second, longer lasting, "traumatic neurosis" consisted of sleep disturbance and autonomic changes, including rapid or labile pulse, hyperactive patellar reflexes, tremor, and fatigue.

A landmark study of the Coconut Grove fire in Boston in 1943 established the feasibility of systematic investigation into the psychological effects of major disasters (1). The following two decades saw the publication of a number of studies in the wake of major disasters, including a tornado in Mississippi in 1952 (23), the 1962 Alaska earthquake (119), the 1956 sinking of the Andrea Doria (71), and the 1968 Bristol floods (18).

In 1950, publication of an article on extreme stress in studies of animals (203) heralded new approaches to research into neuroendocrine mechanisms of stress. This study also first introduced the word *stress* into everyday speech in reference to psychological experiences (118). More recently, the word *trauma* has been used loosely in common parlance to represent anything emotionally upsetting. Having to give a speech in class, being embarrassed by a colleague's comment, and sitting for a difficult examination represent examples of emotionally stressful events sometimes labeled "traumatic" in popular language. Unfortunately, the use of the word *trauma* to describe purely emotionally stressful events has blurred the distinction between emotional stress and precise conceptualization of trauma in general usage.

In the first two editions of the American Psychiatric Association's *Diagnostic and Statistical Manual of Mental Disorders* (*DSM-I* and *DSM-II*), in 1952 and 1968, stress-related disorders were classified as transient situational personality disorders under the names "gross stress reaction" and "transient situational disturbance," respectively (4, 5). It was not until *DSM-III*, the third edition of the diagnostic manual, in 1980 (6), that PTSD was introduced as a specific disorder in its own right, reflecting social and political influences surrounding the American Vietnam War experience (123). PTSD has been one of the most rapidly evolving disorders across subsequent editions of the American diagnostic criteria sets.

The specific definition of a traumatic event for the diagnosis of PTSD has changed across editions of the diagnostic criteria (167). Prior versions of PTSD criteria have defined a traumatic event as one that is likely to evoke subjective distress responses in most people (*DSM-III* and *DSM-III-R*) and an experience that is "outside the range of usual human experience" (p. 236 in *DSM-III* and p. 247 in *DSM-III-R*), and physical threat of death or serious injury (*DSM-IV*) (7). *DSM-5* criteria defined the traumatic event as "involving actual or threatened death, serious injury, or sexual violence" (p. 271) (9). *DSM-IV* added a requirement of subjective individual reaction of "intense fear, helplessness, or horror" (pp. 424 and 428) to the definition of trauma exposure, which was removed from the criteria in *DSM-5* (167).

The definition of trauma exposure has also varied greatly among the editions of the diagnostic criteria. Besides direct personal exposure, other types of exposure in prior versions of the diagnostic criteria have included witnessing trauma to others, learning of trauma exposures of close associates, and sudden destruction of one's home or community. *DSM-5* clarified that witnessed events include only "in person" or eye-witnessed events, adding, however, that exposures through electronic media would qualify if they are work-related exposures to repeated or extreme images (167).

Posttraumatic stress symptoms were originally organized into categories of intrusion and avoidance/denial proposed by Horowitz (96), along with a third category representing hyperarousal. Since the original presentation of the criteria in 1980, the symptoms of the disorder have increased from 12 symptoms in three symptom groups to 20 symptoms in four symptom groups. *DSM-5* split the avoidance/numbing symptom group into two groups, one for avoidance, and another for negative cognitions and mood.

Recent studies have linked PTSD with childhood molestation, depression, anxiety disorders, borderline personality disorder, somatization disorder, multiple personality disorder, smoking, alcohol and drug abuse, irritable bowel syndrome, and just about any label, problem, or disorder imaginable. Much of the academic literature describing the interrelationships of these problems has assumed a causal role of childhood trauma in the pathogenesis of borderline personality and PTSD (87). However, such causal relationships have not been adequately demonstrated in methodologically rigorous studies controlling for confounding effects of other variables associated with childhood trauma in these relationships.

EPIDEMIOLOGY

Because PTSD by definition originates in trauma exposure, the approach to the epidemiology of PTSD logically begins with the epidemiology of trauma exposure. Seminal research on the population prevalence of trauma exposure and PTSD was published in the 1990s. This research has documented that violent trauma is an endemic part of community existence. Lifetime exposure to trauma was reported in 39% of a sample of 1,007 young adults in an urban health maintenance organization (36) and in 90% of 2,188 residents of the Detroit metropolitan area ages 15–45 studied by the same research group (40), 56% of 5,877 noninstitutionalized US civilians ages 15 to 54 in the National Comorbidity Study (104), and 69% of a community sample of 1,000 adults (147). One study found that 21% of people may be exposed to trauma in any one year (147), and another found that 50% may be exposed to trauma over a decade (45). Pratchett and colleagues (178) concluded that "most [of] the US population will, at some point in their life, be exposed to at least 1 traumatic event, with estimates of prevalence ranging from 58% to 92%" (p. 465). Breslau et al. (40) noted that a major contributor to the variation in estimates of trauma prevalence is the reliance on different definitions of trauma that have arisen with extensive changes in PTSD criteria across different editions of the DSM. The most commonly reported types of trauma exposures are witnessing serious or fatal injury (25%), experiencing a life-threatening accident (19%), being in a natural disaster (17%) (104), and learning of the sudden, unexpected death of a loved one (60%) (40).

Trauma does not occur completely at random (152). Not everyone is at equal risk for exposure to trauma (232). Several personal risk factors have been found to increase risk for trauma exposure: lower socioeconomic status, lack of education, early conduct problems, preexisting psychiatric illness, substance abuse, and personality traits such as novelty seeking and risk taking (35, 36, 45, 152). Risk for exposure to assaultive violence is higher among men, younger people, and inner-city urban minorities; and serious accidents and witnessed violence are more prevalent in men (30, 40).

Estimates of the prevalence of PTSD vary with characteristics of the specific traumatic event and the populations affected by it. Some studies have measured the prevalence of PTSD in general populations, and other studies have examined the conditional prevalence of PTSD in samples selected for exposure to trauma. Errors in prevalence estimates can occur in studies of traumatized populations that include many individuals not exposed to trauma, such as in studies of largely unexposed populations after the September 11, 2001 terrorist attacks (32). In those studies, symptoms among the largely unexposed samples cannot, by definition, be considered to represent disaster-related PTSD, and likely consist of emotional distress, symptoms of other disorders, or continuation of preexisting psychopathology (161). Counting symptomatic individuals without qualifying exposures as cases of disaster-related PTSD has resulted in overestimation of the number of potential PTSD cases by several magnitudes, as well as underestimation of the prevalence of disaster-related PTSD among presumably exposed groups (152).

In recent years, diminishing resources for conducting research coupled with concurrent demands for larger samples and low-burden assessment tools have conspired to encourage the substitution of rapid self-report symptom screening measures for the more burdensome full diagnostic assessments of PTSD. This trend has produced a literature that increasingly contains articles reporting on symptoms rather than the diagnosis of PTSD; the distinction has often not been noted and sometimes the symptoms have been represented as PTSD or its equivalent. Breslau and Schultz (45) have cautioned that posttraumatic stress symptoms assessed outside the context of diagnosis are ambiguous and their relationship to PTSD is tenuous. Therefore, cautious reading of the PTSD literature in relation to the methods of assessment is needed for accurate interpretation of this research.

PTSD is far less prevalent than trauma exposure. Historically, most knowledge about human response to traumatic experiences has emerged from research on combat veterans (47, 118) and also survivors of disasters and motor vehicle accidents (33, 148). Because the formal diagnosis of PTSD was not available before 1980, this disorder in its current form could not be studied among returning combat personnel before the Vietnam War. Studies of Vietnam War era combat veterans have estimated that 31% developed PTSD and 15% had current PTSD, but subsequent analyses of data from these studies have offered far lower prevalence figures for PTSD (186). Variability in PTSD prevalence findings among studies of Vietnam veterans has been attributed to substantial methodological differences in research studies (186). Research on more recent cohorts has yielded combat-related PTSD prevalence of 2%–13% among veterans of the Persian Gulf War and 4%–17% among veterans of the more recent conflicts in the Middle East (186). Studies of the Middle East conflict have found the prevalence of PTSD to be associated with deployment to Iraq compared to deployment to Afghanistan, but not to active duty compared to reserve or National Guard personnel (90). Recent studies have used symptom checklists rather than full diagnostic assessments, reducing confidence in the accuracy of the estimates of prevalence (130, 186).

The first population PTSD prevalence data were gathered beginning in 1980 in St. Louis and North Carolina as part of the Epidemiologic Catchment Area (ECA) study, using the Diagnostic Interview Schedule, a structured interview providing estimates of psychiatric diagnosis conforming to accepted diagnostic criteria. The lifetime rates of PTSD recorded in the ECA study were 1%–2% (55, 85). Subsequent population studies have estimated the lifetime PTSD prevalence at 8%–9% (36, 104).

The conditional probability of PTSD among people exposed to traumatic events has been reported to be 24% (36) and 9% (40) in population studies by Breslau's group and 14% in the National Comorbidity Study (104). The reported likelihood of PTSD following traumatic events has varied according to the type of event. In the 1991 Breslau et al. study, the type of event most associated with PTSD was rape, with a 49% rate of PTSD. Other types of trauma had somewhat lower rates of associated PTSD: being badly beaten (32%), sexual assault without rape (24%), and serious accident or injury (17%). In the National Comorbidity Study (104), incidents most likely to lead to PTSD were rape (49%) and military combat (39%); far less likely to result in PTSD were witnessing serious or fatal injury (6%) and experiencing a natural disaster (5%).

Disasters present unique opportunities for studies of trauma, because populations may be exposed to disaster trauma more at random, with little regard for preexisting personal characteristics, compared to other types of trauma (152). Thus, disaster studies may avoid the confounding effects of predisposing risk factors for trauma exposure with mental health sequelae of trauma. A recent study of 811 directly exposed survivors of 10 different disasters by the same research team using consistent methods, including full diagnostic assessment, compared mental health effects of survivors of a plane crash into a hotel, a tornado, an earthquake, a firestorm, floods, multiple-shooting incidents, and the Oklahoma City bombing (160). The prevalence of PTSD related to these disasters ranged from none to about one-third, averaging 16%. In this series of disasters, the highest prevalence of PTSD was 35% of survivors of a plane crash into a hotel, and 34% of Oklahoma City bombing survivors. Another study by this research group, also using consistent methods, examined survivors of the 9/11 attacks on the World Trade Center in New York City, finding a 35% prevalence of disaster-related PTSD (164). These findings seem to suggest a ceiling of PTSD prevalence of about one-third of directly exposed survivors of the most severe disasters.

Two individual characteristics have repeatedly emerged as robust predictors of PTSD: gender and preexisting psychopathology. General population women are more prone than men to develop PTSD, by a factor of about 2 (31, 36, 37, 85, 95, 104, 160, 178, 199). (This generalization does not appear to apply specifically, however, to female military veterans, whose combat-related PTSD prevalence appears to match that of their male counterparts (197).) Breslau (31) noted that research has yet to uncover the exact reasons behind the sex difference in the conditional risk of PTSD; it appears to be unrelated to women's greater prevalence of sexual assault, previous trauma exposures, preexisting depressive or anxiety disorders, or gender-related reporting bias. Breslau and colleagues (40) concluded that research findings suggest an inherent vulnerability to PTSD among women exposed to trauma. Preexisting psychopathology is strongly associated with PTSD, with approximately twice the likelihood, in trauma-exposed populations (59, 88, 160, 199). Specifically, preexisting personality characteristics predict PTSD (36, 59, 151, 154, 199, 233).

Intensity of trauma exposure and severity of trauma-related injury have not been as strongly or reliably found to be associated with PTSD (88, 160, 199). Breslau's group (46) has concluded that exposures to extremely severe stressors and to milder stressors do not differ in the amount of prediction of PTSD contributed by preexisting psychopathology or other predispositions. Other potential predictors of PTSD have been inconsistently reported: age, intelligence, education, race/ethnicity, marital status, prior trauma or adversity, and involvement in litigation or compensation seeking (59, 88, 148, 187).

The conditional definition of PTSD based on exposure to trauma means that two sets of risk factors are involved with the occurrence of PTSD, one involving risk for trauma exposure and the other involving risk for development of psychopathology after trauma exposure (35). Risk factors for trauma exposure must be differentiated from risk factors for PTSD in trauma-exposed individuals to infer causality. For example, a review by DiGangi et al. (59) of studies with prospective assessment completed prior to trauma exposure and assessment again after trauma exposure concluded that many factors historically thought to be consequences of trauma may actually also represent risk factors for exposure to trauma. Therefore, mental health problems observed after trauma may in turn represent preexisting risk factors for the trauma exposure, creating a tautology obscuring the determination of causal relationships. It follows from this reasoning that not all mental health problems that are found to occur in association with trauma exposure are necessarily caused by the trauma (156). Practitioners are encouraged to consider other causal possibilities rather than assuming that all mental health problems identified in individuals with trauma histories are a direct result of the traumatic experience.

CLINICAL PICTURE

Posttraumatic stress symptoms are very common after exposure to substantial trauma. Most disaster trauma survivors describe one or more emotional responses consistent with the diagnostic list of posttraumatic stress symptoms. Among directly exposed survivors of the Oklahoma

City bombing, 96% endorsed at least one posttraumatic stress symptom. Intrusive memories of the event and hyperarousal symptoms such as insomnia, difficulty concentrating, and enhanced startle or jumpiness were especially common (158). Members of disaster-affected communities who were not personally exposed, as well as people of other communities affected only remotely such as by hearing news broadcast coverage of a disaster, may also acknowledge similar symptoms (201, 202, 206).

Less commonly encountered posttraumatic stress symptoms are avoidance and numbing symptoms (29, 158). Psychogenic amnesia and restricted range of affect are especially infrequent (158). Avoidance and numbing symptoms, despite their low prevalence, however, are the defining features of PTSD criteria and serve as a marker for the disorder (42, 44, 158, 230). In the Oklahoma City bombing study, 94% of directly exposed survivors with three or more avoidance and numbing symptoms met full criteria for the diagnosis of PTSD (158). Avoidance and numbing symptoms were also associated with other indicators of illness: preexisting psychopathology, postdisaster disorders, functional impairment, seeking treatment, taking medication, and consuming alcohol or drugs to cope.

Symptoms of intrusive re-experience and hyperarousal are so commonly reported that they may be considered the norm, or *normative* (i.e., described by most people). These common re-experience and hyperarousal symptoms would not be assumed to be evidence of illness in the absence of prominent avoidance and numbing responses, but rather emotional distress of nonpathological proportion. Analysis by Breslau and colleagues (44) confirmed that posttraumatic stress symptoms below the level qualifying for a diagnosis of PTSD do not represent the type of pathological process experienced by patients meeting PTSD criteria, discrediting the validity of partial or subthreshold posttraumatic stress syndrome concepts.

A recurring theme in descriptions of PTSD in various settings is the finding of extensive psychiatric comorbidity. The majority of individuals with PTSD are found to have comorbid psychiatric disorders (28, 29, 74, 104, 112, 158), most commonly major depressive disorder, anxiety disorders, and substance use disorders.

Borderline and antisocial personality and somatoform comorbidities have been described in association with PTSD in populations selected from treatment settings, but these syndromes have typically been found to predate the traumatic exposure rather than arising anew after exposure to trauma (67, 149, 157, 158, 174, 182). Research with survivors of the Oklahoma City bombing, a disaster that did not specifically target individuals with preexisting risk factors such as personality characteristics, found that personality abnormalities assessed with the Temperament and

Character Inventory were associated with approximately double the likelihood of PTSD (151, 154). In this study, individuals with borderline temperament were especially prone to PTSD. The newest revision of the diagnostic criteria for PTSD in *DSM-5* added verbal and physical aggression toward others, reckless and self-destructive behavior, and extreme negative self-cognitions to the criteria, representing features of antisocial and borderline personality disorder presentations. These additions to the criteria may reflect the features of some patient populations with PTSD rather than characteristics of PTSD (167).

PTSD has been linked with dissociation, a condition considered by some to result from early psychologically traumatic experiences (56, 60, 73, 209). In clinical settings, dissociative symptoms are commonly observed in patients with comorbid personality disorders of the "Cluster B" ("dramatic, emotional, or erratic") (9) (p. 646) group (234), in which a history of childhood abuse and adversity is prevalent (129, 144, 198). Dissociative disorders are not among the disorders observed to arise after disasters (73). Prevalence of dissociative symptoms has typically been reported without mention of dissociative disorders. The clinical significance and validity of "dissociative" symptoms after disaster exposure have not been adequately determined.

Some researchers have concluded that the comorbidity of other psychiatric disorders with PTSD is merely a consequence of overlap of criteria for other psychiatric disorders (78, 79, 179) (most notably major depressive, generalized anxiety, and phobic disorders) and not truly co-occurring psychopathology. This difficulty appears to be an artifact of the methods of diagnostic assessment used; diligent assessment of PTSD according to diagnostic criteria that require anchoring the symptoms to a qualifying trauma exposure, that is, "beginning or worsening after the traumatic event(s) occurred" (9) (p. 271), should eliminate this difficulty. Inability to differentiate the symptoms of PTSD from other disorders would clearly present a challenge to the validity and reliability of the diagnosis of PTSD.

In clinical practice, the frequent comorbidity of other psychiatric disorders with PTSD (104, 199) points to the utility of continuing the search for psychiatric disorders after PTSD is assessed. Diagnostic comorbidity with PTSD represents a marker for severity of illness and disability, and identifies cases that merit special attention (157). The comorbid disorders may be at least as important as PTSD itself to the treatment, course, and outcome of PTSD.

Breslau and colleagues have investigated the associations of major depressive disorder and substance use disorders with PTSD (30, 38, 39). Their studies found that while these disorders were associated with PTSD, they were not associated with exposure to trauma without the development of PTSD. They concluded from their results that exposure to traumatic events per se does not increase the risk for these other disorders, but rather that PTSD could represent a causal risk factor for these other disorders or, alternatively, that PTSD and these other disorders might co-occur because of shared vulnerability factors other than traumatic exposure.

Acute stress disorder is a diagnosis that was developed to provide a diagnostic category in the first month after trauma exposure, before a diagnosis of PTSD can be applied. It first appeared in diagnostic criteria in *DSM-IV* in 1994. Research to establish the diagnostic validity of acute stress disorder presently falls far short of progress in the incomplete body of work on diagnostic validity of PTSD (143, 166). Because many people with acute stress disorder do not develop PTSD and only about half of people with PTSD start off with acute stress disorder, this diagnosis appears to have limited utility for predicting PTSD (50).

BIOLOGICAL FINDINGS

The introduction of PTSD as an established psychiatric disorder in formal diagnostic criteria in *DSM-III* in 1980 opened new doors to scientific advancements in understanding the disorder. Research findings into PTSD have advanced quickly since this time. Part of this work has investigated the biology of fear conditioning and related neural circuitry that is common to animals and humans, allowing translation of animal research to humans in ways not feasible for research on other mental disorders, such as schizophrenia and bipolar disorder, that lack corresponding animal models (126). According to Yehuda and LeDoux (232), animal studies of cued fear conditioning provide a representative model for the conceptualization of human PTSD, which is hypothesized to represent the failure to recover from normal fear learning. The application of these animal models has facilitated the mapping of phenotypic differences in fear to specific brain circuits and cellular, synaptic, molecular, and genetic mechanisms.

A logical starting point in attempting to understand the biology of PTSD is with the neurobiology of the stress response and fear conditioning. Fear responses to trauma are primarily mediated through the neural circuitry of the limbic system, the part of the brain that is responsible for the processing of emotions. Components of the limbic system that are principally involved in fear circuitry include the amygdala, prefrontal cortex (PFC), and hippocampus, with additional input from the parahippocampal gyrus, orbitofrontal cortex, sensorimotor cortex, thalamus, and anterior cingulate cortex (84, 126, 195).

Trauma exposure memory is encoded and stored in the hippocampus, which directs activation of fear memories (83). New memories are consolidated at the cellular level into long-term storage of stable memories. When memory is retrieved from long-term storage for active recollection, however, the reactivated memory trace enters a labile state in which changes to its content may occur. The reactivated memory is then reconsolidated to long-term memory for permanent storage, but if the memory trace is modified during this process, it will be saved with any revisions made during its malleable phase (219). In short, memories can be changed simply by the process of recalling and entertaining their content.

Perception of threat of danger activates the amygdala, which projects to the midbrain and brainstem to generate rapid autonomic, endocrine, and hyperarousal and hypervigilance responses (84). Hippocampal communications to the amygdala contribute to the shaping of the amygdala's trauma-related emotional responses. The hippocampus also provides input into the medial prefrontal cortex (mPFC) for contextual interpretation and executive determinations that in turn exert inhibitory control over the amygdala's response to the trauma (84, 195). The mPFC feeds back to the hippocampus and inhibits the amygdala to mediate extinction of conditioned fear responses (84).

The amygdala and brainstem stimulate the hypothalamic-pituitary-adrenal (HPA) axis, a system that plays a pivotal role in the biology of stress responses. In response to a stressor, the hypothalamic paraventricular nucleus secretes corticotropin-releasing factor (CRF), which then signals the anterior pituitary to release adrenocorticotropin (ACTH) that in turn prompts the adrenal glands to release glucocorticoids. Glucocorticoids stimulate metabolic, immune, and brain functions that drive physiological responses and direct stress-related behaviors (126). The glucocorticoids produced through HPA axis activity in turn exert negative feedback control on HPA axis functions at various levels (126). This negative feedback represents an autoregulatory mechanism to help return the system to its baseline once an acute stressor is no longer present (232). Inhibition of HPA axis activity is exerted by the PFC and hippocampus.

Fear conditioning is a well-known phenomenon that involves the pairing of a neutral stimulus, such as a particular sound, with a stressful unconditioned stimulus (US), such as a shock to a body part. The US by itself elicits an unconditioned response (UR), such as fear and arousal, but when it is paired with the neutral stimulus, the neutral stimulus becomes a conditioned stimulus (CS) that by itself elicits a conditioned response (CR) with fear and arousal (232). Both UR and CR involve amygdala functions. CS and US pathways converge in the lateral nucleus of the amygdala, which specializes in synaptic plasticity. Subsequent CS exposure prompts the transfer of this activity to the central amygdala, which communicates with the hypothalamus and brainstem to prompt the release of catecholamines, ACTH, and cortisol to direct autonomic, hormonal, arousal, and behavioral responses. As a result, sympathetic activity increases and parasympathetic activity decreases, and end-organ responses include increased heart rate, blood pressure, respiratory rate, and sweating to support the body's ability to mount an effective response to danger (232). Brain function plasticity involved in the development of PTSD is conducted through functions of brain-derived neurotropic factor (BDNF), glutamate functions via N-methyl-D-aspartate (NMDA), and gamma-aminobutyric acid (GABA).

Fear learning is evolutionarily advantageous to the organism and the species (84, 232). Fear learning can, however, become so overly generalized that it not only does not confer any advantage but becomes maladaptive. If, for example, learned fear extends to harmless situations, inappropriate autonomic hyperarousal responses can result (84). There is some evidence that neural processing of trauma exposure memory may involve associative overgeneralization coupled with lack of inhibition of responses to related but harmless stimuli (220). The pathology of PTSD appears to represent abnormal neurobiological processing of acquired fear responses, or it may arise from failure to recover from the acute changes in the brain and body that occur with fear learning (232). Glucocorticoids appear to have a role in extinction of fear memories that could potentially be utilized to intervene in this process for development of novel PTSD treatments (58).

Understanding the neurobiology of PTSD requires differentiation of the elements of normal physiological fear responses from the psychopathology represented in PTSD (232). Thus, to fully understand PTSD, it must be differentiated from nonpathological response to trauma exposure (232).

Various neurobiological abnormalities have been documented in association with PTSD. Research has demonstrated that abnormalities in several brain structures known to be involved in in fear learning are implicated in the development and maintenance of posttraumatic symptoms and PTSD (122, 195). A principal finding in PTSD is excessive activation of the amygdala, coupled with an underactive mPFC that is insufficient to inhibit the amygdala's vigorous response to threat of danger (195, 232). Reduced volume of the hippocampus is a cardinal feature of PTSD (27, 84, 232). Another important finding with PTSD is low cortisol levels with increased sensitivity of the HPA axis to negative glucocorticoid feedback (84, 232). An important function of cortisol is to dampen the response of the sympathetic nervous system to stress, thus contributing to return to the pre-stressor baseline and protection from PTSD (232). PTSD has also been found to be associated with persistently increased levels of catecholamines and heightened autonomic activity (232). Unchecked adrenaline contributes to consolidation of trauma memory to produce stronger and more distressing memories of the trauma that provoke intrusive memories which in turn perpetuate hyperarousal symptoms, ultimately leading to avoidance responses (232) that mark the psychopathology of PTSD.

Yehuda and LeDoux (232) cautioned that biological findings associated with PTSD do not necessarily imply that biological differences in PTSD are causal to the disorder. For example, it has been concluded that the stress-induced glucocorticoid activity of PTSD causes hippocampal damage and loss of volume through toxic effects on dendritic functions and neurogenesis (84). Prospective longitudinal studies of individuals with acute trauma exposure, however, have failed to demonstrate changes in hippocampal volume over time, suggesting that lower hippocampal volume represents a preexisting risk factor for PTSD rather than a result of the disorder (232).

NATURAL HISTORY

Definitions of onset and remission for PTSD have not been uniformly defined or consistently measured, resulting in wide variation in measurement of these concepts and noncomparable data across studies (159). Currently there is considerable confusion as to whether onset and remission of PTSD, respectively, represent the time points of the first appearance and final disappearance of *any* posttraumatic stress symptoms or the time points that the full diagnostic criteria for PTSD are first fulfilled and most recently met (12).

Historically, onset of PTSD has been defined as beginning with "onset of symptoms" in diagnostic nomenclature (p. 429) (8), and a long history of epidemiological research has identified the onset of a psychiatric disorder as the point at which any symptoms of the disorder begin (191). Definition of full remission from a psychiatric disorder in American diagnostic nomenclature has historically referred to the disappearance of all symptoms of the disorder, and partial remission has been defined as continuing symptoms that have fallen below the diagnostic threshold (8). The procedure for determining onset and remission of psychiatric disorders over decades of use of structured diagnostic interviews has been to determine whether diagnostic criteria of a disorder were ever met, and then to identify when the symptoms first occurred (for onset) and whether or when the symptoms most recently disappeared (for remission) (191).

The definition of onset as the time when the first symptoms start is referred to as a "symptom-based definition," and the definition of onset as the time when the diagnostic threshold is met is referred to as a "diagnostic threshold-based definition" (159). Most investigators using structured diagnostic interviews for PTSD have followed the definition of symptom-based onset and remission provided by these instruments, and investigators using symptom scales have generally followed diagnostic threshold-based definitions of onset and remission of the disorder, inherent to the different methods used by these tools for determining onset and remission (based on first and most recent symptoms for diagnostic interviews, and based on crossing diagnostic threshold between separate symptom scale assessments at different time points). Compared to studies using diagnostic threshold-based definitions, studies using symptom-based definitions of onset and remission generally find a far lower prevalence of delayed-onset PTSD and less optimistic rates of remission from PTSD (159).

From *DSM-III* through *DSM-IV-TR*, the diagnostic criteria for PTSD used a symptom-based definition of onset. *DSM-5* provides no formal definitions of onset for psychiatric disorders in general or for individual disorders, including PTSD. However, *DSM-5* added a new specifier for "delayed expression" of PTSD, defined as "full diagnostic criteria are not met until at least 6 months after the event") (p. 272), indicating a shift from the symptom-based conceptualization of PTSD onset in earlier versions of the criteria to a diagnostic-threshold basis in *DSM-5*. Because of PTSD's unusual construction as a conditional disorder following trauma exposure, the timing of the onset of the disorder in relation to the traumatic event is of considerable relevance to this diagnosis.

PTSD and its symptoms have been found to start very quickly after exposure to trauma. In a combined dataset from studies of 716 directly exposed survivors of 10 different disasters, 71% of the survivors with PTSD had onset of symptoms the same day as the disaster and 97% had onset within 1 month; no cases began after 6 months (159). A study of 42 inpatients admitted to a trauma ward for serious injuries determined that 59% developed PTSD as assessed by structured diagnostic interview at 1 month. These patients were prospectively interviewed daily over the first month after their trauma incidents. Posttraumatic stress symptoms for the entire sample began by 5–7 days after the incident on average and reached saturation by about 2 weeks (230). Intrusion and hyperarousal symptoms began much more rapidly (approximately 70% on the first post-trauma day) than avoidance and numbing symptoms (approximately 15% on the first post-trauma day). The presence of three or more avoidance/numbing symptoms at 1 week identified most of the patients who went on to develop a 1-month diagnosis of PTSD, and by 2 weeks, the lack of these symptoms significantly identified most of those who did not develop PTSD by 1 month.

Delayed-onset PTSD defined in *DSM-IV-TR* as symptoms beginning 6 months or later after trauma exposure has been described in specific populations. These populations include professional groups such as military personnel and combat veterans, firefighters, rescue workers, utility workers, and police, with the disorder beginning sometimes even decades after the traumatic event (99, 223). In most studies reporting delayed-onset PTSD, symptoms of the disorder were present in more than 90% of cases during the early post-trauma period, well before the declared onset of the disorder (223). A pattern of accumulating earlier symptoms has also been observed in delayed-onset PTSD in military veterans, as well as association with a severe life stressor in the year before the delayed onset of PTSD (13).

PTSD tends to follow a relatively chronic course, lasting, on average, 2–5 years in general populations (40, 104). The study of 716 disaster survivors by North and Oliver (159) found that only 39% of those with PTSD had remitted by about 18 months. Over a 7-year period, only 37% of directly exposed survivors of the Oklahoma City bombing with PTSD had achieved remission, and the time course for remission from PTSD was significantly slower than that for new major depression episodes that began after the disaster (162). Even for survivors who did not develop PTSD, posttraumatic stress symptoms were initially highly prevalent, dropping off quickly and then plateauing, with nearly 40% continuing to report symptoms at 7 years. There is some evidence that women have a more chronic PTSD course than that of men (34, 40), but other disaster studies have not found predictors of remission or chronicity, including female sex (159, 162).

COMPLICATIONS

PTSD is well documented to be associated with reduced functioning and quality of life (64, 106, 138, 225, 228). Posttraumatic stress symptoms, however, do not necessarily follow the same path as functional status and quality of life in the course of recovery from trauma (95, 162). In a study of 824 trauma center patients, those who developed PTSD reported significantly lower well-being than those without the disorder (95). A follow-up study of the Oklahoma City bombing survivors by North et al. (162) found that PTSD was significantly associated with functional impairment in the first few postdisaster months. By 7 years, however, functional impairment problems had largely resolved, regardless of PTSD remission or chronicity (162).

Increased substance use has been observed after major catastrophes such as the September 11, 2001 attacks (155, 227), although increased substance use has not always been observed after such incidents (155), and the significance and context of trauma-related changes in substance use requires further interpretation and investigation. Substance use disorders are well documented in association with PTSD (188, 196), and circumspect consideration of these associations is appropriate.

In attempting to explain apparent associations of substance use and substance use disorders with trauma and PTSD, a "self-medication" hypothesis for coping with distress through substances has been invoked (24, 105, 132, 176, 222, 226). There are two problems with assumptions of substance use as "self-medication" of trauma-related distress. First, most substance use disorders observed after disaster trauma exposure have been found to have developed before the disaster (157, 158, 168, 176, 227). In some cases, a preexisting substance use disorder was found to actually increase the risk for encountering trauma (150–152, 157). Second, although studies on substance use disorders and disaster have found increased substance use after disaster, this increase in use has been found to be relatively small (155, 226, 227) and to not regularly translate into new substance use disorders (150, 155, 165). Additionally, because rationalization of excessive substance use is well appreciated as an inherent part of the clinical manifestations of substance use disorders (25), claims by individuals with these disorders that they use substances to medicate their posttraumatic distress should be interpreted in this context.

PTSD is well documented to be associated with risk for suicidal behaviors (177, 183) and suicide (205), but some studies have found that associated psychiatric comorbidities such as depression and alcohol dependence are the underlying source of these relationships (77, 120, 185, 192, 218), and others have pointed to preexisting risk factors such as PTSD related to prior trauma and preexisting suicidality (146, 169). Yet other studies have separated the effects of PTSD from those of trauma exposure, finding that PTSD but not trauma exposure is associated with suicidality (75, 77). Regardless, this research indicates the need to assess risk for suicide among individuals with PTSD, especially in the presence of psychiatric comorbidities and preexisting psychopathology (183, 185). It has been pointed out that suicidal behaviors and completed suicide are two different phenomena, and that the association of PTSD and suicidal behaviors may not extend to completed suicide (175).

Major disasters afford opportunities to compare pre- and postdisaster statistics on suicide in affected populations. The development of new psychiatric disorders such as PTSD and major depression, well documented to develop after disasters (158, 160, 163), could logically be considered a potential source of suicide risk. A number of studies have examined suicide rates in relation to earthquakes, and the results have varied. Suicides have been reported to increase (170) and to decrease (145, 217) after earthquakes, and other studies have found mixed effects, with suicide rates decreasing in men and increasing in women (97, 171), decreasing initially and rising later (172), or increasing with severe earthquakes but decreasing with milder earthquakes (128). Two studies found no change in suicide rates in New York City after the September 11, 2001 attacks (136, 180), and one study reported an increase in suicides in New Orleans after Hurricane Katrina (216). After surviving a disaster, most people express gratitude for having survived and a greater appreciation of the value of life, rather than focusing on desires to end their lives (133, 134).

Research in the last dozen years has identified an association of cardiovascular disease (61) and metabolic syndrome with PTSD (86, 100, 225). A recent meta-analysis of nine studies including a total of 9,673 individuals with PTSD and 6,852 population controls found risk for metabolic syndrome to be nearly double in those with PTSD, at 39%. In addition, abdominal obesity was found in 49%, hyperglycemia in 36%, hypertriglyceridemia in 46%, and hypertension in 77% (194). Although metabolic syndrome clearly represents an important medical comorbidity to be addressed in relation to PTSD, causal associations within this relationship are unclear; the extent to which the experience of trauma and/or PTSD may lead to metabolic syndrome, or the extent to which metabolic syndrome may predispose to trauma and/or PTSD, or the possibility of shared vulnerability factors in these two conditions has not been determined.

FAMILY STUDIES

Family studies have demonstrated that PTSD runs in families, but family studies cannot sort out genetic and environmental contributions to the familiality of the disorder. Twin studies are needed to sort out the roles of genetic and environmental contributors to the disorder, but they cannot implicate the specific genes involved. Molecular genetic studies are needed to identify the genes determining risk for PTSD (110, 113, 116).

PTSD in families has been studied more through family history research (asking probands about their family members) than with the more methodologically reliable and exacting family research (directly examining family members) methods. Research on families has demonstrated not only that PTSD runs in families, but that PTSD also accompanies other disorders in families, especially depressive, anxiety, and substance use disorders (111, 113), and that genetic risk for psychopathology is not disorder-specific (200). Most of the available knowledge about genetic heritability of PTSD comes from twin studies, which have found the disorder to be moderately heritable (2, 10) with about one-third of the variance in risk for PTSD to be genetically contributed (110).

Understanding familial risk for PTSD has been complicated by demonstrated contributions of genetic factors to significant risk for exposure to trauma (110). Heritable preexisting personal characteristics such as personality and major psychopathology have been shown to increase risk for trauma exposure (10, 36, 113). Even mixed-handedness in a co-twin, in a study of identical twin pairs discordant for combat exposure in Vietnam, was found to be a risk factor for combat exposure trauma, which in turn mediated the relationship with PTSD (76). Abnormalities in twins with PTSD shared with their unaffected co-twins, such as smaller hippocampal volume and lower general intellectual ability and specific cognitive deficits, suggest preexisting vulnerabilities to PTSD. Abnormalities in twins with PTSD but not in their identical co-twins, such as exaggerated psychophysiological responsiveness, may represent consequences of PTSD or trauma exposure (116). Studies controlling for exposure to trauma have found that genetic factors remain contributory to PTSD independent of trauma exposure (110). A study by Amstadter et al. (10) of Norwegian twins from a national registry found that about one-third of variance in PTSD symptom liability can be attributed to familial factors, with about 80% of this variance being specific to risk for PTSD after exposure and the remaining fraction overlapping with the liability for trauma exposure.

Molecular genetic studies have generally examined candidate genes of the dopaminergic and serotonergic systems, HPA axis markers, and the adrenergic system (110). Because of the conditional nature of PTSD based on an environmental exposure (trauma), understanding its heritability requires the disentanglement of environmental and genetic factors. The conditional basis of PTSD in trauma exposure makes this disorder an ideal candidate for research on gene–environment (G×E) interactions (110). Only a few G×E studies of PTSD have been conducted (110). In a study of Florida hurricane survivors that examined the 5-HTTLPR polymorphism of the serotonin transporter SLC6A4 gene, the short (low-expression) allele variant of 5-HTTLPR increased risk relative to the long (high-expression) allele for hurricane-related PTSD, but only under conditions of high trauma exposure in the hurricane and low social support (107). A study of Rwandan refugees with severe trauma exposure and 81% meeting full criteria for PTSD found that those who were homozygous for the 5-HTTLPR short allele had 100% likelihood of PTSD regardless of the amount of trauma exposure, but risk for PTSD among carriers of the long allele was increased in proportion to the amount of trauma they had experienced (114). A study of low-income African American patients identified G×E interactions between severity of child abuse (but not adult trauma) and polymorphisms of the glucocorticoid-regulating gene FKBP5 (21).

DIFFERENTIAL DIAGNOSIS

PTSD must be differentiated from conditions that suggest or mimic it, because the appropriate response to emotional sequelae of trauma requires the selection of interventions that are appropriate to individual needs. Emotional distress, which is nearly ubiquitous in people intensely exposed to severe trauma, and may be substantial in the early post-trauma phases, must be differentiated from PTSD. Time may help to sort out immediate distress from psychopathology destined to represent PTSD. Symptoms not meeting PTSD criteria in relation to trauma may represent normal experiences, emotional distress of nondiagnostic proportion, or response to other life stressors. Symptoms in people not exposed to trauma may represent any of these or part of preexisting psychopathology or response to other stressors.

Physiological reactivity to reminders of a traumatic event and exaggerated startle responses of PTSD resemble features of panic attacks in panic disorder, including tachycardia and palpitations, sweating, and tremor. Symptoms of PTSD that also occur in generalized anxiety disorder include feeling "keyed up" or "on edge" and sleep disturbance. Symptoms of PTSD reminiscent of major depressive disorder are loss of interest, sleep disturbance, cognitive distortions regarding self-worth and guilt, psychomotor agitation, and difficulty concentrating. Some PTSD symptoms such as flashbacks and emotional numbing appear similar to dissociative syndromes, and others such as self-destructive behavior and aggression toward others suggest features of borderline personality disorder and antisocial personality disorder, respectively. A key to differentiation of posttraumatic stress symptoms from symptoms of these other disorders is the temporal and/or conceptual anchoring of the symptoms to the trauma exposure. If the symptoms were present before the trauma without significant worsening afterward, they likely represent symptoms of disorders other than PTSD related to the specific trauma. Of course, posttraumatic stress symptoms reported by people not related to a qualifying trauma exposure would not be considered contributory to a diagnosis of PTSD.

Well-known characteristics of somatization disorder and borderline personality disorder are the habitual endorsement of multiple symptoms of many psychiatric disorders by individuals who do not meet criteria for those disorders (121, 153). Patients with somatization and borderline personality disorders commonly endorse posttraumatic stress symptoms. This can result in apparent high comorbidities between these disorders and PTSD (11). Somatization and borderline personality disorders are associated with chaotic and dysfunctional family backgrounds with many opportunities for trauma exposure in childhood. These disorders are also characterized by exaggerated reporting styles and suggestibility that may provide fertile ground for elaboration of posttraumatic stress symptom complaints. For individuals with somatization or borderline personality disorder who also meet criteria for PTSD, the course of treatment of the latter disorder without recognizing the former disorders is likely to be tumultuous, complicated, and unsuccessful (15, 51, 81). However, there is evidence that provision of treatment focused on stabilizing suicidal and self-injurious behaviors of borderline personality psychopathology can promote readiness of patients with comorbid PTSD to receive and benefit from trauma-focused therapy (81).

PTSD must also be distinguished from malingering, which is well documented in association with circumstances of potential financial compensation, such as in civil litigation and disability benefits (3, 135). In these settings, the occurrence of malingering has the potential to distort academic and clinical understanding of PTSD (3). Keys to identifying malingering in patients presenting with trauma-related psychopathology such as PTSD are competent interviewing techniques, collection of various sources of collateral information, and psychometric and physiological testing (3).

CLINICAL MANAGEMENT

Both psychotherapy and pharmacotherapy are recognized as providing benefit for PTSD (68, 92, 109). Research to date has not determined whether pharmacotherapy or psychotherapy alone or in combination is superior for the treatment of PTSD (68, 89, 92, 212). Patient preference in choosing treatment as well as weighing of potential advantages and disadvantages related to different choices are important to take into account (92, 212). Some patients would prefer to avoid medications and the potential for side effects and adverse effects of pharmacotherapy (66). Other patients find that the commitment to attending multiple therapy sessions and the amount of effort and discomfort that may be involved in psychotherapy may not be most suitable for their situation. A disadvantage to pharmacotherapy for PTSD is the likelihood that the benefits of treatment will not be sustained once the medication is stopped (66).

The mainstay of pharmacotherapy for PTSD is selective serotonin reuptake inhibitors (SSRIs), including fluoxetine, sertraline, and paroxetine, and serotonin norepinephrine reuptake inhibitors (SNRIs), such as venlafaxine (92, 102, 109, 213). The only two antidepressants approved by the U.S. Food and Drug Administration (FDA) for the treatment of PTSD, however, are sertraline and paroxetine (16, 102). The older tricyclic antidepressants (TCAs), such as amitriptyline and imipramine, and monoamine oxidase inhibitors (MAOIs), including phenelzine, have also been demonstrated to have efficacy, but their less favorable side-effect and safety profiles make them unsuitable as primary agents for the treatment of PTSD (92, 102, 109). Military veterans, especially those with chronic PTSD, may be less responsive than civilians to antidepressant medications (66, 102, 212, 213).

Mood stabilizers such as carbamazepine and divalproex have garnered little evidence of efficacy for PTSD (109). Antipsychotic medications, including the atypical agent risperidone (117), have little evidence to support their use as monotherapy or adjunctive therapy for PTSD (92, 109). Benzodiazepines are not recommended for PTSD not only because they are ineffective but also because of their liability for tolerance, abuse, and dependence (92, 102, 109).

Some adjunctive medications targeting specific posttraumatic stress symptoms have been found to provide some benefit. Prazosin, an alpha-1 adrenergic antagonist, has been shown effective for reducing nightmares and sleep disturbances (92, 109). Guanfacine, an alpha-2 adrenergic agonist, has been found to dampen trauma-related noradrenergic overactivity but has not been shown to be effective for PTSD (16, 102). Propranolol, a beta-adrenergic antagonist, has been paired with memory reactivation procedures in attempts to interfere with memory reconsolidation processes theorized to contribute to posttraumatic psychopathology (48, 49, 103), but clinical trials of this agent have not demonstrated significant benefit for prevention or treatment of PTSD (102, 211).

Psychotherapies used for PTSD include both trauma-focused and non-trauma-focused approaches (212). It is unclear whether focusing on the traumatic experience is necessary for recovery from PTSD (93, 212). The best evidence for PTSD psychotherapy has been identified for trauma-focused approaches, especially prolonged exposure and cognitive therapies (17, 66, 109, 212), but this may be an artifact of the recent emphasis on funding for this research (94). Exposure therapy helps patients with their traumatic experience by having them confront it directly with controlled introduction to fear-related situations through imaginal or graded in vivo exposure to achieve desensitization or habituation to fear cues (109, 212). Cognitive therapy seeks to modify dysfunctional thoughts, beliefs, and expectations by challenging and replacing maladaptive cognitions with more realistic and helpful cognitions (109, 212). A form of cognitive therapy developed specifically for individuals exposed to trauma is cognitive processing therapy (CPT) (212). These therapies were developed for individual treatment, and their application in group therapy has not been found to be sufficiently effective (94).

Research on these trauma-focused therapies has recently been criticized for very small symptom improvement, with most patients still meeting criteria for PTSD after completing treatment (94). Another problem with current psychotherapy, particularly among military veterans with PTSD, is poor participation in psychotherapy for the disorder (94). A difficulty with the application of trauma-related therapies is that psychological stability is needed for successful participation in the therapy (109). Patients without sufficient psychological stability include individuals with prominent avoidance and numbing profiles, who may have poor tolerance of procedures involving confrontation with trauma reminders inherent in trauma-focused therapies. For these patients, preliminary application of supportive therapy and pharmacotherapy may ultimately provide the psychological stability needed for advancement to trauma-related therapies (22).

Eye movement desensitization and reprocessing (EMDR) therapy for PTSD involves patient discussion of emotionally disturbing material in conjunction with a therapist-applied external stimulus, typically maneuvers to elicit lateral eye movements (212). Although this treatment has been found effective, dismantling studies have not demonstrated the eye moments to be instrumental in the therapeutic effects. Rather, addressing the traumatic memory, cognitive processing, and rehearsal of coping and mastery skills are considered the functionally operative elements of this technique (212). Other therapies with less evidence that are used for patients with PTSD include supportive therapy, motivational interviewing (techniques aimed at reducing resistance to change), and Seeking Safety (techniques for developing skills for emotional regulation and substance abstinence) (109).

Psychological debriefing became a popular tool for post-trauma intervention around the globe, especially for employees of fire stations and hospitals, with little evidence supporting its efficacy. Psychological debriefing has not been demonstrated to prevent or treat PTSD (109). However, psychological debriefing was not designed for these purposes, but rather to provide emotional processing, education, reassurance, and social support (161). Research suggests that this intervention may actually interfere with recovery and worsen PTSD, especially among individuals with prominent avoidance and numbing profiles who may poorly tolerate shared recollections of the trauma in a group setting (109, 142). Current recommendations are that participation in debriefing interventions should not be made mandatory at workplaces, and that individuals with psychopathology should not participate in debriefing and instead be referred to formal treatment (161).

An important principle in psychiatric assessment and management of PTSD is that the disorder more often than not presents with comorbid disorders that may be at least as important as the PTSD in determining clinical outcome and choice of treatment. Therefore, clinicians should continue the search for other disorders even after considering the diagnosis of PTSD. Cases of PTSD with psychiatric comorbidity can be expected to have more severe symptoms and greater functional disability than PTSD-only cases (125, 158). Comorbid disorders can be treated in conjunction with treatment of PTSD, and many of the medications used in the treatment of PTSD are also effective for anxiety disorders and major depression that may accompany PTSD.

In the treatment of patients with psychiatric problems related to histories of childhood abuse and maltreatment, it is recommended that psychiatric disorders be diagnosed and treated in the usual manner as described in other chapters of this text. Although childhood abuse is a potentially important problem for individual patients, its recognition should not circumvent the complete assessment and treatment of psychiatric disorders and should not overshadow recognition of the multiple early background and family problems of many patients with this history. Psychotherapists are cautioned to avoid assumptions of direct causality from childhood abuse to current problems or psychiatric disorders (41, 43, 231).

REFERENCES

1. Adler, A. Neuropsychiatric complications in victims of Boston's Coconut Grove disaster. JAMA, *123*:1098–1101, 1943.

2. Afifi, T. O., Asmundson, G. J., Taylor, S., and Jang, K. L. The role of genes and environment on trauma exposure and posttraumatic stress disorder symptoms: a review of twin studies. Clin. Psychol. Rev., *30*:101–112, 2010.
3. Ali, S., Jabeen, S., and Alam, F. Multimodal approach to identifying malingered posttraumatic stress disorder: a review. Innov. Clin. Neurosci., *12*:12–20, 2015.
4. American Psychiatric Association. *Diagnostic and Statistical Manual: Mental Disorders*, 1st edition. Washington, DC: Author, 1952.
5. American Psychiatric Association. *Diagnostic and Statistical Manual of Mental Disorders*, 2nd edition. Washington, DC: Author, 1968.
6. American Psychiatric Association. *Diagnostic and Statistical Manual of Mental Disorders*, 3rd edition. Washington, DC: Author, 1980.
7. American Psychiatric Association. *Diagnostic and Statistical Manual of Mental Disorders*, 4th edition. Washington, DC: Author, 1994.
8. American Psychiatric Association. *Diagnostic and Statistical Manual of Mental Disorders*, 4th text revision edition. Washington, DC: Author, 2000.
9. American Psychiatric Association. *Diagnostic and Statistical Manual for Mental Disorders*, 5th edition. Washington, DC: Author, 2013.
10. Amstadter, A. B., Aggen, S. H., Knudsen, G. P., Reichborn-Kjennerud, T., and Kendler, K. S. A population-based study of familial and individual-specific environmental contributions to traumatic event exposure and posttraumatic stress disorder symptoms in a Norwegian twin sample. Twin Res. Hum. Genet., *15*:656–662, 2012.
11. Amstadter, A. B., Aggen, S. H., Knudsen, G. P., Reichborn-Kjennerud, T., and Kendler, K. S. Potentially traumatic event exposure, posttraumatic stress disorder, and Axis I and II comorbidity in a population-based study of Norwegian young adults. Soc. Psychiatry Psychiatr. Epidemiol., *48*:215–223, 2013.
12. Andrews, B., Brewin, C. R., Philpott, R., and Stewart, L. Delayed-onset posttraumatic stress disorder: a systematic review of the evidence. Am. J. Psychiatry, *164*:1319–1326, 2007.
13. Andrews, B., Brewin, C. R., Stewart, L., Philpott, R., and Hejdenberg, J. Comparison of immediate-onset and delayed-onset posttraumatic stress disorder in military veterans. J. Abnorm. Psychol., *118*:767–777, 2009.
14. Babinski, J., and Froment, J. *Hysteria or Pithiatism and Reflect Nervous Disorders in the Neurology of War*. London: University of London Press, 1918.
15. Becker, D. When she was bad: borderline personality disorder in a posttraumatic age. Am. J. Orthopsychiatry, *70*:422–432, 2000.
16. Belkin, M. R., and Schwartz, T. L. Alpha-2 receptor agonists for the treatment of posttraumatic stress disorder. Drugs Context, *4*:212286, 2015.
17. Benedek, D. M., Friedman, M. J., Zatzick, Z., and Ursano, R. J. Guideline watch (March 2009): practice guideline for the treatment of patients with acute stress disorder and posttraumatic stress disorder. FOCUS, *VII*:204–213, 2009.
18. Bennett, G. Bristol floods 1968: controlled survey of effects on health of local community disaster. Br. J. Med., *3*:454–458, 1970.
19. Bensheim, H. Die K.Z. Neurose rassisch Verfolgter: Ein Beitrag zur Psychopathologie der Neurosen [The concentration camp neurosis of the racially persecuted: a contribution on the psychopathology of neuroses]. Der Nervenarzt, *31*:462–469, 1960.
20. Benton, G. H. "War" neurosis and allied conditions in ex-service men: as observed in the United States Public Health Service Hospitals for Psychoneurotics. JAMA, *17*:360–365, 1931.

21. Binder, E. B., Bradley, R. G., Liu, W., Epstein, M. P., Deveau, T. C., Mercer, K. B., Tang, Y., Gillespie, C. F., Heim, C. M., Nemeroff, C. B., Schwartz, A. C., Cubells, J. F., and Ressler, K. J. Association of FKBP5 polymorphisms and childhood abuse with risk of posttraumatic stress disorder symptoms in adults. JAMA, 299:1291–1305, 2008.

22. Bisson, J. I., Ehlers, A., Matthews, R., Pilling, S., Richards, D., and Turner, S. Psychological treatments for chronic post-traumatic stress disorder. Systematic review and meta-analysis. Br. J. Psychiatry, 190:97–104, 2007.

23. Block, D. A., Silber, E., and Perry, S. E. Some factors in the emotional reaction of children to disaster. Am. J. Psychiatry, 412:416–422, 1956.

24. Boscarino, J. A., Adams, R. E., and Galea, S. Alcohol use in New York after the terrorist attacks: a study of the effects of psychological trauma on drinking behavior. Addict. Behav., 31:606–621, 2006.

25. Bowler, J. L., Bowler, M. C., and James, L. R. The cognitive underpinnings of addiction. Subst. Use Misuse, 46:1060–1071, 2011.

26. Bradford, J. M., and Bradford, E. J. Neurosis in escaped prisoners of war. Br. J. Med. Psychol., 20:422–435, 1947.

27. Bremner, J. D., Elzinga, B., Schmahl, C., and Vermetten, E. Structural and functional plasticity of the human brain in posttraumatic stress disorder. Prog. Brain Res., 167:171–186, 2008.

28. Breslau, N. Outcomes of posttraumatic stress disorder. J. Clin. Psychiatry, 62(Suppl 17):55–59, 2001.

29. Breslau, N. The epidemiology of posttraumatic stress disorder: what is the extent of the problem? J. Clin. Psychiatry, 62:16–22, 2001.

30. Breslau, N. Epidemiologic studies of trauma, posttraumatic stress disorder, and other psychiatric disorders. Can. J. Psychiatry, 47:923–929, 2002.

31. Breslau, N. The epidemiology of trauma, PTSD, and other posttrauma disorders. Trauma Violence Abuse, 10:198–210, 2009.

32. Breslau, N., Bohnert, K. M., and Koenen, K. C. The 9/11 terrorist attack and posttraumatic stress disorder revisited. J. Nerv. Ment. Dis., 198:539–543, 2010.

33. Breslau, N., Chase, G. A., and Anthony, J. C. The uniqueness of the DSM definition of post-traumatic stress disorder: implications for research. Psychol. Med., 32:573–576, 2002.

34. Breslau, N., and Davis, G. C. Posttraumatic stress disorder in an urban population of young adults: risk factors for chronicity. Am. J. Psychiatry, 149:671–675, 1992.

35. Breslau, N., Davis, G. C., and Andreski, A. Risk factors for PTSD-related traumatic events: a prospective analysis. Am. J. Psychiatry, 152:529–535, 1995.

36. Breslau, N., Davis, G. C., Andreski, P., and Peterson, E. Traumatic events and posttraumatic stress disorder in an urban population of young adults. Arch. Gen. Psychiatry, 48:216–222, 1991.

37. Breslau, N., Davis, G. C., Andreski, P., Peterson, E. L., and Schultz, L. R. Sex differences in posttraumatic stress disorder. Arch. Gen. Psychiatry, 54:1044–1048, 1997.

38. Breslau, N., Davis, G. C., Peterson, E. L., and Schultz, L. R. A second look at comorbidity in victims of trauma: the posttraumatic stress disorder-major depression connection. Biol. Psychiatry, 48:902–909, 2000.

39. Breslau, N., Davis, G. C., and Schultz, L. R. Posttraumatic stress disorder and the incidence of nicotine, alcohol, and other drug disorders in persons who have experienced trauma. Arch. Gen. Psychiatry, 60:289–294, 2003.

40. Breslau, N., Kessler, R. C., Chilcoat, H. D., Schultz, L. R., Davis, G. C., and Andreski, P. Trauma and posttraumatic stress disorder in the community: the 1996 Detroit Area Survey of Trauma. Arch. Gen. Psychiatry, 55:626–632, 1998.

41. Breslau, N., Koenen, K. C., Luo, Z., Agnew-Blais, J., Swanson, S., Houts, R. M., Poulton, R., and Moffitt, T. E. Childhood maltreatment, juvenile disorders and adult post-traumatic stress disorder: a prospective investigation. Psychol. Med., 44:1937–1945, 2014.

42. Breslau, N., Lucia, V. C., and Davis, G. C. Partial PTSD versus full PTSD: an empirical examination of associated impairment. Psychol. Med., 34:1205–1214, 2004.

43. Breslau, N., and Peterson, E. L. Assaultive violence and the risk of posttraumatic stress disorder following a subsequent trauma. Behav. Res. Ther., 48:1063–1066, 2010.

44. Breslau, N., Reboussin, B. A., Anthony, J. C., and Storr, C. L. The structure of posttraumatic stress disorder: latent class analysis in 2 community samples. Arch. Gen. Psychiatry, 62:1343–1351, 2005.

45. Breslau, N., and Schultz, L. Neuroticism and post-traumatic stress disorder: a prospective investigation. Psychol. Med., 43:1697–1702, 2013.

46. Breslau, N., Troost, J. P., Bohnert, K., and Luo, Z. Influence of predispositions on post-traumatic stress disorder: does it vary by trauma severity? Psychol. Med., 43:381–390, 2013.

47. Brewin, C. R., Andrews, B., and Valentine, J. D. Meta-analysis of risk factors for posttraumatic stress disorder in trauma-exposed adults. J. Consult. Clin. Psychol., 68:748–766, 2000.

48. Brunet, A., Poundja, J., Tremblay, J., Bui, E., Thomas, E., Orr, S. P., Azzoug, A., Birmes, P., and Pitman, R. K. Trauma reactivation under the influence of propranolol decreases posttraumatic stress symptoms and disorder: 3 open-label trials. J. Clin. Psychopharmacol., 31:547–550, 2011.

49. Brunet, A., Thomas, E., Saumier, D., Ashbaugh, A. R., Azzoug, A., Pitman, R. K., Orr, S. P., and Tremblay, J. Trauma reactivation plus propranolol is associated with durably low physiological responding during subsequent script-driven traumatic imagery. Can. J. Psychiatry, 59:228–232, 2014.

50. Bryant, R. A. Acute stress disorder as a predictor of posttraumatic stress disorder: a systematic review. J. Clin. Psychiatry, 72:233–239, 2011.

51. Classen, C. C., Pain, C., Field, N. P., and Woods, P. Posttraumatic personality disorder: a reformulation of complex posttraumatic stress disorder and borderline personality disorder. Psychiatr. Clin. North Am., 29:87–ix, 2006.

52. Culpin, M. The need for psychopathology. Lancet, 2:725–726, 1930.

53. Da Costa, J. M. On irritable heart: a clinical study of a form of functional cardiac disorder and its consequence. Am. J. Med. Sci., 11:559–567, 1951.

54. Daly, R. J. Samuel Pepys and post-traumatic stress disorder. Br. J. Psychiatry, 143:64–68, 1983.

55. Davidson, J. R. T., Hughes, D., Blazer, D. G., and George, L. K. Post-traumatic stress disorder in the community: an epidemiological study. Psychol. Med., 21:713–721, 1991.

56. Dayan, J., and Olliac, B. From hysteria and shell shock to posttraumatic stress disorder: comments on psychoanalytic and neuropsychological approaches. J. Physiol. Paris, 104:296–302, 2010.

57. Denham, R. H., and Currier, F. P. The traumatic neurosis and the relation to the surgeon. J. Mich. State Med. Soc., 23:299–303, 1924.

58. deQuervain, D., Schwabe, L., and Roozendaal, B. Stress, glucocorticoids and memory: implications for treating fear-related disorders. Nat. Rev. Neurosci., *18*:7–19, 2017.

59. DiGangi, J., Guffanti, G., McLaughlin, K. A., and Koenen, K. C. Considering trauma exposure in the context of genetics studies of posttraumatic stress disorder: a systematic review. Biol. Mood Anxiety Disord., *3*:2, 2013.

60. Dorahy, M. J., Middleton, W., Seager, L., Williams, M., and Chambers, R. Child abuse and neglect in complex dissociative disorder, abuse-related chronic PTSD and mixed psychiatric samples. J. Trauma Dissociation, *17*:223–236, 2016.

61. Edmondson, D., and von Känel, R. Post-traumatic stress disorder and cardiovascular disease. Lancet Psychiatry, *4*:320–329, 2017.

62. Ellenberger, H. F. *The Discovery of the Unconscious*. New York: Basic Books, 1970.

63. Erichsen, J. *On Concussion of the Spine: Nervous Shock and Other Obscure Injuries of the Nervous System* [reprinted in New York: William Wood; 1886, pp. 36–37]. London: Longmans, Green, 1875.

64. Fang, S. C., Schnurr, P. P., Kulish, A. L., Holowka, D. W., Marx, B. P., Keane, T. M., and Rosen, R. Psychosocial functioning and health-related quality of life associated with posttraumatic stress disorder in male and female Iraq and Afghanistan War veterans: the VALOR registry. J. Womens Health (Larchmt.), *4*:1038–1046, 2015.

65. Fischer-Homberger, E. Railway Spine and traumatische Neurose: Seele und Rückenmark [Railway Spine and traumatic neurosis: soul and spine]. Gesnerus, *27*:96–111, 1970.

66. Foa, E. B., Keane, T. M., Friedman, M. J., and Cohen, J. A. Guideline 6. Psychopharmacotherapy for adults. In *Effective Treatments for PTSD: Practice Guidelines from the International Society for Traumatic Stress Studies*, 2nd edition. New York: Guilford Press, pp. 563–567, 2009.

67. Fontana, A., and Rosenheck, R. The role of war-zone trauma and PTSD in the etiology of antisocial behavior. J. Nerv. Ment. Dis., *193*:203–209, 2005.

68. Forbes, D., Creamer, M., Bisson, J. I., Cohen, J. A., Crow, B. E., Foa, E. B., Friedman, M. J., Keane, T. M., Kudler, H. S., and Ursano, R. J. A guide to guidelines for the treatment of PTSD and related conditions. J. Trauma. Stress, *23*:537–552, 2010.

69. Freud, S. The etiology of hysteria. In *The Standard Edition of the Complete Psychological Works of Sigmund Freud, Vol. 3*, Strachey, J. (ed.). London: Hogarth Press, 1962, pp. 186–221, 1896.

70. Freud, S. My views on the part played by sexuality in the aetiology of the neuroses. In *The Standard Edition of the Complete Psychological Works of Sigmund Freud, Volume VII (1901-1905): A Case of Hysteria, Three Essays on Sexuality and Other Works*, Strachey, J. (ed.). London: Hogarth Press, 1962, pp. 269–279, 1906.

71. Friedman, P., and Linn, L. Some psychiatric notes on the Andrea Doria disaster. Am. J. Psychiatry, *114*:426–432, 1957.

72. Frueh, B. C., Smith, D. W., and Barker, S. E. Compensation seeking status and psychometric assessment of combat veterans seeking treatment for PTSD. J. Trauma. Stress, *9*:427–439, 1996.

73. Gaon, A., Kaplan, Z., Dwolatzky, T., Perry, Z., and Witztum, E. Dissociative symptoms as a consequence of traumatic experiences: the long-term effects of childhood sexual abuse. Isr. J. Psychiatry Relat. Sci., *50*:17–23, 2013.

74. Ginzburg, K., Ein-Dor, T., and Solomon, Z. Comorbidity of posttraumatic stress disorder, anxiety and depression: a 20-year longitudinal study of war veterans. J. Affect. Dis., *123*:249–257, 2010.

75. Glaesmer, H., and Braehler, E. The differential roles of trauma, posttraumatic stress disorder, and comorbid depressive disorders on suicidal ideation in the elderly population. J. Clin. Psychiatry, 73:1141–1146, 2012.

76. Goetz, J. M., Pitman, S. R., Tanev, K. S., Pitman, R. K., and Chemtob, C. M. Mixed-handedness in identical twins discordant for combat exposure in Vietnam: relationship to posttraumatic stress disorder. J. Neuropsychiatry Clin. Neurosci., 28:45–48, 2015.

77. Griffith, J. Suicide and war: the mediating effects of negative mood, posttraumatic stress disorder symptoms, and social support among army National Guard soldiers. Suicide Life Threat. Behav., 42:453–469, 2012.

78. Gros, D. F., Price, M., Magruder, K. M., and Frueh, B. C. Symptom overlap in posttraumatic stress disorder and major depression. Psychiatr. Res., 196:267–270, 2012.

79. Grubaugh, A. L., Long, M. E., Elhai, J. D., Frueh, B. C., and Magruder, K. M. An examination of the construct validity of posttraumatic stress disorder with veterans using a revised criterion set. Behav. Res. Ther., 48:909–914, 2010.

80. Hall, J. C. Medical evidence in railway accidents. Br. Med. J., i:216–217, 272–274, 325–327, 1868.

81. Harned, M. S., Jackson, S. C., Comtois, K. A., and Linehan, M. M. Dialectical behavior therapy as a precursor to PTSD treatment for suicidal and/or self-injuring women with borderline personality disorder. J. Trauma. Stress, 23:421–429, 2010.

82. Hawthorne, H. On heart disease in the army. Am. J. Med. Sci., 48:89–92, 1863.

83. Hayes, J. P., LaBar, K. S., McCarthy, G., Selgrade, E., Nasser, J., Dolcos, F., and Morey, R. A. Reduced hippocampal and amygdala activity predicts memory distortions for trauma reminders in combat-related PTSD. J. Psychiatr. Res., 45:660–669, 2011.

84. Heim, C., and Nemeroff, C. B. Neurobiology of posttraumatic stress disorder. CNS Spectr., 14:13–24, 2009.

85. Helzer, J. E., Robins, L. N., and McEvoy, L. Post-traumatic stress disorder in the general population. Findings of the Epidemiologic Catchment Area survey. N. Engl. J. Med., 317:1630–1634, 1987.

86. Heppner, P. S., Crawford, E. F., Haji, U. A., Afari, N., Hauger, R. L., Dashevsky, B. A., Horn, P. S., Nunnink, S. E., and Baker, D. G. The association of posttraumatic stress disorder and metabolic syndrome: a study of increased health risk in veterans. BMC Med., 7:1, 2009.

87. Herman, J., and van der Kolk, B. A. Traumatic antecedents of borderline personality disorder. In *Psychological Trauma*, van der Kolk, B. A. (ed.). Washington, DC: American Psychiatric Press, 1987.

88. Heron-Delaney, M., Kenardy, J., Charlton, E., and Matsuoka, Y. A systematic review of predictors of posttraumatic stress disorder (PTSD) for adult road traffic crash survivors. Injury, 44:1413–1422, 2013.

89. Hetrick, S. E., Purcell, R., Garner, B., and Parslow, R. Combined pharmacotherapy and psychological therapies for post traumatic stress disorder (PTSD). Cochrane Database Syst. Rev., 7:CD007316, 2010.

90. Hines, L. A., Sundin, J., Rona, R. J., Wessely, S., and Fear, N. T. Posttraumatic stress disorder post Iraq and Afghanistan: prevalence among military subgroups. Can. J. Psychiatry, 59:468–479, 2014.

91. Hoffman, J. Erfahrungen über die traumatische Neurose [Experiences with traumatic neurosis]. Berliner Klinische Wochenschrift, 27:655–660, 1890.

92. Hoge, C. W. Interventions for war-related posttraumatic stress disorder: meeting veterans where they are. JAMA, 306:549–551, 2011.

93. Hoge, C. W., and Chard, K. M. A window into the evolution of trauma-focused psychotherapies for posttraumatic stress disorder. JAMA, *319*:343–345, 2018.

94. Hoge, C. W., Lee, D. J., and Castro, C. A. Refining trauma-focused treatments for servicemembers and veterans with posttraumatic stress disorder: progress and ongoing challenges. JAMA Psychiatry, *74*:13–14, 2017.

95. Holbrook, T. L., Hoyt, D. B., Stein, M. B., and Sieber, W. J. Perceived threat to life predicts posttraumatic stress disorder after major trauma: risk factors and functional outcome. J. Trauma. Stress, *51*:287–292, 2001.

96. Horowitz, M. J. *Stress Response Syndromes*. New York: Jason Aronson, 1976.

97. Hyodo, K., Nakamura, K., Oyama, M., Yamazaki, O., Nakagawa, I., Ishigami, K., Tsuchiya, Y., and Yamamoto, M. Long-term suicide mortality rates decrease in men and increase in women after the Niigata-Chuetsu earthquake in Japan. Tohoku J. Exp. Med., *220*:149–155, 2010.

98. Inman, T. G. Some comparisons between war neuroses and those of civilian life. J. Calif. State Med. Soc., *18*:184–186, 1920.

99. Iversen, A. C., van, S. L., Hughes, J. H., Browne, T., Greenberg, N., Hotopf, M., Rona, R. J., Wessely, S., Thornicroft, G., and Fear, N. T. Help-seeking and receipt of treatment among UK service personnel. Br. J. Psychiatry, *197*:149–155, 2010.

100. Jakovljevic, M., Crncevic, Z., Ljubicic, D., Babic, D., Topic, R., and Saric, M. Mental disorders and metabolic syndrome: a fatamorgana or warning reality? Psychiatr. Danub., *19*:76–86, 2007.

101. Janet, P. *The Major Symptoms of Hysteria: 15 Lectures Given in the Medical School of Harvard University*. New York: Macmillan, 1907.

102. Jeffreys, M., Capehart, B., and Friedman, M. J. Pharmacotherapy for posttraumatic stress disorder: review with clinical applications. J. Rehabil. Res. Dev., *49*:703–715, 2012.

103. Kearns, M. C., Ressler, K. J., Zatzick, D., and Rothbaum, B. O. Early interventions for PTSD: a review. Depress. Anxiety, *29*:833–842, 2012.

104. Kessler, R. C., Sonnega, A., Bromet, E., Hughes, M., and Nelson, C. B. Posttraumatic stress disorder in the National Comorbidity Survey. Arch. Gen. Psychiatry, *52*:1048–1060, 1995.

105. Khantzian, E. J. The self-medication hypothesis of substance use disorders: a reconsideration and recent applications. Harv. Rev. Psychiatry, *4*:231–244, 1997.

106. Khati, I., Hours, M., Charnay, P., Chossegros, L., Tardy, H., Nhac-Vu, H. T., Boisson, D., and Laumon, B. Quality of life one year after a road accident: results from the adult ESPARR cohort. J. Trauma Acute Care Surg., *74*:301–311, 2013.

107. Kilpatrick, D. G., Koenen, K. C., Ruggiero, K. J., Acierno, R., Galea, S., Resnick, H. S., Roitzsch, J., Boyle, J., and Gelernter, J. The serotonin transporter genotype and social support and moderation of posttraumatic stress disorder and depression in hurricane-exposed adults. Am. J. Psychiatry, *164*:1693–1699, 2007.

108. Kinzie, J. D., and Goetz, R. R. A century of controversy surrounding posttraumatic stress-spectrum syndromes: the impact on DSM-III and DSM-IV. J. Trauma. Stress, *9*:159–179, 1996.

109. Kirkpatrick, H. A., and Heller, G. M. Post-traumatic stress disorder: theory and treatment update. Int. J. Psychiatry Med., *47*:337–346, 2014.

110. Koenen, K. C., Amstadter, A. B., and Nugent, N. R. Gene–environment interaction in posttraumatic stress disorder: an update. J. Trauma. Stress, *22*:416–426, 2009.

111. Koenen, K. C., Harley, R., Lyons, M. J., Wolfe, J., Simpson, J. C., Goldberg, J., Eisen, S. A., and Tsuang, M. A twin registry study of familial and individual risk

factors for trauma exposure and posttraumatic stress disorder. J. Nerv. Ment. Dis., *190*:209–218, 2002.

112. Koenen, K. C., Moffitt, T. E., Caspi, A., Gregory, A., Harrington, H., and Poulton, R. The developmental mental-disorder histories of adults with posttraumatic stress disorder: a prospective longitudinal birth cohort study. J. Abnorm. Psychol., *117*:460–466, 2008.

113. Koenen, K. C., Nugent, N. R., and Amstadter, A. B. Gene–environment interaction in posttraumatic stress disorder: review, strategy and new directions for future research. Eur. Arch. Psychiatry Clin. Neurosci., *258*:82–96, 2008.

114. Kolassa, I. T., Ertl, V., Eckart, C., Glockner, F., Kolassa, S., Papassotiropoulos, A., de Quervain, D. J., and Elbert, T. Association study of trauma load and SLC6A4 promoter polymorphism in posttraumatic stress disorder: evidence from survivors of the Rwandan genocide. J. Clin. Psychiatry, 71:543–547, 2010.

115. Kramer, S. N. A Sumerian lamentation. In *Ancient Near Eastern Texts Relating to the Old Testament*, Pritchard, J. B. (ed.). Trenton, NJ: Princeton University Press, pp. 455–463, 1969.

116. Kremen, W. S., Koenen, K. C., Afari, N., and Lyons, M. J. Twin studies of posttraumatic stress disorder: differentiating vulnerability factors from sequelae. Neuropharmacology, *62*:647–653, 2012.

117. Krystal, J. H., Rosenheck, R. A., Cramer, J. A., Vessicchio, J. C., Jones, K. M., Vertrees, J. E., Horney, R. A., Huang, G. D., and Stock, C. Adjunctive risperidone treatment for antidepressant-resistant symptoms of chronic military service-related PTSD: a randomized trial. JAMA, *306*:493–502, 2011.

118. Lamprecht, F., and Sack, M. Posttraumatic stress disorder revisited. Psychosom. Med., *64*:222–237, 2002.

119. Langdon, J. R., and Parker, A. H. Psychiatric aspects of the March 7, 1954 earthquake. Alaska Med., *6*:33–35, 1954.

120. Lee, D. J., Liverant, G. I., Lowmaster, S. E., Gradus, J. L., and Sloan, D. M. PTSD and reasons for living: associations with depressive symptoms and alcohol use. Psychiatr. Res., *219*:550–555, 2014.

121. Lenze, E. L., Miller, A., Munir, Z., Pornoppadol, C., and North, C. S. Psychiatric symptoms endorsed by somatization disorder patients in a psychiatric clinic. Ann. Clin. Psychiatry, *11*:73–79, 1999.

122. Liberzon, I., and Sripada, C. S. The functional neuroanatomy of PTSD: a critical review. Prog. Brain Res., *167*:151–169, 2008.

123. Lowe, B., Henningsen, P., and Herzog, W. Post-traumatic stress disorder: history of a politically unwanted diagnosis. Psychother. Psychosom. Med. Psychol., *56*:182–187, 2006.

124. MacKenzie, J. The soldier's heart and war neurosis: a study in symptomatology. Br. Med. J., *Part II*:530–534, 1920.

125. Maes, M., Mylle, J., Delmeire, L., and Altamura, C. Psychiatric morbidity and co-morbidity following accidental man-made traumatic events: incidence and risk factors. Eur. Arch. Psychiatry Clin. Neurosci., *250*:156–162, 2000.

126. Mahan, A. L., and Ressler, K. J. Fear conditioning, synaptic plasticity and the amygdala: implications for posttraumatic stress disorder. Trends Neurosci., *35*:24–35, 2012.

127. Mathers, A. T. The psychoneuroses in wartime. Can. Med. Assoc. J., *47*:103–111, 1942.

128. Matsubayashi, T., Sawada, Y., and Ueda, M. Natural disasters and suicide: evidence from Japan. Soc. Sci. Med., *82*:126–133, 2013.

129. McCrory, E., De Brito, S. A., and Viding, E. The link between child abuse and psychopathology: a review of neurobiological and genetic research. J. R. Soc. Med., 105:151–156, 2012.

130. McDonald, S. D., and Calhoun, P. S. The diagnostic accuracy of the PTSD checklist: a critical review. Clin. Psychol. Rev., 30:976–987, 2010.

131. McDougall, W. *Outline of Abnormal Personality*. New York: Scribner, 1926.

132. McFarlane, A. C., Browne, D., Bryant, R. A., O'Donnell, M., Silove, D., Creamer, M., and Horsley, K. A longitudinal analysis of alcohol consumption and the risk of posttraumatic symptoms. J. Affect. Dis., 118:166–172, 2009.

133. McMillen, J. C. Better for it: how people benefit from adversity. Soc. Work, 44:455–468, 1999.

134. McMillen, J. C., Smith, E. M., and Fisher, R. H. Perceived benefit and mental health after three types of disaster. J. Consult. Clin. Psychiatry, 6:733–739, 1997.

135. McNally, R. J., and Frueh, B. C. Why we should worry about malingering in the VA system: comment on Jackson et al. (2011). J. Trauma. Stress, 25:454–456, 2012.

136. Mezuk, B., Larkin, G. L., Prescott, M. R., Tracy, M., Vlahov, D., Tardiff, K., and Galea, S. The influence of a major disaster on suicide risk in the population. J. Trauma. Stress, 22:481–488, 2009.

137. Micale, M. Charcot and the idea of hysteria in the male: gender, mental science, and medical diagnosis of the late nineteenth century in France. Med. Hist., 34:363–411, 1990.

138. Moergeli, H., Wittmann, L., and Schnyder, U. Quality of life after traumatic injury: a latent trajectory modeling approach. Psychother. Psychosom., 81:305–311, 2012.

139. Moleen, G. A. Nervous disturbances as a result of injury, with special reference to the true and false traumatic neurasthenia. Colorado Med., 21:87–91, 1924.

140. Mott, F. W. *War Neurosis and Shell Shock*. London: Oxford University Press, 1919.

141. Myers, C. S. A contribution to the study of shell shock. Lancet, i:316–320, 1915.

142. Nash, W. P., and Watson, P. J. Review of VA/DOD Clinical Practice Guideline on management of acute stress and interventions to prevent posttraumatic stress disorder. J. Rehabil. Res. Dev., 49:637–648, 2012.

143. National Academy of Sciences Institute of Medicine. *Posttraumatic Stress Disorder: Diagnosis and Assessment*. Washington, DC: National Academy Press, 2006.

144. Newnham, E. A., and Janca, A. Childhood adversity and borderline personality disorder: a focus on adolescence. Curr. Opin. Psychiatry, 27:68–72, 2014.

145. Nishio, A., Akazawa, K., Shibuya, F., Abe, R., Nushida, H., Ueno, Y., Nishimura, A., and Shioiri, T. Influence on the suicide rate two years after a devastating disaster: a report from the 1995 Great Hanshin-Awaji Earthquake. Psychiatry Clin. Neurosci., 63:247–250, 2009.

146. Nock, M. K., Stein, M. B., Heeringa, S. G., Ursano, R. J., Colpe, L. J., Fullerton, C. S., Hwang, I., Naifeh, J. A., Sampson, N. A., Schoenbaum, M., Zaslavsky, A. M., and Kessler, R. C. Prevalence and correlates of suicidal behavior among soldiers: results from the Army Study to Assess Risk and Resilience in Servicemembers (Army STARRS). JAMA Psychiatry, 71:514–522, 2014.

147. Norris, F. H. Epidemiology of trauma: frequency and impact of different potentially traumatic events on different demographic groups. J. Consult. Clin. Psychol., 60:409–418, 1992.

148. Norris, F. H., Friedman, M. J., Watson, P. J., Byrne, C. M., Diaz, E., and Kaniasty, K. 60,000 disaster victims speak: part I. An empirical review of the empirical literature, 1981–2001. Psychiatry, 65:207–239, 2002.

149. North, C. S. Somatization in survivors of catastrophic trauma: a methodological review. Environ. Health Perspect., *110*:637–640, 2002.

150. North, C. S. Assessing the link between disaster exposure and mental illness. In *Mental Health in Public Health*, Cottler, L. B. (ed.). New York: Oxford University Press, pp. 104–117, 2011.

151. North, C. S. An exploration of causality in the development and timing of disaster-related PTSD. In *Psychopathology and Violence*, Widom, C. S. (ed.). New York: Oxford University Press, pp. 219–230, 2012.

152. North, C. S. Current research and recent breakthroughs on the mental health effects of disasters. Curr. Psychiatry Rep., *16*:481, 2014.

153. North, C. S. The classification of hysteria and related disorders: historical and phenomenological considerations. Behav. Sci. (Basel), *5*:496–517, 2015.

154. North, C. S., Abbacchi, A., and Cloninger, C. R. Personality and posttraumatic stress disorder among directly exposed survivors of the Oklahoma City bombing. Compr. Psychiatry, *53*:1–8, 2012.

155. North, C. S., Adinoff, B., Pollio, D. E., Kinge, S., Downs, D. L., and Pfefferbaum, B. Alcohol use disorders and drinking among survivors of the 9/11 attacks on the World Trade Center in New York City. Compr. Psychiatry, *5*:962–969, 2013.

156. North, C. S., Hong, B. A., Surís, A., and Spitznagel, E. L. Distinguishing distress and psychopathology among survivors of the Oakland/Berkeley firestorm. Psychiatry, *71*:35–45, 2008.

157. North, C. S., Kawasaki, A., Spitznagel, E. L., and Hong, B. A. The course of PTSD, major depression, substance abuse, and somatization after a natural disaster. J. Nerv. Ment. Dis., *192*:823–829, 2004.

158. North, C. S., Nixon, S. J., Shariat, S., Mallonee, S., McMillen, J. C., Spitznagel, E. L., and Smith, E. M. Psychiatric disorders among survivors of the Oklahoma City bombing. JAMA, *282*:755–762, 1999.

159. North, C. S., and Oliver, J. Analysis of the longitudinal course of PTSD in 716 survivors of 10 disasters. Soc. Psychiatry Psychiatr. Epidemiol., *48*:1189–1197, 2013.

160. North, C. S., Oliver, J., and Pandya, A. Examining a comprehensive model of disaster-related PTSD in systematically studied survivors of ten disasters. Am. J. Publ. Health, *102*:e40–e48, 2012.

161. North, C. S., and Pfefferbaum, B. Mental health response to community disasters: a systematic review. JAMA, *310*:507–518, 2013.

162. North, C. S., Pfefferbaum, B., Kawasaki, A., Lee, S., and Spitznagel, E. L. Psychosocial adjustment of directly exposed survivors 7 years after the Oklahoma City bombing. Compr. Psychiatry, *52*:1–8, 2011.

163. North, C. S., Pollio, D. E., Hong, B. A., Pandya, A., Smith, R. P., and Pfefferbaum, B. The postdisaster prevalence of major depression relative to PTSD in survivors of the 9/11 attacks on the World Trade Center selected from affected workplaces. Compr. Psychiatry, *60*:119–125, 2015.

164. North, C. S., Pollio, D. E., Smith, R. P., King, R. V., Pandya, A., Surís, A. M., Hong, B. A., Dean, D. J., Wallace, N. E., Herman, D. B., Conover, S., Susser, E., and Pfefferbaum, B. Trauma exposure and posttraumatic stress disorder among employees of New York City companies affected by the September 11, 2001 attacks on the World Trade Center. Dis. Med. Publ. Health Prep., *5*:S205–S213, 2011.

165. North, C. S., Ringwalt, C. L., Downs, D., Derzon, J., and Galvin, D. Postdisaster course of alcohol use disorders in systematically studied survivors of 10 disasters. Arch. Gen. Psychiatry, *68*:173–180, 2011.

166. North, C. S., Surís, A. M., Davis, M., and Smith, R. P. Toward validation of the diagnosis of posttraumatic stress disorder. Am. J. Psychiatry, *166*:34–41, 2009.

167. North, C. S., Surís, A. M., Smith, R. P., and King, R. V. The evolution of PTSD criteria across editions of the DSM. Ann. Clin. Psychiatry, *28*:197–208, 2016.

168. North, C. S., Tivis, L., McMillen, J. C., Pfefferbaum, B., Spitznagel, E. L., Cox, J., Nixon, S., Bunch, K. P., and Smith, E. M. Psychiatric disorders in rescue workers after the Oklahoma City bombing. Am. J. Psychiatry, *159*:857–859, 2002.

169. O'Connor, S. S., Dinsio, K., Wang, J., Russo, J., Rivara, F. P., Love, J., McFadden, C., Lapping-Carr, L., Peterson, R., and Zatzick, D. F. Correlates of suicidal ideation in physically injured trauma survivors. Suicide Life Threat. Behav., *44*:473–485, 2014.

170. Ohto, H., Maeda, M., Yabe, H., Yasumura, S., and Bromet, E. E. Suicide rates in the aftermath of the 2011 earthquake in Japan. Lancet, *385*:1727, 2015.

171. Orui, M., Harada, S., and Hayashi, M. Changes in suicide rates in disaster-stricken areas following the Great East Japan Earthquake and their effect on economic factors: an ecological study. Environ. Health Prev. Med., *19*:459–466, 2014.

172. Orui, M., Sato, Y., Tazaki, K., Kawamura, I., Harada, S., and Hayashi, M. Delayed increase in male suicide rates in tsunami disaster-stricken areas following the Great East Japan Earthquake: a three-year follow-up study in Miyagi Prefecture. Tohoku J. Exp. Med., *235*:215–222, 2015.

173. Page, H. W. *Injuries of the Spine and Spinal Cord without Apparent Mechanical Lesions and Nervous Shock in Their Surgical and Medical Legal Aspects.* London: J. A. Churchill, 1885.

174. Pagura, J., Stein, M. B., Bolton, J. M., Cox, B. J., Grant, B., and Sareen, J. Comorbidity of borderline personality disorder and posttraumatic stress disorder in the U.S. population. J. Psychiatr. Res., *44*:1190–1198, 2010.

175. Panagioti, M., Gooding, P. A., and Tarrier, N. A meta-analysis of the association between posttraumatic stress disorder and suicidality: the role of comorbid depression. Compr. Psychiatry, *53*:915–930, 2012.

176. Pfefferbaum, B., and Doughty, D. E. Increased alcohol use in a treatment sample of Oklahoma City bombing victims. Psychiatry, *64*:296–303, 2001.

177. Pompili, M., Sher, L., Serafini, G., Forte, A., Innamorati, M., Dominici, G., Lester, D., Amore, M., and Girardi, P. Posttraumatic stress disorder and suicide risk among veterans: a literature review. J. Nerv. Ment. Dis., *201*:802–812, 2013.

178. Pratchett, L. C., Pelcovitz, M. R., and Yehuda, R. Trauma and violence: are women the weaker sex? Psychiatr. Clin. North Am., *33*:465–474, 2010.

179. Price, M., and van Stolk-Cooke, K. Examination of the interrelations between the factors of PTSD, major depression, and generalized anxiety disorder in a heterogeneous trauma-exposed sample using DSM-5 criteria. J. Affect. Dis., *186*:149–155, 2015.

180. Pridemore, W. A., Trahan, A., and Chamlin, M. B. No evidence of suicide increase following terrorist attacks in the United States: an interrupted time-series analysis of September 11 and Oklahoma City. Suicide Life Threat. Behav., *39*:659–670, 2009.

181. Putnam, J. J. Recent investigation into the so-called concussion of the spine. Med. Surg. J., *109*:217–220, 1883.

182. Raja, M., Onofri, A., Azzoni, A., Borzellino, B., and Melchiorre, N. Post-traumatic stress disorder among people exposed to the Ventotene street disaster in Rome. Clin. Pract. Epidemol. Ment. Health, *4*:5, 2008.

183. Ramsawh, H. J., Fullerton, C. S., Mash, H. B., Ng, T. H., Kessler, R. C., Stein, M. B., and Ursano, R. J. Risk for suicidal behaviors associated with PTSD, depression, and their comorbidity in the U.S. Army. J. Affect. Dis., *161*:116–122, 2014.

184. Regier, D. A., Narrow, W. E., Clarke, D. E., Kraemer, H. C., Kuramoto, S. J., Kuhl, E. A., and Kupfer, D. J. DSM-5 field trials in the United States and Canada, Part II: test-retest reliability of selected categorical diagnoses. Am. J. Psychiatry, *170*:59–70, 2013.

185. Richardson, J. D., St Cyr, K. C., McIntyre-Smith, A. M., Haslam, D., Elhai, J. D., and Sareen, J. Examining the association between psychiatric illness and suicidal ideation in a sample of treatment-seeking Canadian peacekeeping and combat veterans with posttraumatic stress disorder PTSD. Can. J. Psychiatry, *57*:496–504, 2012.

186. Richardson, L. K., Frueh, B. C., and Acierno, R. Prevalence estimates of combat-related post-traumatic stress disorder: critical review. Aust. N. Z. J. Psychiatry, *44*:4–19, 2010.

187. Roberts, A. L., Gilman, S. E., Breslau, J., Breslau, N., and Koenen, K. C. Race/ethnic differences in exposure to traumatic events, development of post-traumatic stress disorder, and treatment-seeking for post-traumatic stress disorder in the United States. Psychol. Med., *41*:71–83, 2011.

188. Roberts, N. P., Roberts, P. A., Jones, N., and Bisson, J. I. Psychological interventions for post-traumatic stress disorder and comorbid substance use disorder: a systematic review and meta-analysis. Clin. Psychol. Rev., *38*:25–38, 2015.

189. Robins, E., and Guze, S. B. Establishment of diagnostic validity in psychiatric illness: its application to schizophrenia. Am. J. Psychiatry, *126*:983–987, 1970.

190. Robins, L. N. Steps toward evaluating post-traumatic stress reaction as a psychiatric disorder. J. Appl. Soc. Psychol., *20*:1674–1677, 1990.

191. Robins, L. N., and Regier, D. A. *Psychiatric Disorders in America: The Epidemiologic Catchment Area Study*. New York: The Free Press, 1991.

192. Rojas, S. M., Bujarski, S., Babson, K. A., Dutton, C. E., and Feldner, M. T. Understanding PTSD comorbidity and suicidal behavior: associations among histories of alcohol dependence, major depressive disorder, and suicidal ideation and attempts. J. Anxiety Disord., *28*:318–325, 2014.

193. Rosen, G. M., and Lilienfeld, S. O. Posttraumatic stress disorder: an empirical evaluation of core assumptions. Clin. Psychol. Rev., *28*:837–868, 2008.

194. Rosenbaum, S., Stubbs, B., Ward, P. B., Steel, Z., Lederman, O., and Vancampfort, D. The prevalence and risk of metabolic syndrome and its components among people with posttraumatic stress disorder: a systematic review and meta-analysis. Metabolism, *64*:926–933, 2015.

195. Rougemont-Bucking, A., Linnman, C., Zeffiro, T. A., Zeidan, M. A., Lebron-Milad, K., Rodriguez-Romaguera, J., Rauch, S. L., Pitman, R. K., and Milad, M. R. Altered processing of contextual information during fear extinction in PTSD: an fMRI study. CNS Neurosci. Ther., *17*:227–236, 2011.

196. Ruglass, L. M., Lopez-Castro, T., Cheref, S., Papini, S., and Hien, D. A. At the crossroads: the intersection of substance use disorders, anxiety disorders, and posttraumatic stress disorder. Curr. Psychiatry Rep., *16*:505, 2014.

197. Runnals, J. J., Garovoy, N., McCutcheon, S. J., Robbins, A. T., Mann-Wrobel, M. C., and Elliott, A. Systematic review of women veterans' mental health. Womens Health Issues, *24*:485–502, 2014.

198. Samuels, J. Personality disorders: epidemiology and public health issues. Int. Rev. Psychiatry, *23*:223–233, 2011.

199. Sareen, J. Posttraumatic stress disorder in adults: impact, comorbidity, risk factors, and treatment. Can. J. Psychiatry, 59:460–467, 2014.

200. Sartor, C. E., Grant, J. D., Lynskey, M. T., McCutcheon, V. V., Waldron, M., Statham, D. J., Bucholz, K. K., Madden, P. A., Heath, A. C., Martin, N. G., and Nelson, E. C. Common heritable contributions to low-risk trauma, high-risk trauma, posttraumatic stress disorder, and major depression. Arch. Gen. Psychiatry, 69:293–299, 2012.

201. Schlenger, W. E., Caddell, J. M., Ebert, L., Jordan, B. K., Rourke, K. M., Wilson, D., Thalji, L., Dennis, J. M., Fairbank, J. A., and Kulka, R. A. Psychological reactions to terrorist attacks: findings from the National Study of Americans' Reactions to September 11. JAMA, 288:581–588, 2002.

202. Schuster, M. A., Stein, B. D., Jaycox, L., Collins, R. L., Marshall, G. N., Elliott, M. N., Zhou, A. J., Kanouse, D. E., Morrison, J. L., and Berry, S. H. A national survey of stress reactions after the September 11, 2001, terrorist attacks. N. Engl. J. Med., 345:1507–1512, 2001.

203. Selye, H., and Fortier, C. Adaptive reaction to stress. Psychosomat. Med., 12:149–157, 1950.

204. Shay, J. Learning about combat stress through Homer's *Iliad*. J. Trauma. Stress, 4:561–579, 1991.

205. Sher, L., Braquehais, M. D., and Casas, M. Posttraumatic stress disorder, depression, and suicide in veterans. Cleve. Clin. J. Med., 79:92–97, 2012.

206. Silver, R. C., Holman, E. A., McIntosh, D. N., Poulin, M., and Gil-Rivas, V. Nationwide longitudinal study of psychological responses to September 11. JAMA, 288:1235–1244, 2002.

207. Skey, F. C. Compensation for railway injuries. Lancet, ii:161–163, 1865.

208. Sparr, L. F. Legal aspects of posttraumatic stress disorder, uses and abuses. In *Posttraumatic Stress Disorder: Etiology, Phenomenology, and Treatment*, Wolfe, M. E., Mosniam, A. D. (eds.). Washington, DC: American Psychiatric Press, 1990.

209. Spiegel, D. Multiple personality as a post-traumatic stress disorder. Psychiatr. Clin. North Am., 7:101–110, 1984.

210. Spitzer, R. L., First, M. B., and Wakefield, J. C. Saving PTSD from itself in DSM-V. J. Anxiety Disord., 21:233–241, 2007.

211. Steenen, S. A., van Wijk, A. J., van der Heijden, G. J., van Westrhenen, R., de Lange, J., and de Jongh, A. Propranolol for the treatment of anxiety disorders: systematic review and meta-analysis. J. Psychopharmacol., 30:128–139, 2016.

212. Steenkamp, M. M., Litz, B. T., Hoge, C. W., and Marmar, C. R. Psychotherapy for military-related PTSD: a review of randomized clinical trials. JAMA, 314:489–500, 2015.

213. Stein, D. J., Ipser, J., and McAnda, N. Pharmacotherapy of posttraumatic stress disorder: a review of meta-analyses and treatment guidelines. CNS Spectr., 14:25–31, 2009.

214. Stierlin, E. Nervöse und psychische Störungen nach Katastrophen [Nervous and psychological disturbances following catastrophes]. Deutsche Medizinische Wochenschrift, 37:2028–2035, 1911.

215. Stinson, B. Battle fatigue and how it was treated in the Civil War. Civil War Times Illustrated, 4:40–44, 1965.

216. Straif-Bourgeois, S., and Ratard, R. Suicide mortality rates in Louisiana, 1999-2010. J. La. State Med. Soc., 164:274–6, 2012.

217. Stratta, P., and Rossi, A. Suicide in the aftermath of the L'Aquila (Italy) earthquake. Crisis, *34*:142–144, 2013.
218. Surís, A., Link-Malcolm, J., and North, C. S. Predictors of suicidal ideation in veterans with PTSD related to military sexual trauma. J. Trauma. Stress, *24*:605–608, 2011.
219. Surís, A., Smith, J., Powell, C., and North, C. S. Interfering with the reconsolidation of traumatic memory: sirolimus as a novel agent for treating veterans with posttraumatic stress disorder. Ann. Clin. Psychiatry, *25*:33–40, 2013.
220. Triantafyllou, D., North, C. S., Zartman, A., and Roediger, H. L., III. A Deese-Roediger-McDermott study of trauma memory among employees of New York City companies affected by the September 11, 2001, attacks. Ann. Clin. Psychiatry, *27*:165–174, 2015.
221. Trimble, M. R. *Post-traumatic Neurosis from Railway Spine to Whiplash*. Chichester, England: Wiley and Sons, 1981.
222. Ullman, S. E., Filipas, H. H., Townsend, S. M., and Starzynski, L. L. Trauma exposure, posttraumatic stress disorder and problem drinking in sexual assault survivors. J. Stud. Alcohol, *66*:610–619, 2005.
223. Utzon-Frank, N., Breinegaard, N., Bertelsen, M., Borritz, M., Eller, N. H., Nordentoft, M., Olesen, K., Rod, N. H., Rugulies, R., and Bonde, J. P. Occurrence of delayed-onset post-traumatic stress disorder: a systematic review and meta-analysis of prospective studies. Scand. J. Work Environ. Health, *40*:215–229, 2014.
224. van der Kolk, B., and van der Hart, O. Pierre Janet and the breakdown of adaptation in psychological trauma. Am. J. Psychiatry, *146*:1530–1540, 1989.
225. Violanti, J. M., Fekedulegn, D., Hartley, T. A., Andrew, M. E., Charles, L. E., Mnatsakanova, A., and Burchfiel, C. M. Police trauma and cardiovascular disease: association between PTSD symptoms and metabolic syndrome. Int. J. Emerg. Ment. Health, *8*:227–237, 2006.
226. Vlahov, D., Galea, S., Ahern, J., Resnick, H., and Kilpatrick, D. Sustained increased consumption of cigarettes, alcohol, and marijuana among Manhattan residents after September 11, 2001. Am. J. Publ. Health, *94*:253–254, 2004.
227. Vlahov, D., Galea, S., Resnick, H., Ahern, J., Boscarino, J. A., Bucavalas, M., Gold, J., and Kilpatrick, D. Increased use of cigarettes, alcohol, and marijuana among Manhattan, New York, residents after the September 11th terrorist attacks. Am. J. Epidemiol., *155*:988–996, 2002.
228. Westphal, M., Olfson, M., Gameroff, M. J., Wickramaratne, P., Pilowsky, D. J., Neugebauer, R., Lantigua, R., Shea, S., and Neria, Y. Functional impairment in adults with past posttraumatic stress disorder: findings from primary care. Depress. Anxiety, *28*:686–695, 2011.
229. Whiles, H. A study of neurosis among repatriated prisoners of war. Br. Med. J., *2*:697–698, 1945.
230. Whitman, J. B., North, C. S., Downs, D. L., and Spitznagel, E. L. A prospective study of the onset of PTSD symptoms in the first month after trauma exposure. Ann. Clin. Psychiatry, *25*:163–172, 2013.
231. Widom, C. S., and Czaja, S. J. Childhood trauma, psychopathology, and violence: disentangling causes, consequences, and correlates. In *Trauma, Psychopathology, and Violence: Causes, Consequences, or Correlations?*, Widom, C. S. (ed.). New York: Oxford University Press, pp. 291–317, 2012.
232. Yehuda, R., and LeDoux, J. Response variation following trauma: a translational neuroscience approach to understanding PTSD. Neuron, *56*:19–32, 2007.

233. Yoon, S. J., Jun, C. S., An, H. Y., Kang, H. R., and Jun, T. Y. Patterns of temperament and character in patients with posttraumatic stress disorder and their association with symptom severity. Compr. Psychiatry, *50*:226–231, 2009.

234. Zanarini, M. C., Frankenburg, F. R., Jager-Hyman, S., Reich, D. B., and Fitzmaurice, G. The course of dissociation for patients with borderline personality disorder and Axis II comparison subjects: a 10-year follow-up study. Acta Psychiatr. Scand., *118*:291–296, 2008.

CHAPTER 6

cℳɔ

Obsessive-Compulsive Disorder

Obsessions are persistent distressing thoughts, images, or impulses experienced as unwanted and senseless but irresistible. *Compulsions* are repetitive behaviors aimed to prevent or reduce anxiety or distress but not to provide pleasure or gratification. Obsessive-compulsive disorder (OCD) is a chronic illness dominated by obsessions and compulsions occurring in the absence of another psychiatric disorder. "Obsessional neurosis" was a synonym in vogue before *DSM-III* was published in 1980.

HISTORICAL BACKGROUND

The term "obsessional neurosis" apparently originated with Karl Westphal (1833–1890), a German neurologist who wrote about obsessional conditions and phobias. Kraepelin described obsessional neurosis (*Zwangsneurose*) in his textbooks in the early part of the twentieth century, and the same term was adopted by Freud, whose classical description of the clinical picture, published in 1917 (p. 229) (36), follows:

> The obsessional neurosis takes this form: the patient's mind is occupied with thoughts that do not really interest him, he feels impulses which seem alien to him, and he is impelled to perform actions which not only afford him no pleasure but from which he is powerless to desist. The thoughts (obsessions) may be meaningless in themselves or only of no interest to the patient; they are often only absolutely silly.

Recognition of obsessional traits, however, substantially antedated psychiatrists' description of the syndrome. In the early seventeenth century Richard Flecknoe, in discussing "enigmaticall characters," described one such character as an "irresolute Person" (pp. 70–71) (32):

> He hovers in his choice just like an empty ballance without any weight of judgement to incline him to either Scale. Everything he thinks on, is matter of deliberation and he does nothing readily, but what he thinks not on . . . when he begins to consider once, never makes an end. He ha's some dull *Daemon* in him cryes *do not, do not* still, when he is going to do anything . . . . He playes at *shall I, shall I?* so long, till opportunity of doing it be past; and then . . . he repents at leisure.

In the seventeenth century, obsessions were often referred to as "scruples," defined by Jeremy A. Taylor (pp. 262–263) (121) as

> a great trouble of mind preceding from a little motive, and a great indisposition, by which the conscience though sufficiently determined by proper arguments, dares not proceed to action, or if it do, it cannot rest . . . some persons dare not eat for fear of gluttony, they fear that they shall sleep too much, and that keeps them waking, and troubles their heads more and then their scruples increase . . . . When they are married they are afraid to do their duty, for fear it be secretly an indulgence to the flesh, and be to be suspected of carnality, and yet they dare not omit it, for fear they should be unjust, and yet their fear that the very fearing it to be unclean should be a sin, and suspect that if they do not fear so, it is too great a sign they adhere to nature more than to the spirit . . . . Scruple is a little stone in the foot, if you set it upon the ground it hurts you; if you hold it up you cannot go forward; it is a trouble where the trouble is over, a doubt when doubts are resolved . . . very often it hath no reason at all for its inducement.

The content of obsessions, today as in years past, is often religious. In his treatise *Of Religious Melancholy* (80), published in 1692, John Moore described (pp. 208–210) such obsessions as follows: "Naughty, and sometimes Blasphemous thoughts start up in their Minds, while they are exercised in the worship of God [despite] all their Endeavors to stifle and suppress them." In fact, he wrote, "the more they struggle with them, the more they increase." Bishop Moore had difficulty understanding this state as the sufferers were "mostly good People," whereas "bad men . . . rarely know any Thing of these kinds of Thoughts." Like others, he argued that this was good reason "to judge them to be Distempers of the Body rather than Faults of the Mind" (pp. 208–210). He was particularly concerned about the phobic avoidances that could result from such obsessions and wrote, "I exhort you not to quit your Employment ... for no business at all, is as bad for you as too much: and there is always more Melancholy to be found in a Cloyster, than in the Marketplace" (p. 215).

The obsessional fear of suffering from syphilis was also well recognized as a manifestation of mental illness by the clergy and later by psychiatrists. In the past, the word *superstition* was often used to describe obsessive behaviors by today's conventions. Samuel Johnson apparently had this in mind when he wrote that "the superstitious are often melancholic, and the melancholic almost always superstitious" (p. 373) (63). As will be noted later, obsessions are common in depressive states and vice versa.

EPIDEMIOLOGY

Obsessive-compulsive disorder was once considered rare, but studies in the mid-1980s suggested that the disorder may affect 2% of the general population, making it one of the more common forms of serious psycho-pathology (64, 102, 104). Comparison of prevalence rates of OCD in seven countries found the rates to be remarkably consistent, falling in the 1%–2% range (99). Subsequent studies have continued to find OCD in the 2% range (110), which verges on 30 years of a stable finding. Only a small proportion of OCD patients visit psychiatrists. Less than 5% of psychiatric inpatients and outpatients receive the diagnosis. Primary care settings see this disorder at much lower frequency than population studies suggest (125). According to some studies, OCD occurs more frequently in women than in men (9, 102). When compared with all other psychiatric patients, those with OCD reportedly differ in the following ways: 1) they belong to higher social classes, 2) they make higher scores on intelligence tests, and 3) they have a higher educational level (53, 73, 102, 109).

CLINICAL PICTURE

When medical attention is finally sought for OCD (often years after the illness began), it may be because of depression, acute anxiety, exacerbation of obsessions, or social incapacity resulting from any of these conditions (14, 72, 97). The onset of symptoms often seems associated with a life event: the death of a relative, a sexual conflict, overwork, or pregnancy (53, 73). Just as often, however, no precipitating factors can be identified.

Common presenting complaints are the obsessional fears of contamination or injuring oneself or another person, often a child or close relative. Fearful of losing control, these patients may develop avoidances or rituals that lead in turn to social incapacity. They may refuse to leave the house and may avoid sharp objects or may wash repeatedly.

On reflection, they may identify the obsessional idea as illogical, but not always. Sometimes the ideas are not, strictly speaking, illogical (e.g., germs do produce disease) and sometimes, even when obviously absurd, the ideas are not viewed as such. What distinguishes an obsession from a delusion is not so much insight (recognizing the idea's absurdity) as the person's struggle against the obsessional experience itself. Individuals with the disorder strive to free themselves from the obsession but cannot, and feel increasingly uncomfortable until the idea temporarily runs its course or the compulsive act has been completed (72).

The frequency of obsessional symptoms in patients with OCD has been studied systematically by many groups, and their results indicate that the illness may assume one or more of the following forms (1, 27, 65):

> *Obsessional ideas:* Thoughts that repetitively intrude into consciousness (words, phrases, rhymes) and interfere with the normal train of thought, causing distress to the person. Often the thoughts are obscene, blasphemous, or nonsensical.
>
> *Obsessional images:* Vividly imagined scenes, often of a violent, sexual, or disgusting nature (images of a child being killed, cars colliding, excrement, parents having sexual intercourse) that repeatedly come to mind.
>
> *Obsessional convictions:* Notions that are often based on the magical formula of thought equals act: "Thinking ill of my son will cause him to die." Unlike delusions, obsessional beliefs are characterized by ambivalence: The person believes and simultaneously does not believe. As Jaspers expressed it, there is a "constant going on between a consciousness of validity and nonvalidity. Both push this way and that, but neither can gain the upper hand" (59).
>
> *Obsessional rumination:* Prolonged, inconclusive thinking about a subject to the exclusion of other interests. The subject is often religion or metaphysics—why and wherefore questions that are as unanswerable, as they are endlessly ponderable. Indecisiveness in ordinary matters is very common: "Which necktie should I wear?" Doubt may lead to extremes in caution, both irksome and irresistible. "Did I turn off the gas?" "Lock the door?" "Write the correct

address?" The individual checks and rechecks, stopping only when exhausted or on checking a predetermined "magical" number of times. Several studies suggest that obsessional doubts—*manie du doute*—may well be the most prominent feature in obsessive-compulsive illness (1, 27, 113). As with other obsessions, ruminations are resisted. The person tries to turn his or her attention elsewhere, but cannot; often the more he or she tries, the more intrusive and distressing the thoughts become.

Obsessional impulses: Typically relates to self-injury (leaping from a window); injury to others (smothering an infant); or embarrassing behavior (shouting obscenities in church).

Obsessional fears: Often of dirt, disease, contamination; of potential weapons (razors, scissors); of being in specific situations or performing particular acts.

Obsessional rituals (compulsions): Repetitive, stereotyped acts of counting, touching, arranging objects, moving, washing, tasting, looking in specific ways. Compulsions may be inseparable from obsessions. About one-quarter of patients display no compulsions (1).

Counting rituals are especially common. The person feels compelled to count letters or words or the squares in a tile floor or to perform arithmetical operations. Certain numbers, or their multiples, may have special significance (the person "must" lay down her pencil three times or step on every fifth sidewalk crack). Other rituals concern the performance of excretory functions and such everyday acts as preparing to go to bed. Also common are rituals involving extremes of cleanliness (handwashing compulsions, relentless emptying of wastebaskets) and complicated routines assuring orderliness and punctuality. Women apparently have a higher prevalence of contamination phobia and of compulsive cleaning behavior than men (27).

According to a study of patients with OCD (14), four kinds of rituals occur most frequently: counting, checking, cleaning, and avoidance rituals. Each occurred in half of the patients. Avoidance rituals were similar to those seen in phobic disorders (see "Differential Diagnosis" section in this chapter). An example can be seen in a patient who avoided anything colored brown. Her inability to approach brown objects greatly limited her activities.

Other less common rituals include slowing, striving for completeness, and extreme meticulousness. With slowing, such simple tasks as buttoning a shirt or tying a shoelace might take up to 15 minutes. Striving for completeness may be seen in dressing also. Asked why he spends so much time with a single button, the patient might reply that he was trying to prove to himself that he had "buttoned the button properly."

A common form of pathological meticulousness is a concern that objects be arranged in a special way. Pencils, for example, may have to be arranged so that the points are directed away from the person. Students may spend so much time arranging pencils, pens, erasers, and so on that they cannot do their work.

Rituals, ridiculous as they may seem to the person, are accompanied by a profound dread and apprehension that assures their performance because they alone give relief. "I'll explode if I don't do it," a patient may say. Occasional patients believe that failure to perform a given ritual will result in harm to themselves or others; often the ritual is as inexplicable to patients as it is to observers.

Obsessional symptoms often are accompanied by a dysphoric mood. The patient may be irritable, tense, or depressed. This may lead to an erroneous diagnosis of a mood disorder because the mood element at the time of examination may overshadow the obsessional content.

Obsessional symptoms rarely occur singly (69). As with most psychiatric illnesses, obsessional disorder presents as a cluster of symptoms that, individually, are variable and inconstant over time but as a group maintain characteristics unique to the illness. Thus a patient may now have one set of obsessional impulses, fears, and rituals and later another set, but the symptoms remain predominantly obsessional.

> R. J. obsessed so much about eating contaminated food that he was 30 pounds underweight. He worried so much that he might gun the accelerator and run people over at an intersection that he always put the car in park. He was so compulsive that he copied serial numbers off dollar bills and dressed and undressed so many times in the morning that it was noon before he was ready to go to work as a school custodian.

Occasionally, however, a single obsession dominates the clinical picture:

> A 35-year-old banker, P. T. had an obsession concerning the length of his trousers. He would buy a pair of trousers but fail to convince himself that they were the correct length. He would then go back to the tailor repeatedly to have them adjusted—returning as many as a dozen times and stopping only when his embarrassment became acute as the tailor became more frustrated. Then he would adjust the length himself. He would stand endlessly before mirrors, trying to decide whether the length was correct. Whenever he crossed his leg and the pant

was hiked up, showing a part of his sock, he worried that there was too much sock showing or too little. Again he would alter the pants.

The obsession made him miserable. He could not concentrate on his work. He repeatedly asked fellow employees whether they thought his pants were too long or too short and was convinced that they thought he was crazy (which perhaps they did). He had legitimate fears of losing his position at the bank. He started staying home more and more, hating himself for succumbing to what he recognized was a foolish fear. But he could not stop the fear. It came to occupy most of his waking hours as he altered between studying the pant leg to see if it should be a millimeter shorter or longer and castigating himself for being a weak and feckless fellow in worrying about such matters.

Although P. T. had mild-to-moderate symptoms of depression, the obsession dominated his clinical picture. It had begun in his early 20s and had persisted more or less intensely since then. He had no other obsessions.

BIOLOGICAL FINDINGS

Neuroimaging studies, including both structural (computed tomography [CT], magnetic resonance imaging [MRI], and voxel-based morphometry) and functional (positron emission tomography [PET], single photon emission computed tomography [SPECT], functional-magnetic resonance imagining [fMRI]) as well as newer techniques (magnetic resonance spectroscope [MRS], diffusion tensor imaging [DTI], near infrared spectroscopy [NIRS], and magnetoencephalography [MEG]) have produced inconsistent results (89). The usual issues of small sample size, mixed samples (diagnoses), treatment, age, and severity of illness prevent confident convergence of findings to allow either causal inference or biological marker.

NATURAL HISTORY

The onset of obsessive-compulsive illness is usually before age 25 (10). The median age of onset in one study (102) was 23, and clear-cut obsessional symptoms often develop by age 15. The illness may begin as early as age 6. Fewer than 15% of cases begin after age 35 (33, 53, 69, 86).

Though the mean age of onset of symptoms is roughly 20 in both sexes, the first psychiatric contact is made on average about 7 years later. If hospitalized, most patients are in their 30s by the time they enter a hospital, and hospitalization for the first time after age 40 is rare (40).

The mode of onset may be acute or insidious (69). The course of the disorder may be unremitting (with or without social incapacity), episodic, or characterized by incomplete remissions that permit normal social functioning.

In one outpatient study, the majority of patients had episodic courses with exacerbations that usually lasted less than a year (97). Most investigators who study patients requiring hospitalization, however, have found the course to be steady, with exacerbations often attributed to fatigue or medical illness and with a tendency for the severity of the illness to wane gradually over many years (53, 73).

Patients with mild obsessional symptoms requiring only outpatient therapy appear to have a rather good prognosis; as many as 60%–80% are asymptomatic or improved 1–5 years after diagnosis (59, 97). The prognosis is not as good for hospitalized patients, who comprise a more severely ill group. One-third or fewer are improved symptomatically on reexamination several years after discharge; two-thirds or more, however, are functioning as well socially as before hospitalization (53, 69). Between 5% and 10% of clear-cut cases of OCD do have a course marked by progressive social incapacity (100). Favorable prognosis is reported to be associated with three factors: 1) mild or atypical symptoms, including predominance of phobic-ruminative ideas and absence of compulsions (53, 69); 2) short duration of symptoms before treatment is begun (97); and 3) good premorbid personality without childhood symptoms or abnormal personality traits (69, 70).

COMPLICATIONS

Depression—often indistinguishable symptomatically from depression diagnosed as major depressive disorder—is probably the most common complication of obsessional disorder. Failure to marry also may be a complication of OCD. Additionally, those who marry appear to be more likely than married people in the general population to experience substantial marital maladjustment (19, 77). Further, fertility rates appear to be reduced among people with OCD (88). Despite the frequency with which suicide may figure in obsessional thinking (44, 53), completed suicide is rare in these patients, less than 1%.

Patients with OCD sometimes fear they will injure someone by an impulsive act. They fear they will lose control in some manner and embarrass themselves. They worry about becoming addicted to drugs prescribed by their physician. These fears are generally unwarranted (21). There is little evidence that OCD predisposes to homicide, criminal behavior, alcoholism, or drug addiction (53, 69).

Finally, people with OCD may fear they will "lose" their minds, become totally disabled, or need chronic hospitalization. None of these events is a common complication of OCD. If schizophrenia is clearly ruled out at the beginning, schizophrenia probably develops in these individuals no more often than in anyone else. Patients with OCD infrequently become totally disabled, and they usually do not require long-term hospitalization (44, 53, 97).

FAMILY AND GENETIC STUDIES

Initial family studies of OCD were limited by substantial methodological difficulties, but they suggested a greater frequency of obsessional illness in families of OCD patients than in families of other patients or the general population (10, 56). Additional studies (82, 92) have strongly supported the familial nature of OCD. There is also substantial evidence of a link to Tourette syndrome (60, 71, 93). About half of people with Tourette syndrome also have obsessive-compulsive symptoms. In one study, relatives of patients with Tourette syndrome had an increased rate of OCD, regardless of whether the Tourette probands had OCD symptoms. Surprisingly, no increase in other anxiety disorders was found among the family members of Tourette patients (93). The association between OCD and Tourette syndrome is firmly established, but family studies of the disorders yield conflicting results.

Studies of twins with obsessional illness indicate that monozygotic twins are more concordant for OCD than dizygotic twins (55, 102). About 80%–90% of monozygotic twins are concordant for OCD compared to a concordance rate in dizygotic twins of no more than 50% and probably much lower (16, 54). Later studies have indeed found somewhat lower concordance. This does not prove the existence of genetic factors in obsessional illness; all of the twin pairs were raised together and identical twins may emulate each other more than fraternal twins. Unfortunately, there have been no published adoption studies. Of note, in instances where twins have little contact, environmental explanations seem implausible, as illustrated by the following case histories adapted from a published report (78).

The "W" twins. Jean, a housewife, developed her symptoms at age 24 when she acquired a fear of contamination by dirt with severe washing and cleansing rituals. At the time of her referral for hospitalization 3 years later she was washing her hands between 60 and 80 times per day, spending 12 hours a day cleaning and disinfecting her house, and using up to 20 quarts of liquid disinfectant a week. Her daughter, aged 2.5 years, was not toilet trained and was restricted to one room of the house in order to avoid spread of contamination, and her husband had been obliged to give up sports for fear that his soiled sports clothes would introduce dirt to their home. When she was admitted to the hospital, the skin on her hands was roughened, red, cracked, and bleeding.

Jill, the co-twin, a social worker, developed her symptoms at age 22 when she and Jean were leading separate lives and had little contact with each other. Her traits of neatness and cleanliness became more pronounced, and she developed rituals concerned with washing up the dishes and utensils, which had to be started immediately when a meal was finished; any delay resulted in severe anxiety. The washing of the dishes and utensils had to proceed in a specific order, and failure to comply with the routine, or an attempt by others to relieve her of her task, provoked great discomfort. She attempted to resist carrying out her rituals, which she considered silly and unnecessary, but the time spent on them increased and interfered with her social life.

Their father, a retired clerk, was fastidiously neat and orderly in his habits, but neither he nor other family members had received psychiatric treatment. The twins' early development and childhood were unremarkable, and at school both did well academically. They attended separate universities. Both were normally outgoing and sociable and both had personality traits of orderliness, determination, and conscientiousness. Neither had suffered any previous illness and they only learned of their similar obsessional problems after Jean began treatment.

The "K" twins. Linda, a secretary, began having obsessional thoughts at age 25 when she felt envious of a roommate who had formed a close relationship with a man. Aware of her envy and associated guilt, she began to think of imaginary pleasant scenes of herself with her friend, but within a few weeks these thoughts became recurrent, intrusive, difficult to resist, and were no longer associated with relief of unpleasant feelings. Obsessional thoughts troubled her to a varying degree for several years, with exacerbations during times of stress or unhappiness. Often she would have to repeat a conversation in her mind and, if interrupted before it was completed, she felt bound to repeat the whole conversation again. Sometimes she was compelled to touch an object to signify completion of an obsessional thought and this sometimes had a magical aspect; for example, if the object was a clock, the numbers indicating the time became her "lucky numbers" for the rest of the day.

Ann, the co-twin, an actress, also developed obsessional thoughts in her mid-20s. She was not in regular contact with Linda at this time, and only years later learned of her similar difficulties. Ann also used "good thoughts" to counter anxiety, which was usually caused by parental disapproval of her career. The thoughts soon developed an obsessional quality and were associated with compulsive behavior. For example, if a "bad thought" occurred to her while speaking on the telephone, after the call ended she felt compelled to repeat the conversation and create "good thoughts." If she passed a shop window and could not recall its contents, she would have to go back and check them. She also spent hours arranging clothing in her wardrobe according to the color or type of garment. Although she considered her obsessions to be irrational, any attempts to resist them gave rise to the fears of impending disaster.

The father was an accountant described as being "compulsively neat." Their mother had older twin sisters who both had a lifelong phobia of birds.

As noted, twin and family studies strongly implicate a genetic etiology for OCD (3, 81, 115). Few details of the genetic nature of this disorder have been elucidated (90), and no specific genes (or alleles) for OCD have been identified (81). Multiple new molecular genetic methodologies, including segregation analysis, linkage analyses, and association studies, have been applied in attempts to map (with replication) the heritability of OCD (3, 15, 25, 41, 46, 81, 127) with very limited success.

DIFFERENTIAL DIAGNOSIS

Obsessions occur in children, in healthy adults, and in patients with a variety of psychiatric and medical illnesses. The rituals and superstitions of children—avoidance of sidewalk cracks, insistence on a given routine, carrying of amulets and charms—may resemble the compulsive acts of OCD, but with a difference: Children usually do not complain about these acts, which seem natural to them and produce little distress. Further, obsessional children do not view the behavior as unreasonable.

Only a small proportion of children manifesting obsessional behavior can be classified by usual standards as having an obsessional disorder. It is not known whether children who are exceptionally ritualistic and superstitious have a greater risk of developing OCD than their less obsessional peers.

Many adults with OCD give a history of obsessional symptoms in childhood (40, 73, 109), but the commonness of such symptoms and

the influence of retrospective distortion make such data hard to interpret. Adults with OCD commonly cite phobias and rituals as childhood
symptoms (53, 69, 73). They rarely give a history of stealing, truancy, or
tantrums in childhood (69, 73).

Obsessional personality, currently termed "obsessive-compulsive personality disorder" (OCPD) in *DSM-5*, remains more a description than a diagnosis. People with OCPD are punctual, orderly, scrupulous, meticulous,
and dependable. They are seen as rigid, stubborn, pedantic, and something
of a bore. They have trouble making up their minds, but once their minds
are made up, they are single-minded and obstinate (78). Complaints about
the OCPD label have focused on a lack of core symptoms (49), Shea and
colleagues (114) showed that almost 60% of individuals diagnosed with
OCPD on a structured diagnostic interview using *DSM-IV* criteria no longer
met the diagnosis 12 months later.

Many individuals with OCD have obsessional personalities antedating
the illness (69, 97, 109), although one study (10) found no relationship
between OCD and obsessional personality. The proportion of patients with
obsessional personalities who develop OCD, depression, or other psychiatric illness is not known.

Phobias are commonly associated with OCD, and many patients with
OCD have anxiety symptoms. Obsessional phobias have a compulsive
quality and are almost always accompanied by rituals as well as other obsessional phenomena (69). The phobias of phobic disorders, by contrast,
are characterized primarily by simple avoidance of the anxiety-provoking
object or situation.

Obsessions and depression occur together so commonly that discriminating symptom from illness may be difficult. The difficulty is
compounded by the fact that people with OCD may develop depressive
symptoms as florid as those seen in major depression or bipolar illness.
During the depression the obsessional symptoms may remain unchanged,
worsen, or disappear. Similarly, after the depression lifts, the obsessions
may be worse, better, or unchanged (the last being the most common
outcome) (38).

Episodes of depression, in a substantial number of cases, are
accompanied by obsessions (38). These are usually ruminative in nature,
characterized by guilt and self-deprecation, and mild by comparison with
the depressed mood. In more atypical depressions, however, obsessions
may dominate the picture. According to one study, one-third of patients
with major depression have obsessional personality traits premorbidly and
during remissions (72). Obsessional traits apparently precede depression
as often as they precede OCD (72).

OCD in some instances may be as cyclical as bipolar disorder, with alternating remissions and exacerbations having no apparent relation to life events (53, 73, 97). The episodicity may suggest a mood disorder. Some clinicians treat patients with cyclical obsessions as if they had depressive illness, that is, with antidepressant drugs or electrotherapy.

In distinguishing between OCD and major depressive disorder, the following points may be helpful: Compared with patients with major depression and bipolar disorder who have obsessional symptoms, OCD patients who develop a depression do so at an earlier age, have more depressive episodes in their history, exhibit obsessional symptoms episodically during each depression, have a lower rate of attempted suicide, and lack a history of mania (38).

Family history is of diagnostic value when it includes clear-cut depressive episodes, mania, suicide, or alcoholism, which are found more regularly in the families of patients with major depression than in the families of patients with any other illness (126).

Mistaking OCD for schizophrenia is not unusual, especially in the early stages of the illness. Error may arise from difficulty in distinguishing obsessions from delusions and from equating bizarreness or disablement with schizophrenia. Early onset and insidious development are common in both illnesses.

Schizophrenia is characterized by delusions, hallucinations, and *formal* thought disorder (*form* referring to the flow and connections of thought). Obsessive-compulsive disorder is primarily a disorder of thought *content*. The speech of patients with OCD is understandable; only their ideas are weird. The fact that people with OCD recognize their ideas are weird is one of the chief distinctions between OCD and schizophrenia. According to one study, obsessions occur in schizophrenia in about 3% of cases, usually early in the course and almost always in the paranoid type (119). When obsessions and schizophrenia symptoms occur together, schizophrenia is usually the appropriate diagnosis.

Obsessions have been observed in the following medical conditions: encephalitis lethargia, especially during oculogyric crises; early stages of dementia; post-encephalitic states; hearing loss with tinnitus; and hypothyroidism (40). Each of these conditions may be accompanied by the sense that one's mind is working independently, that it is not an integrated part of oneself (72), and by repetitive behavior resembling compulsions. However, the "forced thinking" and "organic orderliness" (39) occasionally observed in brain-damaged patients are said to be less well organized than those that occur in OCD, and they also lack the sense of internal compulsion that distinguishes OCD.

The hallmarks of acute of chronic brain syndromes—confusion, disorientation, memory loss—are not seen in OCD. Their presence makes the diagnosis comparatively simple. Past history; neurological examination; blood, urine, and spinal fluid studies; plus special imaging techniques help establish the specific cause.

CLINICAL MANAGEMENT

The data on OCD justify a certain measure of optimism about its natural course. Spontaneous improvement often occurs, and the patient can be informed of this. Patients can be reassured that their impulses to commit injury or socially embarrassing acts almost certainly will not be carried out and that they will not—as they often fear—lose their mind. Persons who need to be hospitalized can be assured that the hospitalization is unlikely to be a long one.

OCD is rarely helped by psychotherapy alone. "Insight" therapy may even be contraindicated. A quote by Noonan (83) as cited by Salzman and Thaler (p. 290) (111) indicates that "a searching, interpretive, in-depth approach in many instances facilitates an introspective obsessive stance" (75). Pessimism about psychotherapy for OCD is reflected by the scarcity of quality research testing its efficacy.

Over the last 50 years four major treatments (and neurosurgery) have emerged as offering substantial effectiveness for OCD: clomipramine, selective serotonin-reuptake inhibitors (SSRSs), and two behavioral therapeutic approaches. The gold standard for treatment of obsessional illness has been clomipramine, which was identified in 1967 (30) and consistently found to be effective in randomized controlled trials (4, 5, 57, 75, 122). Clomipramine structurally is considered a tricyclic antidepressant but it is also a serotonin-norepinephrine reuptake inhibitor (SNRI). Use of this medication has been limited by its side-effect profile (anticholinergic, antihistaminic, and anti-alpha-1 adrenergic effects) and potential lethality in overdose. While speculation abounds, the mechanism of action in OCD remains unknown. Many other medications have been tried over time, including other tricyclic antidepressants, antipsychotic medications (described later), monoamine oxidase inhibitors (MAOIs), and lysergic diethyl amide (LSD-25) (58) without noted success in large-scale or replication studies.

Introduction of the SSRIs, beginning in the 1980s, allowed a focus on the role of serotonin in OCD. Multiple SSRIs, including fluoxetine, fluvoxamine, sertraline, paroxetine, citalopram, and escitalopram, have been studied for treatment of OCD. Reviews of SSRI treatment studies have consistently revealed that 40%–70% of OCD patients have a significant response to their first SSRI treatment (61, 95, 101, 117). Noteworthy also are the limited side-effect profiles and general acceptance of the SSRIs. The mechanism of action for these medications remains unclear. Studies of blood serotonin concentration in OCD patients have produced mixed results, one (45) showing that OCD patients had *higher* pretreatment blood levels of serotonin than controls. This contradicts the idea that the mechanism of action of SSRIs is to *increase* serotonin levels. Imaging studies suggest that SSRIs may normalize cerebral metabolism, said to be subnormal in OCD (8, 120). Although OCD patients respond to SSRIs, the improvement usually does not include complete remission (18, 101), supporting the need for conjunctive (or alternative) therapies as well as adjunctive approaches. Pharmacological response includes reduction in the frequency of symptoms and an improvement in quality of life. Discontinuation of the medication can result in relapse (18, 86, 91, 103).

The third and fourth major interventions involve behavior therapy. According to learning theory, obsessional thoughts are conditioned responses paired to an anxiety-provoking stimulus. Compulsions are established when the individual discovers that the compulsive act reduces the anxiety attendant on obsessional thought. The reduction in anxiety reinforces the compulsive act.

The techniques of behavior therapy are manifold, but their application to OCD usually involves a single principle: The patient must be exposed to the fear-inducing stimulus. After repeated exposure and refraining from the compulsion it presents, the fear disappears because, at bottom, it is unfounded. As fear subsides, so do the obsessions and compulsions. The various techniques for achieving this goal bear such names as desensitization, implosion, paradoxical intention, operant shaping, and cognitive rehearsal (6, 17, 20, 29, 33, 62). Meyer (79) is generally credited as being the first to use lengthy exposure (EX) to distressing situations and objects coupled with strict ritual prevention (RP).

Many studies indicate that behavior therapy (particularly with EX/RP) produces relief from compulsive rituals in many patients; the relief is maintained for at least 2–3 years following treatment (76, 118). Behavior therapy may take up to 30 sessions in the therapist's office plus self-exposure homework, sometimes with relatives cooperating as exposure cotherapists. Unfortunately, some patients are too apprehensive to submit to such an ordeal. Others are too depressed. A pure cognitive component (fourth intervention) is sometimes added to challenge the false beliefs, thereby reducing relapse by supporting the patient.

Given the failure of any one single agent or intervention to provide complete sustained responses, the last two decades have witnessed substantial efforts to clarify and offer guidance through systematic reviews and meta-analyses of the recommended treatments (clomipramine, SSRIs, exposure and cognitive behavioral therapies) (66, 87, 106, 107, 116) as well as publication of guidelines (67, 68, 85, 108). Although the guidelines overlap, their focus not surprisingly differs somewhat. Additionally, in response to the incomplete and unsatisfactory symptom suppression (or treatment refractoriness), there has been a drive to develop pharmacological augmentation strategies.

Benzodiazepines relieve anxiety associated with obsessions and are often instituted at the outset of treatment before other pharmacological and behavioral interventions are in place. As opposed to clomipramine and the SSRIs, the benzodiazepines do not reduce obsessional thinking, and their combination with SSRIs has not been shown to enhance response long term compared with placebo (23, 51). Use of benzodiazepines, particularly chronically, must also be tempered with potential for physiological dependence that reduces the anti-anxiety effect and risks associated with frank withdrawal.

Augmentation of OCD pharmacotherapy with an antipsychotic agent has become one of the most common approaches to OCD symptom reduction. Meta-analyses (11, 26) support this approach, with no particular agent (typical or atypical) being advanced. If no improvement is obtained after an adequate trial, significant consideration should be given to discontinuing the antipsychotic medication because of the significant risks of metabolic syndrome (50) and tardive dyskinesia, among others.

In summary, the literature clearly indicates that behavior therapy (exposure therapy with relapse prevention) is the most effective treatment for compulsive rituals and that one older and the newer antidepressants (with or without augmentation for treatment resistance) are helpful for treating obsessions and compulsions. Behavior therapy has one distinct advantage over medications: The improvement persists after the treatment ends. Studies continue to agree that clomipramine and the SSRIs are effective only while the medication is being taken.

Commonplace in psychiatry have been trials of repurposing agents from other areas of medicine, including attempts to augment treatment for OCD (and other psychiatric illnesses). Most have established safety with some early evidence of success in open or small trials including N-acetylcysteine (94), memantine (37), ondansetron (48), celecoxib (112), lamotrigine (13), riluzole (28, 96), and ketamine (12, 105).

Electroconvulsive therapy (ECT) has been tried in OCD with historically generally poor outcomes. However, two studies reported somewhat favorable results. One study (109) suggested that ECT is less effective for depression if comorbid OCD is present. In this series, half the patients with OCD who received ECT improved and half did not. The second study (74) reported cautious positive findings in the treatment of OCD with (and without) depression. A systematic review in 2015 (34) reported on collected case reports/series (no randomized controlled trials identified), finding a significantly positive response (greater than 60% in 265 cases), particularly in those with later onset of the illness, no depression, and severe OCD.

Other brain stimulation techniques continue to be evaluated for treatment of refractory OCD, such as vagal nerve stimulation, transcranial magnetic stimulation (TMS), and deep brain stimulation (24, 42, 52, 98). Early findings were mixed. Small sample sizes and difficulties in methodological design have limited available data addressing the effectiveness of these techniques, which are not approved for treatment of OCD by the Food and Drug Administration (FDA) (24). However, the FDA in 2009 granted a humanitarian device exemption (35) for a neuromodulation device that was regarded as somewhat controversial (31). Recent systematic reviews with meta-analyses (2, 124) have reported TMS as superior to sham in OCD, but larger sample sizes in controlled trials remain necessary.

Several follow-up studies (7, 22, 43, 47, 123) have indicated that various neurosurgical procedures (anterior cingulotomy, limbic leucotomy, anterior capsulotomy, or subcaudate tractotomy) produce symptomatic improvement in OCD superior to that which occurs spontaneously. The individual surgical procedures have recently been reviewed (43).

Efforts recently have progressed in earnest to establish an international consensus guideline for the neurosurgical approach to psychiatric illness (84). Even so, there is general agreement that, if used at all, surgical intervention should be reserved for those severely ill with OCD who have failed all reasonable treatments and are totally disabled by the disease.

REFERENCES

1. Akhtar, S., Wig, N. N., Varma, V. K., Pershad, D., and Verma, S. K. A phenomenological analysis of symptoms in obsessive-compulsive neurosis. Br. J. Psychiatry, *127*:342–348, 1975.
2. Alonso, P., Cuadras, D., Gabriels, L., Denys, D., Goodman, W., Greenberg, B. D., Jimenez-Ponce, F., Kuhn, J., Lenartz, D., Mallet, L., Nuttin, B., Real, E., Segalas, C., Schuurman, R., du Montcel, S. T., and Menchon, J. M. Deep brain stimulation for obsessive-compulsive disorder: a meta-analysis of treatment outcome and predictors of response. PLoS One, *10*:e0133591, 2015.

3. Alsobrook II, J. P., Leckman, J. F., Goodman, W. K., Rasmussen, S. A., and Pauls, D. L. Segregation analysis of obsessive-compulsive disorder using symptom-based factor scores. Am. J. Med. Genet., 88:669–675, 1999.

4. Ananth, J. Clomipramine in obsessive-compulsive disorder: a review. Psychosomatics, 24:723–727, 1983.

5. Ananth, J., Pecknold, J. C., Van Den Steen, M., and Engelsmann, F. Double-blind comparative study of clomipramine and amitriptyline in obsessive neurosis. Prog. Neuropsychopharmacol., 5:257–262, 1981.

6. Baer, L. Behavior therapy for obsessive compulsive disorder in the office-based practice. J. Clin. Psychiatry, 54(Suppl):15, 30, 1993.

7. Baer, L., Rauch, S. L., Ballantine, Jr. T., Martuza, R., Cosgrove, R., Cassem, E., Giriunas, I., Manzo, P. A., Dimino, C., and Jenike, M. A. Cingulotomy for intractable obsessive-compulsive disorder. Arch. Gen. Psychiatry, 52:384–394, 1995.

8. Baxter Jr, L. R., Schwartz, J. M., Bergman, K. S., Szuba, M. P., Guze, B. H., Mazziotta, J. C., Alazraki, A., Selin, C. E., Ferng, H.-K., Munford, P., and Phelps, M. E. Caudate glucose metabolic rate changes with both drug and behavior therapy for obsessive-compulsive disorder. Arch. Gen. Psychiatry, 49:681–689, 1992.

9. Bebbington, P. E. Epidemiology of obsessive-compulsive disorder. Br. J. Psychiatry, 173:2–6, 1998.

10. Black, D. W., Noyes Jr, R., Pfohl, B., Goldstein, R. B., and Blum, N. Personality disorder in obsessive-compulsive volunteers, well comparison subjects, and their first-degree relatives. Am. J. Psychiatry, 150:1226–1232, 1993.

11. Bloch, M. H., Landeros-Weisenberger, A., Kelmendi, B., Coric, V., Bracken, M. B., and Leckman, J. F. A systematic review: antipsychotic augmentation with treatment refractory obsessive-compulsive disorder. Mol. Psychiatry, 11:622–632, 2006.

12. Bloch, M. H., Wasylink, S., Landeros-Weisenberger, A., Panza, K. E., Billingslea, E., Leckman, J. F., Krystal, J. H., Bhagwagar, Z., Sanacora, G., and Pittenger, C. Effects of ketamine in treatment-refractory obsessive-compulsive disorder. Biol. Psychiatry, 72:964–970, 2012.

13. Bruno, A., Mico, U., Pandolfo, G., Mallamace, D., Abenavoli, E., Di, N. F., D'Arrigo, C., Spina, E., Zoccali, R. A., and Muscatello, M. R. Lamotrigine augmentation of serotonin reuptake inhibitors in treatment-resistant obsessive-compulsive disorder: a double-blind, placebo-controlled study. J. Psychopharmacol., 26:1456–1462, 2012.

14. Burke, K. C., Burke Jr, J. D., Regier, D. A., and Rae, D. S. Age at onset of selected mental disorders in five community populations. Arch. Gen. Psychiatry, 47:511–518, 1990.

15. Camarena, B., Aguilar, A., Loyzaga, C., and Nicolini, H. A family-based association study of the 5-HT-1Dbeta receptor gene in obsessive-compulsive disorder. Int. J. Neuropsychopharmacol., 7:49–53, 2004.

16. Carey, G., and Gottesman, I. I. Twin and family studies of anxiety, phobic, and obsessive disorders. In *Anxiety: New Research and Changing Concepts*, Klein, D. F., Rabkin, J. G. (eds.). New York: Raven, pp. 117–136, 1981.

17. Carney, R. M. Behavior therapy and the anxiety disorders: some conceptual and methodological issues. Psychiatr. Dev., 3:65–81, 1985.

18. Catapano, F., Perris, F., Masella, M., Rossano, F., Cigliano, M., Magliano, L., and Maj, M. Obsessive-compulsive disorder: a 3-year prospective follow-up study of patients treated with serotonin reuptake inhibitors OCD follow-up study. J. Psychiatr. Res., 40:502–510, 2006.

19. Cillicilli, A. S., Telcioglu, M., Askin, R., Kaya, N., Bodur, S., and Kucur, R. Twelve-month prevalence of obsessive-compulsive disorder in Konya, Turkey. Compr. Psychiatry, 45:367–374, 2004.

20. Cobb, J. Behaviour therapy in phobic and obsessional disorders. Psychiatr. Dev., 1:361–365, 1983.

21. Coryell, W. Obsessive-compulsive disorder and primary unipolar depression: comparisons of background, family history, course, and mortality. J. Nerv. Ment. Dis., 169:220–224, 1981.

22. Cosgrove, G. R., and Rauch, S. L. Psychosurgery. Neurosurg. Clin. N. Am., 6:167–176, 1995.

23. Crockett, B. A., Churchill, E., and Davidson, J. R. A double-blind combination study of clonazepam with sertraline in obsessive-compulsive disorder. Ann. Clin. Psychiatry, 16:127–132, 2004.

24. Dell'Osso, B., Altamura, A. C., Allen, A., and Hollander, E. Brain stimulation techniques in the treatment of obsessive-compulsive disorder: current and future directions. CNS Spectr., 10:966–979, 983, 2005.

25. Dickel, D. E., Veenstra-VanderWeele, J., Bivens, N. C., Wu, X., Fischer, D. J., Etten-Lee, M., Himle, J. A., Leventhal, B. L., Cook, E. H., Jr., and Hanna, G. L. Association studies of serotonin system candidate genes in early-onset obsessive-compulsive disorder. Biol. Psychiatry, 61:322–329, 2007.

26. Dold, M., Aigner, M., Lanzenberger, R., and Kasper, S. Antipsychotic augmentation of serotonin reuptake inhibitors in treatment-resistant obsessive-compulsive disorder: an update meta-analysis of double-blind, randomized, placebo-controlled rrials. Int. J. Neuropsychopharmacol., 18, 2015.

27. Dowson, J. The phenomenology of severe obsessive-compulsive neurosis. Br. J. Psychiatry, 131:75–78, 1977.

28. Emamzadehfard, S., Kamaloo, A., Paydary, K., Ahmadipour, A., Zeinoddini, A., Ghaleiha, A., Mohammadinejad, P., Zeinoddini, A., and Akhondzadeh, S. Riluzole in augmentation of fluvoxamine for moderate to severe obsessive-compulsive disorder: randomized, double-blind, placebo-controlled study. Psychiatry Clin. Neurosci., 70:332–341, 2016.

29. Fals-Stewart, W., Marks, A. P., and Schafer, J. A comparison of behavioral group therapy and individual behavior therapy in treating obsessive-compulsive disorder. J. Nerv. Ment. Dis., 181:189–193, 1993.

30. Fernandez, C. E., and Lopez-Ibor, A. J. Use of monochlorimipramine in psychiatric patients who are resistant to other therapy. Actas Luso. Esp. Neurol. Psiquiatr., 26:119–147, 1967.

31. Fins, J. J., Mayberg, H. S., Nuttin, B., Kubu, C. S., Galert, T., Sturm, V., Stoppenbrink, K., Merkel, R., and Schlaepfer, T. E. Misuse of the FDA's humanitarian device exemption in deep brain stimulation for obsessive-compulsive disorder. Health Aff. (Millwood), 30:302–311, 2011.

32. Flecknoe, R. *Rich. Flecknoe's œnigmatical characters being rather a new work, than new impression of the old*. London: R. Wood, 1665.

33. Foa, E. B., Steketee, G. S., and Ozarow, B. J. Behavior therapy with obsessive-compulsives: from theory to treatment. In *Obsessive-Compulsive Disorders: Psychological and Pharmacological Treatments*, Mavissakalian, M. (ed.). New York: Plenum, pp. 49–129, 1985.

34. Fontenelle, L. F., Coutinho, E. S., Lins-Martins, N. M., Fitzgerald, P. B., Fujiwara, H., and Yucel, M. Electroconvulsive therapy for obsessive-compulsive disorder: a systematic review. J. Clin. Psychiatry, 76:949–957, 2015.

35. Food and Drug Administration. Letter to Patrick C. Johnson, Medtronic Neuromodulation, from Donna-Bea Tillman, director, Office of Device Evaluation. Silver Spring, MD: Centers for Device and Radiologic Health, 2009.

36. Freud, S. *A General Introduction to Psycho-analysis*, Riviere, J. (trans.). New York: Liveright, 1937.

37. Ghaleiha, A., Entezari, N., Modabbernia, A., Najand, B., Askari, N., Tabrizi, M., Ashrafi, M., Hajiaghaee, R., and Akhondzadeh, S. Memantine add-on in moderate to severe obsessive-compulsive disorder: randomized double-blind placebo-controlled study. J. Psychiatr. Res., 47:175–180, 2013.

38. Gittelson, N. L. The phenomenology of obsessions in depressive psychosis. Br. J. Psychiatry, 112:261–264, 1966.

39. Goldstein, K. *After Effects of Brain Injuries in War. Their Evaluation and Treatment.* New York: Grune & Stratton, 1942.

40. Goodwin, D. W., Guze, S. B., and Robins, E. Follow-up studies in obsessional neurosis. Arch. Gen. Psychiatry, 20:182–187, 1969.

41. Grados, M. A., Walkup, J., and Walford, S. Genetics of obsessive-compulsive disorders: new findings and challenges. Brain Dev., 25(*Suppl* 1):S55–S61, 2003.

42. Greenberg, B. D., Malone, D. A., Friehs, G. M., Rezai, A. R., Kubu, C. S., Malloy, P. F., Salloway, S. P., Okun, M. S., Goodman, W. K., and Rasmussen, S. A. Three-year outcomes in deep brain stimulation for highly resistant obsessive-compulsive disorder. Neuropsychopharmacology, 31:2384–2393, 2006.

43. Greenberg, B. D., Rauch, S. L., and Haber, S. N. Invasive circuitry-based neurotherapeutics: stereotactic ablation and deep brain stimulation for OCD. Neuropsychopharmacology, 35:317–336, 2010.

44. Grimshaw, L. The outcome of obsessional disorder: a follow-up study of 100 cases. Br. J. Psychiatry, 111:1051–1056, 1965.

45. Hanna, G. L., Yuwiler, A., and Cantwell, D. P. Whole blood serotonin in juvenile obsessive-compulsive disorder. Biol. Psychiatry, 29:738–744, 1991.

46. Hasler, G., Kazuba, D., and Murphy, D. L. Factor analysis of obsessive-compulsive disorder YBOCS-SC symptoms and association with 5-HTTLPR SERT polymorphism. Am. J. Med. Genet. B Neuropsychiatr. Genet., 141:403–408, 2006.

47. Hay, P., Sachdev, P., Cumming, S., Smith, J. S., Lee, T., Kitchener, P., and Matheson, J. Treatment of obsessive-compulsive disorder by psychosurgery. Acta Psychiatr. Scand., 87:197–207, 1993.

48. Heidari, M., Zarei, M., Hosseini, S. M., Taghvaei, R., Maleki, H., Tabrizi, M., Fallah, J., and Akhondzadeh, S. Ondansetron or placebo in the augmentation of fluvoxamine response over 8 weeks in obsessive-compulsive disorder. Int. Clin. Psychopharmacol., 29:344–350, 2014.

49. Hertlet, S. C. Understanding obsessive-compulsive personality disorder. SAGE Open, 3, 2013.

50. Hirschtritt, M. E., Bloch, M. H., and Mathews, C. A. Obsessive-compulsive disorder: advances in diagnosis and treatment. JAMA, 317:1358–1367, 2017.

51. Hollander, E., Kaplan, A., and Stahl, S. M. A double-blind, placebo-controlled trial of clonazepam in obsessive-compulsive disorder. World J. Biol. Psychiatry, 4:30–34, 2003.

52. Husted, D. S., and Shapira, N. A. A review of the treatment for refractory obsessive-compulsive disorder: from medicine to deep brain stimulation. CNS Spectr., 9:833–847, 2004.

53. Ingram, I. M. Obsessional illness in mental hospital patients. J. Ment. Sci., 107:382–402, 1961.
54. Inouye, E. Similarity and dissimilarity of schizophrenia in twins. In *Proceedings of the 3rd World Congress on Psychiatry*. Montreal: University of Toronto Press, 1963.
55. Insel, T. R. Similar and dissimilar manifestations of obsessive-compulsive neurosis in monozygotic twins. Am. J. Psychiatry, 131:1171–1175, 1965.
56. Insel, T. R. Obsessive-compulsive disorder. Psychiatr. Clin. North Am., 8:105–117, 1985.
57. Insel, T. R., Murphy, D. L., Cohen, R. M., Alterman, I., Kilts, C., and Linnoila, M. Obsessive-compulsive disorder: a double-blind trial of clomipramine and clorgyline. Arch. Gen. Psychiatry, 40:605–612, 1983.
58. Insel, T. R., and Winslow, J. T. Neurobiology of obsessive compulsive disorder. Psychiatr. Clin. North Am., 15:813–824, 1992.
59. Jaspers, K. *General Psychopathology*. Chicago: University of Chicago Press, 1963.
60. Jenike, M. A. Obsessive compulsive disorder: a question of a neurologic lesion. Compr. Psychiatry, 25:298–304, 1984.
61. Jenike, M. A., Baer, L., Minichiello, W. E. (eds.). *Obsessive-Compulsive Disorders: Practical Management*, 3rd edition. St. Louis: Mosby, 1998.
62. Jenike, M. A., and Rausch, S. L. Managing the patient with treatment-resistant obsessive compulsive disorder: current strategies. J. Clin. Psychiatry, 55(Suppl):11–17, 1994.
63. Johnson, S. In *Johnson: Select Works*, Milnes, A. (ed.). London: Oxford, 1879.
64. Karno, M., Golding, J. M., Sorenson, S. B., and Burnam, M. A. The epidemiology of obsessive-compulsive disorder in five US communities. Arch. Gen. Psychiatry, 45:1094–1099, 1988.
65. Khanna, S., and Channabasavanna, S. M. Phenomenology of obsessions in obsessive-compulsive neurosis. Psychopathology, 21:12–18, 1988.
66. Kobak, K. A., Greist, J. H., Jefferson, J. W., Katzelnick, D. J., and Henk, H. J. Behavioral versus pharmacological treatments of obsessive compulsive disorder: a meta-analysis. Psychopharmacology (Berl)., 136:205–216, 1998.
67. Koran, L., and Simpson, H. Guideline Watch (March 2013): Practice Guideline for the Treatment of Patients with Obsessive Compulsive Disorder. Arlington, VA: American Psychiatric Association, 2013.
68. Koran, L. M., Hanna, G. L., Hollander, E., Nestadt, G., and Simpson, H. B. Practice guideline for the treatment of patients with obsessive-compulsive disorder. Am. J. Psychiatry, 164:5–53, 2007.
69. Kringlen, E. Obsessional neurotics: a long-term follow-up. Br. J. Psychiatry, 111:709–722, 1965.
70. Langfeldt, G. Studier av Tvangsfernomenenes forelomist, genese, klinik og prognose. Norsk Laegeforen, 13:822–850, 1938.
71. Leckman, J. F., and Cohen, D. J. Recent advances in Gilles de la Tourette syndrome: implications of clinical practice and future research. Psychiatr. Dev., 1:301–316, 1983.
72. Lewis, A. J. Problems of obsessional illness. Proc. R. Soc. Med., 29:325–336, 1936.
73. Lo, W. H. A follow-up study of obsessional neurotics in Hong Kong Chinese. Br. J. Psychiatry, 113:823–832, 1967.
74. Maletzky, B., McFarland, B., and Burt, A. Refractory obsessive compulsive disorder and ECT. Convuls. Ther., 10:34–42, 1994.
75. Marks, I. M. Review of behavioral psychotherapy, I: obsessive-compulsive disorders. Am. J. Psychiatry, 138:584–592, 1981.

76. Marks, I. M., Hodgson, R., and Rachman, S. Treatment of chronic obsessive-compulsive neurosis by in-vivo exposure. A two-year follow-up and issues in treatment. Br. J. Psychiatry, *127*:349–364, 1975.

77. Matsunaga, H., Kiriike, N., Matsui, T., Miyata, A., Iwasaki, Y., Fujimoto, K., Kasai, S., and Kojima, M. Gender differences in social and interpersonal features and personality disorders among Japanese patients with obsessive-compulsive disorder. Compr. Psychiatry, *41*:266–272, 2000.

78. McGuffin, P., and Mawson, D. Obsessive-compulsive neurosis: two identical twin pairs. Br. J. Psychiatry, *137*:285–287, 1980.

79. Meyer, V. Modification of expectations in cases with obsessional rituals. Behav. Res. Ther., *4*:273–280, 1966.

80. Moore, J. Of religious melancholy: a sermon preach'd before the Queen at Whitehall, March the 6th, 1692. In *Three Hundred Years of Psychiatry, 1535-1860* (orig. pub. 1692), Hunter, D., Malcalpine, I. (eds.). Cambridge, UK: Cambridge University Press, ch. VI, pp. 193–222, 1963.

81. Nestadt, G., Lan, T., Samuels, J., Riddle, M., Bienvenu, O. J., III, Liang, K. Y., Hoehn-Saric, R., Cullen, B., Grados, M., Beaty, T. H., and Shugart, Y. Y. Complex segregation analysis provides compelling evidence for a major gene underlying obsessive-compulsive disorder and for heterogeneity by sex. Am. J. Hum. Genet., *67*:1611–1616, 2000.

82. Nestadt, G., Samuels, J., Riddle, M., Bienvenu III, J., Liang, K.-Y., LaBuda, M., Walkup, J., Grados, M., and Hoehn-Saric, R. A family study of obsessive-compulsive disorder. Arch. Gen. Psychiatry, *57*:358–363, 2000.

83. Noonan, J. R. An obsessive-compulsive reaction treated by induced anxiety. Am. J. Psychother., *25*:293–299, 1971.

84. Nuttin, B., Wu, H., Mayberg, H., Hariz, M., Gabriels, L., Galert, T., Merkel, R., Kubu, C., Vilela-Filho, O., Matthews, K., Taira, T., Lozano, A. M., Schechtmann, G., Doshi, P., Broggi, G., Regis, J., Alkhani, A., Sun, B., Eljamel, S., Schulder, M., Kaplitt, M., Eskandar, E., Rezai, A., Krauss, J. K., Hilven, P., Schuurman, R., Ruiz, P., Chang, J. W., Cosyns, P., Lipsman, N., Voges, J., Cosgrove, R., Li, Y., and Schlaepfer, T. Consensus on guidelines for stereotactic neurosurgery for psychiatric disorders. J. Neurol. Neurosurg. Psychiatry, *85*:1003–1008, 2014.

85. OCD Clinical Practice Review Task Force. Clinical Practice Review for OCD. Silver Spring, MD: Anxiety and Depression Association of America, 2015.

86. Orloff, L. M., Battle, M. A., Baer, L., Ivanjack, L., Pettit, A. R., Buttolph, M. L., and Jenike, M. A. Long-term follow-up of 85 patients with obsessive-compulsive disorder. Am. J. Psychiatry, *151*:441–442, 1994.

87. Ost, L. G., Havnen, A., Hansen, B., and Kvale, G. Cognitive behavioral treatments of obsessive-compulsive disorder. A systematic review and meta-analysis of studies published 1993–2014. Clin. Psychol. Rev., *40*:156–169, 2015.

88. Parkin, R. Obsessive-compulsive disorder in adults. Int. Rev. Psychiatry, *9*:73–82, 1997.

89. Parmar, A., and Sarkar, S. Neuroimaging studies in obsessive compulsive disorder: a narrative review. Indian J. Psychol. Med., *38*:386–394, 2016.

90. Pato, M. T., Schindler, K. M., and Pato, C. N. The genetics of obsessive-compulsive disorder. Curr. Psychiatry Rep., *3*:163–168, 2001.

91. Pato, M. T., Zohar-Kadouch, R., Zohar, J., and Murphy, D. L. Return of symptoms after discontinuation of clomipramine in patients with obsessive-compulsive disorder. Am. J. Psychiatry, *145*:1521–1525, 1988.

92. Pauls, D. L., Alsobrook II, J. P., Goodman, W., Rasmussen, S., and Leckman, J. F. A family study of obsessive-compulsive disorder. Am. J. Psychiatry, 152:76–84, 1995.

93. Pauls, D. L., Leckman, J. F., and Cohen, D. J. Evidence against a genetic relationship between Tourette's syndrome and anxiety, depression, panic and phobic disorders. Br. J. Psychiatry, 164:215–221, 1994.

94. Paydary, K., Akamaloo, A., Ahmadipour, A., Pishgar, F., Emamzadehfard, S., and Akhondzadeh, S. N-acetylcysteine augmentation therapy for moderate-to-severe obsessive-compulsive disorder: randomized, double-blind, placebo-controlled trial. J. Clin. Pharm. Ther., 41:214–219, 2016.

95. Pigott, T. A., and Seay, S. M. A review of the efficacy of selective serotonin reuptake inhibitors in obsessive-compulsive disorder. J. Clin. Psychiatry, 60:101–106, 1999.

96. Pittenger, C., Bloch, M. H., Wasylink, S., Billingslea, E., Simpson, R., Jakubovski, E., Kelmendi, B., Sanacora, G., and Coric, V. Riluzole augmentation in treatment-refractory obsessive-compulsive disorder: a pilot randomized placebo-controlled trial. J. Clin. Psychiatry, 76:1075–1084, 2015.

97. Pollitt, J. Natural history of obsessional states: a study of 150 cases. Br. Med. J., 1:194–198, 1957.

98. Prasko, J., Paskova, B., Zalesky, R., Novak, T., Kopecek, M., Bares, M., and Horacek, J. The effect of repetitive transcranial magnetic stimulation (rTMS) on symptoms in obsessive compulsive disorder. A randomized, double blind, sham controlled study. Neuro. Endocrinol. Lett., 27:327–332, 2006.

99. Rasmussen, S. A., and Eisen, J. L. Epidemiology of obsessive compulsive disorder. J. Clin. Psychiatry, 51(Suppl):10–13, 1990.

100. Rasmussen, S. A., and Eisen, J. L. The epidemiology and clinical features of obsessive compulsive disorder. Psychiatr. Clin. North Am., 15:743–758, 1992.

101. Rasmussen, S. A., Eisen, J. L., and Pato, M. T. Current issues in the pharmacologic management of obsessive compulsive disorder. J. Clin. Psychiatry, 54:4–9, 1993.

102. Rasmussen, S. A., and Tsuang, M. T. The epidemiology of obsessive compulsive disorder. J. Clin. Psychiatry, 45:450–457, 1984.

103. Ravizz, L., Barzega, G., Bellino, S., Bogetto, F., and Maina, G. Drug treatment of obsessive-compulsive disorder (OCD): long-term trial with clomipramine and selective serotonin reuptake inhibitors (SSRIs). Psychopharmacol. Bull., 32:167–173, 1996.

104. Robins, L. N., Helzer, J. E., Weissman, M. M., Orvaschel, H., Gruenberg, E., Burke, J. D., and Regier, D. A. Lifetime prevalence of specific psychiatric disorders in three sites. Arch. Gen. Psychiatry, 41:949–958, 1984.

105. Rodriguez, C. I., Kegeles, L. S., Levinson, A., Feng, T., Marcus, S. M., Vermes, D., Flood, P., and Simpson, H. B. Randomized controlled crossover trial of ketamine in obsessive-compulsive disorder: proof-of-concept. Neuropsychopharmacology, 38:2475–2483, 2013.

106. Romanelli, R. J., Wu, F. M., Gamba, R., Mojtabai, R., and Segal, J. B. Behavioral therapy and serotonin reuptake inhibitor pharmacotherapy in the treatment of obsessive-compulsive disorder: a systematic review and meta-analysis of head-to-head randomized controlled trials. Depress. Anxiety, 31:641–652, 2014.

107. Rosa-Alcazar, A. I., Sanchez-Meca, J., Rosa-Alcazar, A., Iniesta-Sepulveda, M., Olivares-Rodriguez, J., and Parada-Navas, J. L. Psychological treatment of obsessive-compulsive disorder in children and adolescents: a meta-analysis. Span. J. Psychol., 18:E20, 2015.

108. Royal College of Psychiatrists of the National Collaborating Centre for Mental Health. National Clinical Practice Guideline, No. 31. Obsessive-compulsive disorder: core interventions in the treatment of obsessive-compulsive disorder and body dysmorphic disorder. London: British Psychological Society, 2006.

109. Rüdin, G. Ein Beitrag zur Frage der Zwangskrankheit, insbesondere ihrer heriditären Beziehungen. Arch. Psychiatr. Nervenkr., *191*:14–54, 1953.

110. Ruscio, A. M., Stein, D. J., Chiu, W. T., and Kessler, R. C. The epidemiology of obsessive-compulsive disorder in the National Comorbidity Survey Replication. Mol. Psychiatry, *15*:53–63, 2010.

111. Salzman, L., and Thaler, F. H. Obsessive-compulsive disorders: a review of the literature. Am. J. Psychiatry, *138*:286–296, 1981.

112. Sayyah, M., Boostani, H., Pakseresht, S., and Malayeri, A. A preliminary randomized double-blind clinical trial on the efficacy of celecoxib as an adjunct in the treatment of obsessive-compulsive disorder. Psychiatry Res., *189*:403–406, 2011.

113. Schildre, P. Depersonalization. In *Introduction to Psychoanalytic Psychiatry*. Nervous and Mental Disease Monograph, Series 50, Schildre, P., Gluek, B. (eds.). New York: Nervous and Mental Disease Publishing, 1928.

114. Shea, M. T., Stout, R., Gunderson, J., Morey, L. C., Grilo, C. M., McGlashan, T., Skodol, A. E., Dolan-Sewell, R., Dyck, I., Zanarini, M. C., and Keller, M. B. Short-term diagnostic stability of schizotypal, borderline, avoidant, and obsessive-compulsive personality disorders. Am. J. Psychiatry, *159*:2036–2041, 2002.

115. Shugart, Y. Y., Samuels, J., Willour, V. L., Grados, M. A., Greenberg, B. D., Knowles, J. A., McCracken, J. T., Rauch, S. L., Murphy, D. L., Wang, Y., Pinto, A., Fyer, A. J., Piacentini, J., Pauls, D. L., Cullen, B., Page, J., Rasmussen, S. A., Bienvenu, O. J., Hoehn-Saric, R., Valle, D., Liang, K. Y., Riddle, M. A., and Nestadt, G. Genomewide linkage scan for obsessive-compulsive disorder: evidence for susceptibility loci on chromosomes 3q, 7p, 1q, 15q, and 6q. Mol. Psychiatry, *11*:763–770, 2006.

116. Soomro, G. M., Altman, D., Rajagopal, S., and Oakley-Browne, M. Selective serotonin re-uptake inhibitors (SSRIs) versus placebo for obsessive compulsive disorder (OCD). Cochrane Database Syst. Rev., CD001765, 2008.

117. Stein, D. J., Andersen, E. W., Tonnoir, B., and Fineberg, N. Escitalopram in obsessive-compulsive disorder: a randomized, placebo-controlled, paroxetine-referenced, fixed-dose, 24-week study. Curr. Med. Res. Opin., *23*:701–711, 2007.

118. Steketee, G., and Frost, R. O. Obsessive-compulsive disorder. In *Comprehensive Clinical Psychology, Vol. 6. Adults: Clinical Formulation and Treatment*, Salkovskis, P. (ed.). New York: Pergamon, 1998.

119. Stengel, E. A study of some clinical aspects of the relationship between obsessional neurosis and psychotic reaction types. J. Ment. Sci., *91*:129, 1945.

120. Swedo, S. E., Pietrini, P., Leonard, H. L., Schapiro, M. B., Rettew, D. C., Goldberger, E. L., Rapoport, S. I., Rapoport, J. L., and Grady, C. L. Cerebral glucose metabolism in childhood-onset obsessive-compulsive disorder. Arch. Gen. Psychiatry, *49*:690–694, 1992.

121. Taylor, J. *Duktor Dubitantium, or the Role of Conscience*. London: Royston, 1660.

122. Thoren, P., Asberg, M., Cronholm, B., Jornestedt, L., and Traskman, L. Clomipramine treatment of obsessive-compulsive disorder. I. A controlled clinical trial. Arch. Gen. Psychiatry, *37*:1281–1285, 1980.

123. Tippin, J., and Henn, F. A. Modified leukotomy in the treatment of intractable obsessional neurosis. Am. J. Psychiatry, *139*:1601–1603, 1982.

124. Trevizol, A. P., Shiozawa, P., Cook, I. A., Sato, I. A., Kaku, C. B., Guimaraes, F. B., Sachdev, P., Sarkhel, S., and Cordeiro, Q. Transcranial magnetic stimulation for obsessive-compulsive disorder: an updated systematic review and meta-analysis. J. ECT, 32:262–266, 2016.

125. Veldhuis, J., Dieleman, J. P., Wohlfarth, T., Storosum, J. G., van Den Brink, W., Sturkenboom, M. C., and Denys, D. Incidence and prevalence of "diagnosed OCD" in a primary care, treatment seeking, population. Int. J. Psychiatry Clin. Pract., 16:85–92, 2012.

126. Winokur, G., Clayton, P. J., and Reich, T. *Manic Depressive Illness*. St. Louis: C.V. Mosby, 1969.

127. Wolff, M., Alsobrook, J. P., and Pauls, D. L. Genetic aspects of obsessive-compulsive disorder. Psychiatr. Clin. North Am., 23:535–544, 2000.

CHAPTER 7

⟨ᴏⱽᴏ⟩

Eating Disorders

The major eating disorders are anorexia nervosa and bulimia nervosa.
Anorexia nervosa is characterized by peculiar attitudes toward eating
and weight that lead to obsessive refusal to eat, profound weight loss, and,
when the disorder occurs in girls, persistent amenorrhea. Bulimia refers
to a behavior of gorging of food, typically followed by induced vomiting or
purging. Bulimia is seen in many patients with anorexia nervosa, but it is
the predominant clinical feature in bulimia nervosa (39).

HISTORICAL BACKGROUND

In 1689 Richard Morton published a monograph entitled *Phthisiologia,
or, a Treatise of Consumptions* (67). One of its early chapters, "Nervous
Phthisis," contains case histories of the illness we recognize today as anorexia nervosa. An example follows (pp. 8–9):

> Mr. Duke's Daughter is *St. Mary Axe*, in the Year 1684 and the Eighteenth Year
> of her Age, in the Month of *July* fell into a total suppression of her Monthly
> Courses from a multitude of Cares and Passions of her Mind, but without
> any Symptoms of the Green-Sickness following upon it. From which time her
> Appetite began to abate, and her Digestion to be bad; her Flesh also began to be
> flaccid and loose, and her looks pale, with other Symptoms usual in Universal
> Consumption of the Habit of the Body, and by the extreme and memorable cold
> Weather which happened the Winter following, this Consumption did seem to
> be not a little improved; for that she was wont by her studying at Night, and
> continual poring upon Books, to expose her self both Day and Night to the

injuries of the Air, which was at that time extremely cold, not without some manifest Prejudice to the System of her Nerves. The Spring following, by the Prescription of some Empirik, she took a *Vomit*, and after that I know not what Steel Medicine, but without any Advantage. So from that time loathing all sorts of Medicaments, she wholly neglected the care of herself for two full Years, till at last being brought to the last degree of *Marasmus*, or Consumption, and thereupon subject to frequent Fainting Fits, she apply'd her self to me for Advice.

I do not remember that I did ever in all my Practice see one, that was conversant with the Living so much wasted with the greatest degree of Consumption (like a Skeleton only clad with Skin) yet there was no Fever, but on the contrary a coldness of the whole Body; no Cough, or difficulty of Breathing nor an appearance of any other Distemper of the Lungs, or of any other Entrail; No Looseness, or any other sign of a Colliquation, or Preternatural expence of the Nutritious Juices. Only her Appetite was diminished, and her Digestion uneasy, with Fainting Fits, which did frequently return upon her. Which symptoms I did endeavor to relieve by the outward application of *Aromatick* Bags made to the Region of the Stomack, and by *Stomach-Plaisters*, as also by the internal use of bitter Medicines, *Chalybeates*, and Juleps made of *Cephalick* and *Antihysterick Waters*, sufficiently impregnated with *Spirit of Salt Armoniack*, and *Tincture of Castor*, and other things of that Nature. Upon the use of which she seemed to be much better, but being quickly tired with Medicines, she beg'd that the whole Affair might be committed again to Nature, whereupon, consuming every day more and more, she was after three Months taken with a Fainting Fit, and dyed.

Another vivid and accurate description was presented in 1908 by Dejerine and Gauckler (18), as cited by Cowles (p. 8) (16):

It sometimes happens that a physician has patients—they are more apt to be women—whose appearance is truly shocking. Their eyes are brilliant. Their cheeks are hollow, and their cheek bones seem to protrude through the skin. Their withered breasts hang from the walls of their chests. Every rib stands out. Their shoulder blades appear to be loosened from their frame. Every vertebra shows through the skin. The abdominal wall sinks in below the floating ribs and forms a hollow like a basin. The thighs and the calves of their legs are reduced to a skeleton. One would say it was the picture of an immured nun, such as the old masters have portrayed. These women appear to be fifty or sixty years old. Sometimes they seem to be sustained by some unknown miracle of energy; their voices are strong and their steps firm. On the other hand they often seem almost at the point of death and ready to draw their last breath.

Are they tuberculous or cancerous patients, or muscular atrophies in the last stages, these women whom misery and hunger have reduced to this frightful gauntness? Nothing of the kind. Their lungs are healthy; there is no sign of any organic affection. Although they look so old, they are young women, girls, sometimes children. They may belong to good families and be surrounded by every care. These patients are what are known as mental anorexics, who, without having any physical lesions, but by the association of various troubles, all having a psychic origin, have lost a quarter, a third, and sometimes a half of their weight. The affection which has driven them to this point may have lasted months, sometimes years. Let it go on too long and death will occur either from inanition or from secondary tuberculosis. However, it is a case of nothing but a purely psychic affection of which the mechanisms are of many kinds.

Gull (38) and Lasègue (59) described the syndrome independently in 1873. The English term for the illness has been "anorexia nervosa," the French *l'anorexie hysterique*, and the German *Pubertaetsmagersucht*. Of these, the last, literally meaning "adolescent pursuit of thinness," is probably most precise. It is this relentless pursuit of thinness that especially distinguishes anorexia nervosa from other illnesses associated with loss of weight.

Older historical accounts of patients wasting to the point of death do not usually provide enough information to permit distinguishing between cases of anorexia nervosa, tuberculosis, or panhypopituitarism. Some early photographs of alleged pituitary disease, illustrating markedly wasted patients, probably represent cases of anorexia nervosa (see section "Differential Diagnosis" later in this chapter).

EPIDEMIOLOGY

Anorexia nervosa is not a common illness. A recent review of the prevalence of eating disorders provided an estimated population prevalence of 1%, and the incidence rate is approximately 10 per 100,000 population per year (79). Bulimia nervosa is somewhat more common than anorexia nervosa (79). The incidence of both anorexia nervosa and bulimia nervosa appear to have increased during the middle of the last century (29, 79, 80). Most large teaching hospitals admit several cases each year.

Anorexia nervosa occurs much more frequently in females than in males. Probably 90% of cases are females (26, 29, 51, 56, 80). A similar female preponderance is seen in bulimia nervosa (26, 79). Anorexia nervosa has long been characterized as an illness of mainly middle-class and upper-class Caucasian girls (56). Analysis of referrals to a national specialist treatment center for anorexia nervosa provided solid evidence of a higher social class bias; representation of lower social classes had apparently increased in the previous decade, however (79). Reviews of ethnicity in anorexia nervosa have identified equal rates in Caucasians and Hispanics and lower rates among African Americans and Asians.

Eating disorders are apparently overrepresented among professional dance and modeling students and competitive athletes, usually developing after the individuals have begun their training (1, 24, 50, 56, 72). Several studies have suggested that homosexual males may have increased risk for eating disorders (32, 43, 44, 74). A chart review study of 135 male eating disorder patients treated at the Massachusetts General Hospital in Boston identified homosexuality or bisexuality in 42% of 62 male bulimia nervosa patients (13). One report suggested that adoptees may also be a high-risk group for eating disorders (47). Although early reports identified associations of sexual abuse and bulimia nervosa, more recent work suggests that a history of sexual abuse may be a nonspecific risk factor for psychiatric disorders (54, 55).

CLINICAL PICTURE

An eating disorder typically begins with concern about mild obesity and often dieting, followed by negative attitudes toward eating. A disgust for food that is far stronger than hunger develops. As weight loss progresses, patients may lose their hunger. However thin, they still consider themselves fat and continue to lose weight. These patients may lose so much weight that they resemble survivors of concentration camps, but with several differences. Patients with anorexia nervosa are usually alert and cheerful. In addition, they may be overactive. They often engage in strenuous exercise, sometimes in an open effort to keep from gaining weight.

From the onset of the illness, odd behavior relating to food may be seen. Although starving themselves, patients may hoard food secretly or throw it away. To reduce weight, they may abuse laxatives, enemas, and diuretics. Patients may gorge themselves (bulimia), then induce vomiting voluntarily. In some patients, this feature may be the dominant clinical problem (29, 31, 64, 65, 73).

Amenorrhea may begin before, with, or after the disturbance of appetite (2, 55, 73). It is present in most cases. A few patients first develop anorexia nervosa after bearing children, indicating that an undeveloped reproductive system is not an essential feature of the illness. Other physical findings are bradycardia and lanugo (soft, downy body hair).

Physiological abnormalities have been noted in patients with anorexia nervosa (29, 40, 52, 73). Most investigators believe that starvation produces these abnormalities, which include abnormal glucose tolerance; increased serum cholesterol; increased serum carotene levels; diminished urinary 17-ketosteroids, estrogens, and gonadotropins; elevated serum cortisol; low leptin levels; reduced thyroxine and triiodothyronine; and low basal metabolic rate (29, 40, 52, 73). A striking "immaturity" in the pattern of luteinizing hormone secretion has been described that resembles the hormone functioning of prepubertal girls but usually returns to normal after remission of the anorexia nervosa (34, 73). Male anorexia nervosa patients are reported to have low testosterone levels (56, 83).

Numerous studies have examined the personality profiles of patients with eating disorders. Obsessive-compulsive features, perfectionism, neuroticism, negative emotionality, avoidance, harm avoidance, low self-directedness, and low cooperativeness have been described in association with eating disorders (14). Characteristics especially associated with anorexia nervosa are obsessionality, persistence, perfectionism, self-constraint, and low novelty seeking (14, 42, 56, 57, 85). Features specifically associated with bulimia nervosa are impulsivity, intolerance, immaturity, novelty seeking, and borderline personality traits (14, 23, 55, 57, 76). Even among patients who establish sustained healthy eating patterns, characteristics of high harm avoidance, low cooperativeness, and low self-directedness appear to persist (57).

BIOLOGICAL FINDINGS

The cause of eating disorders is not known, though hypotheses involving endocrine, hypothalamic, and psychosocial factors abound (51, 75). Most investigators assume a multifactorial etiology (55, 56). Imaging studies show reduced brain volumes in both anorexia and bulimia nervosa. When normal weight is regained, brain volume resolves partially, but not completely (81). In anorexia nervosa, imaging studies have demonstrated hypometabolism of the frontal cortex before eating and hyperarousal after eating (69, 70), as well as hyperactivity of the caudate, temporal cortex, lentiform nucleus, and brainstem; these abnormalities normalize with effective treatment (19). Bulimia nervosa appears to involve loss of normal asymmetry of brain activity in frontal and prefrontal areas; these abnormalities fail to correct after long-term recovery (41, 86). In both anorexia and bulimia nervosa, reduced serotonin transporter availability in various brain structures is associated with duration of illness and is not restored with recovery from the illness (5–7, 32, 53). Any of these brain findings in eating disorders could represent effects of starvation, brain damage over the course of the illness, or brain differences predisposing to the illness (81).

NATURAL HISTORY

The age of onset of anorexia nervosa ranges from prepuberty to young adulthood, with the mean in the mid-teens (60). Bulimia nervosa typically presents only slightly later on average (60). The onset of eating disorders may be abrupt. Some patients describe possible precipitating events to the illness, such as the death of a relative or a broken engagement (35, 55, 68). On the other hand, many patients can give no reason for the onset of their abnormal eating behaviors. The illness may involve one lengthy episode lasting many months or years, or it may be marked by remissions and exacerbations.

A review of 119 studies encompassing a total of 5,590 patients with anorexia nervosa concluded that as many as half of patients may experience full or nearly full recovery, and one-third more may improve (82). One in five patients, however, follows a chronic, unremitting course (55, 56, 82). A recent follow-up study found that nearly half of patients were still having some episodes at 12 years, and 40% had a poor outcome (31). Although little research has been conducted on the long-term course of bulimia nervosa, one study found a somewhat more favorable outcome for bulimia than for anorexia nervosa (30). A typical time course for both anorexia nervosa and bulimia nervosa encompasses substantial improvement during treatment, worsening in the first 2 years after treatment, and further improvement with stabilization in subsequent years (30, 31).

Some patients with anorexia nervosa have persistent difficulties even after the initial massive weight loss has been resolved. These problems include amenorrhea and irregular menses, sexual maladjustment, large weight fluctuations, and persistent disturbed eating behaviors (31, 55, 82).

More favorable prognosis appears to be related to earlier age at onset (31, 82) and to healthy family functioning (68). Poorer prognosis appears to be related to later age at onset, longer duration of illness, disturbed relationship with parents, vomiting, bulimia, laxative abuse, and greater severity of obsessional and depressive symptoms (21, 29, 31, 68, 82). Few studies have compared outcomes of male and female patients with anorexia, but available data suggest that males fare at least as well as females (8).

There has been disagreement about whether anorexia nervosa is a specific illness or a manifestation of other illnesses (63). The vast majority of patients with eating disorders have high rates of psychiatric comorbidity, most often major depression, but also anxiety and substance use disorders (26, 31, 55, 60, 80). Even in patients without mood disorders, depressive symptoms are common during the course of the eating disorder (31, 55, 60, 80). Occasionally patients' descriptions of previous periods of anorexia nervosa are reminiscent of episodes of depression. Dexamethasone suppression of cortisol secretion is impaired in some patients with anorexia nervosa. Curiously, weight gain in these patients does not appear to normalize their cortisol response to dexamethasone suppression (25, 77). These observations raise questions about whether some cases of anorexia nervosa may be manifestations of an underlying affective illness. It has been argued, however, that the fact that eating disorders do not regularly evolve into major depression or other disorders supports their validity as a diagnostic category (29).

COMPLICATIONS

The most obvious complication of anorexia nervosa is death from starvation. The illness is fatal in 5%–10% of adult cases, with an expected death rate approximately 10 times that of a comparable population group (3, 26, 31, 37, 56). Thus, anorexia nervosa should not be regarded lightly. One-half of deaths are due to eating-disorder complications, especially cardiac complications. One-fourth of deaths among these patients are by suicide (21, 46, 52). The fatality rate in bulimia nervosa is lower than the fatality rate in anorexia nervosa (37, 56).

Long-term sequelae of anorexia nervosa are osteopenia and, particularly among adolescents, growth retardation (26, 52). Among the more common complications of bulimia nervosa are dental erosion from repeated exposure of teeth to gastric acid and painless swelling of the parotid glands (56). Gastric rupture and esophageal tears from binging and purging are fortunately rare (56). Eating disorders tend to improve during pregnancy, and most patients who suffer from these disorders have normal pregnancies. Women with eating disorders, however, have more infertility, Caesarian sections, gestationally small babies, premature delivery, and perinatal mortality than other women (26, 29).

Patients with anorexia nervosa apparently develop psychoses no more often than persons in the general population (31, 71). When psychotic features do develop, they usually appear to be part of coexisting major mood or schizophrenic disorders (17, 49).

FAMILY AND GENETIC STUDIES

Eating disorders appear to run in families. Family studies have demonstrated that family members of individuals with anorexia and bulimia nervosa have a 10- to 20-fold greater likelihood of having these disorders when compared to relatives of unaffected controls (12, 56). Studies in numerous countries have yielded heritability estimates of 28% to 84% for eating disorders (9, 26, 29). Twin studies have demonstrated a concordance rate of 55% in monozygotic twins and 5% in dizygotic twins for anorexia nervosa; less dramatic monozygotic/dizygotic twin concordance differences have been described for bulimia nervosa (46% vs. 26%) (11, 29). Although eating disorders do not appear to be co-inherited with obsessive-compulsive disorder, there is evidence of co-transmission of anorexia nervosa with obsessive-compulsive personality traits (56).

Fairly recent application of genome-wide linkage studies to anorexia nervosa (4, 22, 36) have not reduced the search area. Use of candidate gene studies (10, 45, 78) have not completed replication. Genome association studies are progressing (61) and also await replication.

DIFFERENTIAL DIAGNOSIS

Anorexia nervosa is characterized by unceasing pursuit of thinness and should not be confused with weight loss occurring in the course of illness such as major depression or schizophrenia. Starvation, when it has causes other than anorexia nervosa, is usually accompanied by apathy and inactivity rather than by the alertness and hyperactivity characteristic of anorexia nervosa. Hypopituitarism is seldom associated with the severe cachexia of anorexia nervosa or the strikingly high level of physical activity. Levels of urinary gonadotropins and serum growth hormone are consistently lower in hypopituitarism than in anorexia nervosa (15, 33).

Differential diagnosis of anorexia nervosa and bulimia nervosa includes consideration of medical illness, especially gastrointestinal diseases: celiac disease, inflammatory bowel disease, bowel adenocarcinoma, and gastrointestinal motility disorders such as achalasia (20, 27, 62). Evidence of psychiatric problems should not preclude appropriate investigation to exclude medical sources of digestive symptoms (20). Gastrointestinal disturbances, especially gastric emptying abnormalities, are frequent among patients with eating disorders, but they usually improve with restoration of healthy eating (20).

CLINICAL MANAGEMENT

Treatment of patients with anorexia nervosa is far from satisfactory, and there is little agreement about the best form. Engaging the patient in treatment is a necessary first step (87). Patients with anorexia nervosa are usually unconcerned about their weight loss and seek treatment only at the insistence of concerned family or friends. Patients with bulimia nervosa, however, are often more motivated to seek treatment for symptoms that trouble them (48).

Indicators of need for hospitalization are self-destructiveness and suicide risk, severe interpersonal problems, body weight below 75% of expected, severe symptoms not relieved with outpatient treatment, psychiatric comorbidity requiring hospitalization, and medical complications (26, 55, 82). The early goals in anorexia nervosa therapy are to stabilize medical complications and restore body weight to safer levels. Rarely, constant observation on a locked psychiatric floor and tube feeding is required (29). Multidisciplinary treatment teams that include the medical practitioner, a nutritionist, and a mental health specialist are best suited to manage eating disorders (84).

No medication has been demonstrated to promote weight gain in anorexia nervosa. Although preliminary findings suggested potential for fluoxetine in preventing relapse among patients after adequate weight is restored (29, 87), a recent randomized, double-blind placebo-controlled clinical trial did not demonstrate such benefit. For bulimia nervosa, on the other hand, numerous double-blind, placebo-controlled trials of fluoxetine have demonstrated effectiveness in reduction of binging frequency (55). Although fluoxetine may also reduce associated depressive and anxiety symptoms, its effectiveness is independent of depression (66). Doses larger than those typically used for treatment of depression are required in bulimia nervosa patients (55, 87).

Psychotherapy is an important component of treatment. Numerous randomized, controlled trials have found cognitive-behavioral therapy to be effective (26, 29). The combination of cognitive-behavioral therapy with fluoxetine may be the most beneficial strategy for management of bulimia nervosa (48, 66). Numerous family-based interventions have recently been found useful, especially for adolescents with anorexia nervosa (28, 58).

REFERENCES

1. Abraham, S. Characteristics of eating disorders among young ballet dancers. Psychopathology, 29:223–229, 1996.
2. American Psychiatric Association. *Diagnostic and Statistical Manual for Mental Disorders,* 5th edition. Washington, DC: Author, 2013.
3. Arcelus, J., Mitchell, A. J., Wales, J., and Nielsen, S. Mortality rates in patients with anorexia nervosa and other eating disorders. A meta-analysis of 36 studies. Arch. Gen. Psychiatry, 68:724–731, 2011.
4. Bacanu, S. A., Bulik, C. M., Klump, K. L., Fichter, M. M., Halmi, K. A., Keel, P., Kaplan, A. S., Mitchell, J. E., Rotondo, A., Strober, M., Treasure, J., Woodside, D. B., Sonpar, V. A., Xie, W., Bergen, A. W., Berrettini, W. H., Kaye, W. H., and Devlin, B. Linkage analysis of anorexia and bulimia nervosa cohorts using selected behavioral phenotypes as quantitative traits or covariates. Am. J. Med. Genet. B Neuropsychiatr. Genet., 139B:61–68, 2005.
5. Bailer, U. F., Frank, G. K., Henry, S. E., Price, J. C., Meltzer, C. C., Weissfeld, L., Mathis, C. A., Drevets, W. C., Wagner, A., Hoge, J., Ziolko, S. K., McConaha, C. W., and Kaye, W. H. Altered brain serotonin 5-HT1A receptor binding after recovery from anorexia nervosa measured by positron emission tomography and [carbonyl11C]WAY-100635. Arch. Gen. Psychiatry, 62:1032–1041, 2005.
6. Bailer, U. F., Price, J. C., Meltzer, C. C., Mathis, C. A., Frank, G. K., Weissfeld, L., McConaha, C. W., Henry, S. E., Brooks-Achenbach, S., Barbarich, N. C., and Kaye, W. H. Altered 5-HT(2A) receptor binding after recovery from bulimia-type anorexia nervosa: relationships to harm avoidance and drive for thinness. Neuropsychopharmacology, 29:1143–1155, 2004.
7. Barbarich, N. C., Kaye, W. H., and Jimerson, D. Neurotransmitter and imaging studies in anorexia nervosa: new targets for treatment. Curr. Drug Targets CNS Neurol. Disord., 2:61–72, 2003.
8. Bean, P., Loomis, C. C., Timmel, P., Hallinan, P., Moore, S., Mammel, J., and Weltzin, T. Outcome variables for anorexic males and females one year after discharge from residential treatment. J. Addict. Dis., 23:83–94, 2004.
9. Bulik, C. M. Exploring the gene-environment nexus in eating disorders. J. Psychiatr. Neurosci., 30:335–339, 2005.
10. Bulik, C. M., Slof-Op't Landt, M. C., Van Furth, E. F., and Sullivan, P. F. The genetics of anorexia nervosa. Annu. Rev. Nutr., 27:263–275, 2007.
11. Bulik, C. M., Sullivan, P. F., Wade, T. D., and Kendler, K. S. Twin studies of eating disorders: a review. Int. J. Eat. Disord., 27:1–20, 2000.
12. Bulik, C. M., and Tozzi, F. Genetics in eating disorders: state of the science. CNS Spectr., 9:511–515, 2004.
13. Carlat, D. J., Camargo, C. A., Jr., and Herzog, D. B. Eating disorders in males: a report on 135 patients. Am. J. Psychiatry, 154:1127–1132, 1997.
14. Cassin, S. E., and von Ranson, K. M. Personality and eating disorders: a decade in review. Clin. Psychol. Rev., 25:895–916, 2005.
15. Couzinet, B., Young, J., Brailly, S., Le Bouc, Y., Chanson, P., and Schaison, G. Functional hypothalamic amenorrhoea: a partial and reversible gonadotrophin deficiency of nutritional origin. Clin. Endocrinol. (Oxf.), 50:229–235, 1999.
16. Cowles, E. S. Psychopathology. Medical Record. Weekly Journal of Medicine and Surgery, 93:6–11, 1918.

17. Deckelman, M. C., Dixon, L. B., and Conley, R. R. Comorbid bulimia nervosa and schizophrenia. Int. J. Eat. Disord., 22:101–105, 1997.

18. Dejerine, J., and Gauckler, E. Le Réeducation des faux gastropathies. Presse Méd., 16:225, 1908.

19. Delvenne, V., Goldman, S., De, M., V, Simon, Y., Luxen, A., and Lotstra, F. Brain hypometabolism of glucose in anorexia nervosa: normalization after weight gain. Biol. Psychiatry, 40:761–768, 1996.

20. Desseilles, M., Fuchs, S., Ansseau, M., Lopez, S., Vinckenbosh, E., and Andreoli, A. Achalasia may mimic anorexia nervosa, compulsive eating disorder, and obesity problems. Psychosomatics, 47:270–271, 2006.

21. Deter, H. C., Schellberg, D., Kopp, W., Friederich, H. C., and Herzog, W. Predictability of a favorable outcome in anorexia nervosa. Eur. Psychiatry, 20:165–172, 2005.

22. Devlin, B., Bacanu, S. A., Klump, K. L., Bulik, C. M., Fichter, M. M., Halmi, K. A., Kaplan, A. S., Strober, M., Treasure, J., Woodside, D. B., Berrettini, W. H., and Kaye, W. H. Linkage analysis of anorexia nervosa incorporating behavioral covariates. Hum. Mol. Genet., 11:689–696, 2002.

23. Diaz-Marsa, M., Carrasco, J. L., and Saiz, J. A study of temperament and personality in anorexia and bulimia nervosa. J. Pers. Disord., 14:352–359, 2000.

24. Dotti, A., Fioravanti, M., Balotta, M., Tozzi, F., Cannella, C., and Lazzari, R. Eating behavior of ballet dancers. Eat. Weight. Disord., 7:60–67, 2002.

25. Duclos, M., Corcuff, J. B., Roger, P., and Tabarin, A. The dexamethasone-suppressed corticotrophin-releasing hormone stimulation test in anorexia nervosa. Clin. Endocrinol. (Oxf.), 51:725–731, 1999.

26. Ebeling, H., Tapanainen, P., Joutsenoja, A., Koskinen, M., Morin-Papunen, L., Jarvi, L., Hassinen, R., Keski-Rahkonen, A., Rissanen, A., and Wahlbeck, K. A practice guideline for treatment of eating disorders in children and adolescents. Ann. Med., 35:488–501, 2003.

27. Eberman, L. E., and Cleary, M. A. Celiac disease in an elite female collegiate volleyball athlete: a case report. J. Athl. Train., 40:360–364, 2005.

28. Eisler, I., Simic, M., Russell, G. F., and Dare, C. A randomised controlled treatment trial of two forms of family therapy in adolescent anorexia nervosa: a five-year follow-up. J. Child Psychol. Psychiatry, 48:552–560, 2007.

29. Fairburn, C. G., and Harrison, P. J. Eating disorders. Lancet, 361:407–416, 2003.

30. Fichter, M. M., and Quadflieg, N. Twelve-year course and outcome of bulimia nervosa. Psychol. Med., 34:1395–1406, 2004.

31. Fichter, M. M., Quadflieg, N., and Hedlund, S. Twelve-year course and outcome predictors of anorexia nervosa. Int. J. Eat. Disord., 39:87–100, 2006.

32. Frank, G. K., Kaye, W. H., Meltzer, C. C., Price, J. C., Greer, P., McConaha, C., and Skovira, K. Reduced 5-HT2A receptor binding after recovery from anorexia nervosa. Biol. Psychiatry, 52:896–906, 2002.

33. Gianotti, L., Broglio, F., Ramunni, J., Lanfranco, F., Gauna, C., Benso, A., Zanello, M., Arvat, E., and Ghigo, E. The activity of GH/IGF-I axis in anorexia nervosa and in obesity: a comparison with normal subjects and patients with hypopituitarism or critical illness. Eat. Weight. Disord., 3:64–70, 1998.

34. Gold, M. S., Pottash, A. C., Martin, D., Extein, I., and Howard, E. The 24-hour LH test in the diagnosis and assessment of response to treatment of patients with anorexia nervosa. Int. J. Psychiatry Med., 11:245–250, 1981.

35. Gowers, S. G., North, C. D., Byram, V., and Weaver, A. B. Life event precipitants of adolescent anorexia nervosa. J. Child Psychol. Psychiatry, 37:469–477, 1996.

36. Grice, D. E., Halmi, K. A., Fichter, M. M., Strober, M., Woodside, D. B., Treasure, J. T., Kaplan, A. S., Magistretti, P. J., Goldman, D., Bulik, C. M., Kaye, W. H., and Berrettini, W. H. Evidence for a susceptibility gene for anorexia nervosa on chromosome 1. Am. J. Hum. Genet., 70:787–792, 2002.
37. Gucciardi, E., Celasun, N., Ahmad, F., and Stewart, D. E. Eating disorders. BMC Womens Health, 4(Suppl 1):S21, 2004.
38. Gull, W. W. Anorexia nervosa (apepsia hysterica). Br. Med. J., 2:527, 1873.
39. Gwirtsman, H. E. Bulimic disorders: pharmacotherapeutic and biological studies. Psychopharmacol. Bull., 29:109–114, 1993.
40. Haas, V., Onur, S., Paul, T., Nutzinger, D. O., Bosy-Westphal, A., Hauer, M., Brabant, G., Klein, H., and Muller, M. J. Leptin and body weight regulation in patients with anorexia nervosa before and during weight recovery. Am. J. Clin. Nutr., 81:889–896, 2005.
41. Hagman, J. O., Buchsbaum, M. S., Wu, J. C., Rao, S. J., Reynolds, C. A., and Blinder, B. J. Comparison of regional brain metabolism in bulimia nervosa and affective disorder assessed with positron emission tomography. J. Affect. Disord., 19:153–162, 1990.
42. Halmi, K. A., Sunday, S. R., Strober, M., Kaplan, A., Woodside, D. B., Richter, M., Treasure, J., Berrettini, W. H., and Kaye, W. H. Perfectionism in anorexia nervosa: variation by clinical subtype, obsessionality, and pathological eating behavior. Am. J. Psychiatry, 157:1799–1805, 2000.
43. Hepp, U., Milos, G., and Braun-Scharm, H. Gender identity disorder and anorexia nervosa in male monozygotic twins. Int. J. Eat. Disord., 35:239–243, 2004.
44. Herzog, D. B., Norman, D. K., Gordon, C., and Pepose, M. Sexual conflict and eating disorders in 27 males. Am. J. Psychiatry, 141:989–990, 1984.
45. Hinney, A., Scherag, S., and Hebebrand, J. Genetic findings in anorexia and bulimia nervosa. Prog. Mol. Biol. Transl. Sci., 94:241–270, 2010.
46. Hoek, H. W. Incidence, prevalence and mortality of anorexia nervosa and other eating disorders. Curr. Opin. Psychiatry, 19:389–394, 2006.
47. Holden, N. L. Adoption and eating disorders: a high-risk group? Br. J. Psychiatry, 158:829–833, 1991.
48. Hsu, L. K. Eating disorders: practical interventions. J. Am. Med. Womens Assoc., 59:113–124, 2004.
49. Hudson, J. I., Pope, Jr. H. G., and Jonas, J. M. Psychosis in anorexia nervosa and bulimia. Br. J. Psychiatry, 145:420–423, 1984.
50. Hughes, C. S., and Hughes, S. The female athlete syndrome. Anorexia nervosa—reflections on a personal journey. Orthop. Nurs., 23:252–260, 2004.
51. Jacobi, C., Hayward, C., de Zwaan, M., Kraemer, H. C., and Agras, W. S. Coming to terms with risk factors for eating disorders: application of risk terminology and suggestions for a general taxonomy. Psychol. Bull., 130:19–65, 2004.
52. Katzman, D. K. Medical complications in adolescents with anorexia nervosa: a review of the literature. Int. J. Eat. Disord., 37 Suppl:S52–S59, 2005.
53. Kaye, W. H., Frank, G. K., Bailer, U. F., and Henry, S. E. Neurobiology of anorexia nervosa: clinical implications of alterations of the function of serotonin and other neuronal systems. Int. J. Eat. Disord., 37(Suppl):S15–S19, 2005.
54. Kendler, K. S., Bulik, C. M., Silberg, J., Hettema, J. M., Myers, J., and Prescott, C. A. Childhood sexual abuse and adult psychiatric and substance use disorders in women: an epidemiological and cotwin control analysis. Arch. Gen. Psychiatry, 57:953–959, 2000.

55. Klein, D. A., and Walsh, B. T. Eating disorders. Int. Rev. Psychiatry, 15:205–216, 2003.

56. Klein, D. A., and Walsh, B. T. Eating disorders: clinical features and pathophysiology. Physiol. Behav., 81:359–374, 2004.

57. Klump, K. L., Strober, M., Bulik, C. M., Thornton, L., Johnson, C., Devlin, B., Fichter, M. M., Halmi, K. A., Kaplan, A. S., Woodside, D. B., Crow, S., Mitchell, J., Rotondo, A., Keel, P. K., Berrettini, W. H., Plotnicov, K., Pollice, C., Lilenfeld, L. R., and Kaye, W. H. Personality characteristics of women before and after recovery from an eating disorder. Psychol. Med., 34:1407–1418, 2004.

58. Kotler, L. A., Boudreau, G. S., and Devlin, M. J. Emerging psychotherapies for eating disorders. J. Psychiatr. Pract., 9:431–441, 2003.

59. Lasègue, E. C. De l'anorexia hystérique. Arch. Gen. Med., 21:385, 1873.

60. Lewinsohn, P. W., Striegel-Moore, R. H., and Seeley, J. R. Epidemiology and natural course of eating disorders in young women from adolescence to young adulthood. J. Am. Acad. Child Adolesc. Psychiatry, 39:1284–1292, 2000.

61. Li, D., Chang, X., Connolly, J. J., Tian, L., Liu, Y., Bhoj, E. J., Robinson, N., Abrams, D., Li, Y. R., Bradfield, J. P., Kim, C. E., Li, J., Wang, F., Snyder, J., Lemma, M., Hou, C., Wei, Z., Guo, Y., Qiu, H., Mentch, F. D., Thomas, K. A., Chiavacci, R. M., Cone, R., Li, B., Sleiman, P. A., and Hakonarson, H. A genome-wide association study of anorexia nervosa suggests a risk locus implicated in dysregulated leptin signaling. Sci. Rep., 7:3847, 2017.

62. McClain, C. J., Humphries, L. L., Hill, K. K., and Nickl, N. J. Gastrointestinal and nutritional aspects of eating disorders. J. Am. Coll. Nutr., 12:466–474, 1993.

63. McElroy, S. L., Kotwal, R., Keck, P. E., Jr., and Akiskal, H. S. Comorbidity of bipolar and eating disorders: distinct or related disorders with shared dysregulations? J. Affect. Disord., 86:107–127, 2005.

64. Milos, G., Spindler, A., Schnyder, U., and Fairburn, C. G. Instability of eating disorder diagnoses: prospective study. Br. J. Psychiatry, 187:573–578, 2005.

65. Mitan, L. A. Menstrual dysfunction in anorexia nervosa. J. Pediatr. Adolesc. Gynecol., 17:81–85, 2004.

66. Mitchell, J. E., de Zwaan, M., and Roerig, J. L. Drug therapy for patients with eating disorders. Curr. Drug Targets CNS Neurol. Disord., 2:17–29, 2003.

67. Morton, R. Phthisiologia, or, a Treatise of Consumptions. London: Smith & Walford, 1689.

68. North, C., Gowers, S., and Byram, V. Family functioning and life events in the outcome of adolescent anorexia nervosa. Br. J. Psychiatry, 171:545–549, 1997.

69. Nozoe, S., Naruo, T., Nakabeppu, Y., Soejima, Y., Nakajo, M., and Tanaka, H. Changes in regional cerebral blood flow in patients with anorexia nervosa detected through single photon emission tomography imaging. Biol. Psychiatry, 34:578–580, 1993.

70. Nozoe, S., Naruo, T., Yonekura, R., Nakabeppu, Y., Soejima, Y., Nagai, N., Nakajo, M., and Tanaka, H. Comparison of regional cerebral blood flow in patients with eating disorders. Brain Res. Bull., 36:251–255, 1995.

71. Oldham, J. M., Skodol, A. E., Kellman, H. D., Hyler, S. E., Doidge, N., Rosnick, L., and Gallaher, P. E. Comorbidity of axis I and axis II disorders. Am. J. Psychiatry, 152:571–578, 1995.

72. Ravaldi, C., Vannacci, A., Zucchi, T., Mannucci, E., Cabras, P. L., Boldrini, M., Murciano, L., Rotella, C. M., and Ricca, V. Eating disorders and body image disturbances among ballet dancers, gymnasium users and body builders. Psychopathology, 36:247–254, 2003.

73. Reba, L., Thornton, L., Tozzi, F., Klump, K. L., Brandt, H., Crawford, S., Crow, S., Fichter, M. M., Halmi, K. A., Johnson, C., Kaplan, A. S., Keel, P., LaVia, M., Mitchell, J., Strober, M., Woodside, D. B., Rotondo, A., Berrettini, W. H., Kaye, W. H., and Bulik, C. M. Relationships between features associated with vomiting in purging-type eating disorders. Int. J. Eat. Disord., 38:287–294, 2005.

74. Robinson, P. H., and Holden, N. L. Bulimia nervosa in the male: a report of nine cases. Psychol. Med., 16:895–903, 1986.

75. Romans, S. E., Gendall, K. A., Martin, H. L., and Mullen, P. E. Child sexual abuse and later disordered eating: a New Zealand epidemiological study. Int. J. Eat. Disord., 29:380–392, 2001.

76. Rosenvinge, J. H., Martinussen, M., and Ostensen, E. The comorbidity of eating disorders and personality disorders: a meta-analytic review of studies published between 1983 and 1998. Eat. Weight Disord., 5:52–61, 2000.

77. Schweitzer, I., Szmukler, G. I., Maguire, K. P., Harrison, L. C., Tuckwell, V., and Davies, B. M. The dexamethasone suppression test in anorexia nervosa. The influence of weight, depression, adrenocorticotrophic hormone and dexamethasone. Br. J. Psychiatry, 157:713–717, 1990.

78. Slof-Op 't Landt, M. C., Van Furth, E. F., Meulenbelt, I., Slagboom, P. E., Bartels, M., Boomsma, D. I., and Bulik, C. M. Eating disorders: from twin studies to candidate genes and beyond. Twin Res. Hum. Genet., 8:467–482, 2005.

79. Smink, F. R., van, H. D., and Hoek, H. W. Epidemiology of eating disorders: incidence, prevalence and mortality rates. Curr. Psychiatry Rep., 14:406–414, 2012.

80. Soundy, T. J., Lucas, A. R., Suman, V. J., and Melton, L. J., III. Bulimia nervosa in Rochester, Minnesota from 1980 to 1990. Psychol. Med., 25:1065–1071, 1995.

81. Stamatakis, E. A., and Hetherington, M. M. Neuroimaging in eating disorders. Nutr. Neurosci., 6:325–334, 2003.

82. Steinhausen, H. C. The outcome of anorexia nervosa in the 20th century. Am. J. Psychiatry, 159:1284–1293, 2002.

83. Wabitsch, M., Ballauff, A., Holl, R., Blum, W. F., Heinze, E., Remschmidt, H., and Hebebrand, J. Serum leptin, gonadotropin, and testosterone concentrations in male patients with anorexia nervosa during weight gain. J. Clin. Endocrinol. Metab., 86:2982–2988, 2001.

84. Walsh, J. M., Wheat, M. E., and Freund, K. Detection, evaluation, and treatment of eating disorders the role of the primary care physician. J. Gen. Intern. Med., 15:577–590, 2000.

85. Wonderlich, S. A., Lilenfeld, L. R., Riso, L. P., Engel, S., and Mitchell, J. E. Personality and anorexia nervosa. Int. J. Eat. Disord., 37 Suppl:S68–S71, 2005.

86. Wu, J. C., Hagman, J., Buchsbaum, M. S., Blinder, B., Derrfler, M., Tai, W. Y., Hazlett, E., and Sicotte, N. Greater left cerebral hemispheric metabolism in bulimia assessed by positron emission tomography. Am. J. Psychiatry, 147:309–312, 1990.

87. Zhu, A. J., and Walsh, B. T. Pharmacologic treatment of eating disorders. Can. J. Psychiatry, 47:227–234, 2002.

CHAPTER 8

cVo

Somatization Disorder

For many centuries, patients with unexplained physical complaints received a diagnosis of "hysteria," an older name for the more modern diagnosis of somatization disorder. Building upon the earlier work of Briquet in France (12), Savill in England (75), and Purtell and colleagues in Boston (22, 69), investigators at Washington University in St. Louis (6, 19–21, 33, 37, 39–41, 43–45, 67) carried out a series of studies and proposed that this diagnosis be replaced by two labels for different presentations of these types of symptoms: "Briquet's syndrome" (after the French psychiatrist who described a large series of such patients) and "conversion symptoms." This proposal was designed to eliminate the pejorative implications associated with the diagnosis of hysteria and to avoid the complications of inconsistent use of terminology. Toward the same ends, *DSM-III* introduced the category of "somatoform disorders" in place of the older concepts of hysterical phenomena, substituting the diagnosis of somatization disorder for Briquet's syndrome. It did not, however, fully clarify the categorization of conversion symptoms. (Of note, "somatoform" or "somatization" symptoms refer to physical symptoms without medical basis, in contrast to "somatic" symptoms, which refer to any physical symptom without regard to medical basis.)

The importance of distinguishing between Briquet's syndrome and conversion symptoms continued to be emphasized by the Washington University group. They argued that the former is typically a polysymptomatic disorder that begins early in life (usually in the teens, rarely after the 20s), chiefly affects women, and is characterized by recurrent multiple somatic complaints, often described dramatically. Characteristic features, all unexplained by other known clinical disorders, include varied pains, anxiety symptoms, gastrointestinal disturbances, urinary symptoms, menstrual difficulties, sexual and marital maladjustment, nervousness, mood disturbances, and "pseudoneurological" symptoms (the last often used synonymously with the term "conversion symptoms"). Repeated visits to physicians and clinics, the use of a large number of medications—often at the same time and prescribed by different physicians—and frequent hospitalizations and operations produce a florid medical history (39, 40).

In keeping with this view, "somatization disorder" continued to be the term for Briquet's syndrome in *DSM-IV-TR*. (In citing historical research on this disorder, this chapter will apply a convention of using the terminology of the study's original authors to help readers appreciate the context of the research.)

It should be emphasized, however, that the diagnostic criteria for somatization disorder in *DSM-IV-TR* were less stringent than those for Briquet's syndrome and were proposed to offer a shortcut to the diagnosis (96). As yet, we have few data about the validity of these criteria for somatization disorder from systematic, controlled follow-up and family studies. The findings thus far indicate that the two sets of criteria (for Briquet's syndrome and somatization disorder) select overlapping but somewhat different populations (21, 27).

The St. Louis group proposed that the term "conversion symptom" be reserved for *unexplained symptoms suggesting neurological disease,* such as amnesia, unconsciousness, paralysis, "spells," aphonia, urinary retention, difficulty walking, anesthesia, and blindness—the so-called pseudoneurological or "grand hysterical" symptoms (57). "Unexplained" means only that the history, neurological examination, and diagnostic tests have failed to reveal a satisfactory explanation for the symptoms. Thus used, the term "conversion symptom" has no etiological implication; it refers, in a descriptive way only, to a limited group of symptoms. To provide specificity for this term, unexplained pains and other unexplained medical symptoms that do not suggest neurological disease are not included in the definition. If other unexplained medical symptoms such as headaches, backaches, and abdominal pains were included, conversion symptom would mean any unexplained medical symptom and thus would lose any precision it has (39, 40).

Sometimes a related syndrome occurs as a sudden, short-lived epidemic ("mass hysteria"), characteristically in a school population and most frequently affecting female students (59, 79). Blackouts, dizziness, weakness, headaches, hyperventilation, nausea, and abdominal pain are the usual symptoms, but unusual syndromes such as involuntary movements have occurred in these outbreaks. Such episodes may suggest, but do not involve, hazardous exposures such as suspected airborne toxins. The pathogenesis of these episodes is thought to involve suggestibility, fear, and social spread. Long-term follow-up of the affected children has not been reported, but the short-term prognosis appears to be very good.

To recapitulate: Conversion symptoms comprise a limited group of individual symptoms suggesting neurological disease. "Somatization disorder" or "Briquet's syndrome" refers to a polysyndromic (many organ systems), polysymptomatic (many symptoms) syndrome that often includes conversion symptoms.

One major criticism of the definition of Briquet's syndrome or somatization disorder is that practically everyone experiences many symptoms characteristic of the syndrome. It is true that most people have experienced headaches, fatigue, anorexia, nausea, diarrhea, vomiting, nervousness, and varied pains. But few report such symptoms when their physicians take a medical history. Most people interpret the physician's questions to mean significant symptoms; they report only symptoms that are recent, recurrent, or otherwise troublesome. Furthermore, the physician evaluates the patient's responses, overlooking symptoms that are not recent, recurrent, or disabling to elicit symptoms that led the patient to consult a physician, take medicines, or alter usual routines. In addition, there are some symptoms that will be considered significant regardless of qualifying features, such as blindness and paralysis. These criteria—ones that physicians ordinarily use to evaluate symptoms—are the same as those applied in the studies of Briquet's syndrome or somatization disorder cited. By these criteria, very few people report enough medically unexplained symptoms to warrant a diagnosis of somatization disorder.

A second major line of criticism has been the complex and burdensome nature of the diagnostic criteria (viz. 25 of 59 possible symptoms for Feighner criteria, 13 of 39 possible symptoms for *DSM-III-R* criteria, and a 4-2-1-1 symptom algorithm for *DSM-IV* criteria), leading to nonuse of the criteria (96, 98).

These criticisms and other issues led the DSM-V Workgroup on Somatic Symptom Disorders (29) to radically change the approach to the somatoform disorders. For *DSM-5* (4), the associated chapter title changed to "Somatic Symptom and Related Disorders," and many changes were made. The diagnosis of somatization disorder was removed and a new label was created—somatic symptom disorder—which was advanced to theoretically subsume a number of disorders including somatization disorder (3). Substantive concerns were raised early about the somatic symptom disorder label (35) because of the false-positive problem (mislabeling subjects with a mental disorder) (28, 36) and the direct harm to patients

(36, 47) that have continued over years (87, 88). Validation has not been forthcoming. Therefore, the decision was made to retain this chapter with new research updates and review, because it contains the most recent data on the previously accepted and well-validated diagnosis of somatization disorder (Briquet's syndrome).

Of paramount importance, and as noted in the next section, because this illness has existed for thousands of years, merely changing the label and developing new criteria for it will not change the disease. See also Chapter 1 for a fuller discussion of recent diagnostic considerations.

HISTORICAL BACKGROUND

The concept of hysteria, which probably originated in Egypt, is at least 4,000 years old. The name *hysteria* has been in use since the time of Hippocrates. The original Egyptian approach to hysteria was perhaps the most fanciful. Believing that physical displacement of the uterus caused the varied symptoms, physicians treated the patient by trying to attract the "wandering uterus" back to its proper site. Sweet-smelling substances were placed in the region of the vagina to attract the errant organ back home; unpleasant materials were ingested or inhaled to drive it away from upper body wanderings (85).

Egyptian and Greek physicians applied the diagnosis whenever they believed that unusual symptoms were caused by a displaced uterus, but the available records do not provide explicit diagnostic criteria. This state of affairs persisted, although various speculations about pathogenesis have been offered over the centuries (78). In particular, witchcraft, demonology, and sorcery were associated with hysteria in the Middle Ages (85). Mysterious symptoms, spells, and odd behavior were frequently considered manifestations of supernatural, evil influences. Patients with this disorder were sometimes perceived as either possessing an active evil spirit (witch, sorceress, or demon) or as the passive victim of such an evil being. Since the Middle Ages there have been speculations of many kinds about the cause of hysteria. Such speculations have included ideas about neurological weakness, neurological degeneration, the effects of various toxins, and disturbances of what Mesmer called "animal magnetism" (63).

Hysteria became Freud's central concern during the early years of psychoanalysis (11). That interest had developed while Freud was working in Paris with Charcot, who was treating hysteria with hypnosis. The psychoanalytic concept of conversion as an ego defense mechanism, referring to unconscious conversion of "psychic energy" into physical symptoms, ultimately led to the identification of conversion symptoms with hysteria in psychoanalytic practice. Many psychoanalysts considered hysteria a simulation of illness designed to work out unconscious conflicts, partially through seeking attention and "secondary gain." "Secondary gain" refers to efforts to attain potential advantages of illness such as sympathy and support, including financial support from relatives and friends, and being excused from various duties (100).

This view led easily to the attitude, widely held by physicians though seldom stated openly, that hysteria is a term of opprobrium to be applied whenever the patient's complaints are not explained or when the demands appear excessive. The most fully developed version of this view is the concept of the hysterical personality. Here, the emphasis is on immature, histrionic, manipulative, seductive, and attention-seeking behavior regardless of the presenting complaint of present illness. In the absence of specific diagnostic criteria and systematic studies, however, use of the term "hysteria" has been inconsistent and confusing. There is considerable evidence that conversion symptoms, somatization disorder, and hysterical personality are different, although any combination of these three is frequently present in the same individual (16, 17, 49).

The syndromatic approach to the diagnosis of hysteria began in 1859 when the French physician Pierre Briquet published his monograph, *Traits clinique et thérapeutique á l'hystérie* (12, 55, 56). Similar descriptions of the syndrome were provided in 1909 by the English physician Savill (75) and in 1951 by the American psychiatrists Purtell, Cohen, and Robins (69). A series of studies by Guze and colleagues refined and clarified the concept of hysteria as a syndrome (39, 40, 42, 67, 94). In a systematic study of women diagnosed as "having a hysterical personality or as being hysterics," Blinder (8) confirmed the clinical description and familiar characteristics described in this chapter.

EPIDEMIOLOGY

A study in an urban community (90) indicated the prevalence of somatization disorder to be 0.4%. Assuming that nearly all of the cases occurred in women, and correcting for the sex distribution of the sample, the prevalence in urban women was just under 1% according to this report. A meta-analysis by Creed and Barsky showed a prevalence of 0.4% (range, 0.03%–0.84%) in a population-based sample (25). In studies of hospitalized, postpartum women with uncomplicated pregnancies and deliveries, the prevalence of the syndrome was between 1% and 2% (33, 62). Women with Briquet's syndrome have been found to be significantly more likely to have an earlier birth order than women with other psychiatric disorders (60).

There is a generally held view that somatization and conversion symptoms are more common among less sophisticated people. One group of investigators found that higher education (1 or more years of college) was significantly less common in patients with conversion symptoms— with or without Briquet's syndrome—than in patients without conversion symptoms. Patients with Briquet's syndrome have been found to have lower education compared to other psychiatric patients as a group (44). Several investigators have reported that "hysterical neurosis, conversion type" is much more frequent in nonwhites than in whites and is highest in the lowest socioeconomic classes (82, 83).

A history of conversion symptoms is commonly found in systematic interviews of hospitalized, normal, postpartum women (33), hospitalized medically ill women (93), and male and female psychiatric outpatients (44). On average, about one-quarter of such patients give a history of conversion symptoms. A history of conversion symptoms may be elicited from patients with any psychiatric disorder, but two conditions are most often associated with such a history: Briquet's syndrome and antisocial personality disorder.

All studies outside of military populations have reported that the great majority of patients with a diagnosis of hysteria (using a variety of diagnostic criteria) have been women (26, 46, 51, 72, 82). Nearly all men with symptoms resembling hysteria in women have had histories of associated compensation factors, such as litigation following injuries, consideration for veterans' and other pensions, disability payments, or serious legal difficulties (74). In 1975, a British anthropological psychiatrist predicted that sociopathy should predominate in men and hysteria in women, based on theories of the persistence of preliterate "magical thinking" in modern society (15).

In summary, a history of conversion symptoms can be found among psychiatric patients of either sex who have any psychiatric disorder. However, such a history is most likely to be associated with somatization disorder in women or sociopathy in men. Somatization disorder is much less common than conversion symptoms; it is seen infrequently among men; and, like conversion symptoms, it is infrequently associated with higher education.

CLINICAL PICTURE

When first seen by a psychiatrist, the typical patient with somatization disorder is a married woman in her 30s. Her history is often delivered in a dramatic, complicated fashion. She usually presents with multiple vague complaints to her general physician, and a straightforward history of the present illness is difficult, if not impossible, to elicit. Frequently, the physician has difficulty deciding when the current illness began or even why the patient presented. Table 8.1 presents the most common symptoms reported by patients with somatization disorder. Not only do they report large numbers of these and other symptoms, but also the symptoms are distributed widely throughout all or nearly all organ systems. It is this range of symptoms ("polysyndromic") in addition to their number ("polysymptomatic") that defines somatization disorder.

The dramatic, colorful, exaggerated description of symptoms is best conveyed by quoting patients, though it should be noted that not all patients show this trait to the same degree. The following quotations are from Purtell et al. (69):

> *Vomiting*: "I vomit every ten minutes. Sometimes it lasts for two to three weeks at a time. I can't even take liquids. I even vomit water. I can't stand the smell of food."
>
> *Food intolerance*: "I can't eat pastries. Always pay for it. I can't eat steak now. I throw up whole milk. I always throw up the skins of tomatoes. Pudding made with canned milk makes me sick. I have to use fresh milk."
>
> *A trance*: "I passed out on the bathroom floor during my period and was still on the floor when they found me the next morning."
>
> *Weight change*: "I can lose weight just walking down the street. I can hold my breath and lose weight. I was down to 65 pounds at one time."
>
> *Dysmenorrhea*: "I can't work. Every month I am in bed for several days. I have had to have morphine hypos. There is a throbbing pain in the legs as if the blood doesn't circulate. Can't go to the bathroom as I faint. It's murder! I want to die. It affects my nervous system."
>
> *Sexual indifference*: "Have never been interested." "It's not a normal thing to me. Disgusting. My husband has never bothered me." "It's just a part of my married life. I have to do it." "I was only disappointed. Never really enjoyed it, but I had to please my husband." "I have no feelings. It's just a duty."

TABLE 8.1 THE FREQUENCY OF SYMPTOMS IN HYSTERIA

Symptom	%	Symptom	%	Symptom	%
Dyspnea	72	Weakness	84	Dyspareunia	52
Palpitation	60	Weight loss	28	Back pain	88
Chest pain	72	Sudden fluctuations in weight	16	Joint pain	84
Dizziness	84	Anorexia	60	Extremity pain	84
Headache	80	Nausea	80	Burning pains in rectum, vagina, mouth	28
Anxiety attacks	64	Vomiting	32	Other bodily pain	36
Fatigue	84	Abdominal pain	80	Depressed feelings	64
Blindness	20	Abdominal bloating	68	Phobias	48
Paralysis	12	Food intolerances	48	Vomiting all 9 months of pregnancy	20
Anesthesia	32	Diarrhea	20	Nervous	92
Aphonia	44	Constipation	64	Had to quit working because felt bad	44
Lump in throat	28	Dysuria	44	Trouble doing anything because felt bad	72
Fits or convulsions	20	Urinary retention	8	Cried a lot	60
Faints	56	Dysmenorrhea (pre-pregnancy only)	4	Felt life was hopeless	28
Unconsciousness	16	Dysmenorrhea (premarital only)	8	Always sickly (most of life)	40
Amnesia	8	Dysmenorrhea (other)	48	Thought of dying	48
Visual blurring	64	Menstrual irregularity	48	Wanted to die	36
Visual hallucination	12	Excessive menstrual bleeding	48	Thought of suicide	28
Deafness	4	Sexual indifference	44	Attempted suicide	12
Olfactory hallucination	16	Frigidity (absence of orgasm)	24		

Adapted from M. Perley and S. B. Guze (67).

Dyspareunia: "Every time I had intercourse I swelled up on one side. It's sore and burns, and afterwards is very painful." "I hate it. I have a severe pain on the right side and have to go to bed for a day."

Presenting complaints: "I am sore all over. I can't explain it. I have been sick all my life. Now I am alone since my husband died, and the doctor said I must come for help. It has taken $10,000 to keep me alive. This is my 76th hospitalization." "I have been taking care of my invalid mother and I get very little rest or sleep." "My father came here for a checkup on his diabetes and insisted that I come along. I had a nervous breakdown a long time ago and have never gotten around to being really well."

The gynecologist, the neurologist, and the psychiatrist are likely to see somatization disorder patients with more focused complaints: the gynecologist because of menstrual pain, irregularity, lapses, or dyspareunia; the neurologist because of headaches, "spells," or other conversion symptoms; the psychiatrist because of suicide attempts, depression, or marital discord. But even these specialists find it difficult to obtain straightforward histories from patients with somatization disorder.

Among the characteristic recurrent or chronic symptoms of somatization disorder, pains are very prominent: headaches, chest pain, abdominal pain, back pain, and joint pain. Abdominal, pelvic, and back pain in association with menstrual or sexual difficulties account for frequent gynecological surgery: dilatation and curettage, uterine suspension, and salpingo-oophorectomy. Abdominal pain, back pain, dysuria, and dyspareunia account for frequent catheterization and cystoscopy. Abdominal pain, indigestion, bowel difficulties, and vomiting are associated with frequent gastrointestinal X-ray examinations and rectal and gallbladder surgery.

Repeated hospitalization and surgery are characteristic of these conditions (22). Because of the dramatic and persistent symptoms, patients are hospitalized for observation, tests, and treatment of a wide variety of medical and surgical conditions that may be mimicked by somatization disorder.

Nervousness and somatic anxiety symptoms (palpitation, dyspnea, chest pain, dizziness, fatigue, tremulousness) are frequent. When chest pain is prominent, it may lead to a diagnosis of heart disease, supported only by nonspecific deviations in the electrocardiogram. The same nervousness and anxiety symptoms, especially when associated with globus (lump in throat) or weight loss, may lead to thyroid studies and a diagnosis of thyroid abnormalities. Moodiness, irritability, depression, suicidal ideation, and suicide attempts are common and lead to psychiatric hospitalization of patients with somatization disorder (24). Somatization disorder accounts for a substantial minority of suicide attempts (76) but rarely leads to suicide (71).

Menstrual symptoms and sexual indifference or frigidity are so characteristic that a diagnosis of Briquet's syndrome or somatization disorder should be made with care if the menstrual and sexual histories are normal. Marital discord related to sexual indifference and frigidity leads to separation or divorce for many of these patients (42).

Recent studies emphasize a point recognized in the past—that somatization disorder is a "psychoform" condition as well as a "somatoform" disorder (52, 63, 66, 77, 91). These patients report a wide range of psychological or emotional symptoms in additional to physical symptoms.

The question of malingering frequently arises in discussions about these patients. Although often suspected, malingering is difficult to prove. Nevertheless, malingering and factitious lesions are striking features in some cases (70). Factitious fever produced by heating thermometers with matches or friction, skin lesions produced by self-injections, and hemoptysis and hematuria produced by pricking fingers and adding blood to sputum or urine may take months or years to recognize. An occasional patient will confide that a given symptom or sign was produced artificially in the past but will insist that it is now real.

The long-recognized association of antisocial personality and Briquet's syndrome within families and within the same individual (6, 13, 14, 19–21, 43, 45, 81, 93) is of great interest. (The relationship of these two disorders in families is discussed in the "Family Studies" section.) A number of the clinical features of both disorders may be clinically tied together within individuals. Many delinquent or antisocial adolescent girls develop somatization disorder as adults (73); many patients with somatization disorder give a history of delinquent or antisocial behavior earlier in life (45, 54); the medical histories of delinquent children indicate an increased prevalence of medical contacts (53); and many convicted women felons present with a mixed picture of sociopathy and somatization (19, 20). Thus, school delinquency, repeated fighting, running away from home, poor work record, poor marital history, sexual promiscuity, heavy drinking, and police trouble are events found in the histories of many, though not all, women with somatization disorder (81). It may be pertinent that Eysenck has concluded from his studies of personality that both patients with hysteria and patients with psychopathic personalities are "extroverted neurotics," an additional possible reason for associating the two conditions (32).

Somatization disorder may be present in many patients demonstrating full or partial manifestations of dissociative identity disorder (formerly termed "multiple personality disorder") (9, 66). Though dissociative identity disorder is considered a rare phenomenon, the reported frequency increased dramatically in the 1980s and 1990s (66), attributed to widespread attention in the professional and popular news media (10, 38). Similarly, somatization disorder can also be diagnosed in some patients who meet the criteria for borderline personality disorder. In fact, evidence from a number of studies suggests that somatization disorder, borderline personality, and dissociative disorders may represent manifestations of a common underlying psychopathology with its manifestations varying in prominence and severity over time and with different circumstances (9, 38, 48, 63, 66, 91). The extensive overlap of clinical features across these disorders suggests the old tale of several blind men drawing different conclusions about an elephant from the different parts of the animal's body each touches.

Another characteristic feature of somatization disorder is the tendency of many patients to give inconsistent histories (41); thus, symptoms that lead to hospitalization on one occasion are denied on another (61). Though this inconsistency has not been studied systematically, it may be related to the patient's perception of the physician's response to her and her desire to influence the physician's judgment about her illness.

Patients with somatization disorder do not often confide all their symptoms in a single interview, and thus it is usually necessary to obtain sufficient information by consulting medical records, questioning collateral sources, and observing the evolution of symptom complaints over time (58). These patients may incorrectly attribute their symptoms to medical illness, obscuring the pattern of multiple medically unexplained symptoms that is characteristic of somatization disorder (18, 58). The difficulties in obtaining information needed for the diagnosis commonly lead to underrecognition of the disorder in clinical practice. To detect cases, a high index of suspicion for the diagnosis must be maintained and systematic effort made to track down the necessary information (30, 34, 84).

During periods of emotional stress, the speech patterns of patients with somatization disorder can deteriorate into disorganized and confused discourse that may simulate cognitive processes of psychosis. These speech patterns in somatization disorder can, however, be differentiated from the formal disturbances of logic and syntax observed in schizophrenia and mania (5, 31, 99). North and colleagues systematized abnormal speech patterns into specific elements (e.g., circumstantiality, vagueness, and loss of goal) collectively termed "nonpsychotic formal thought disorder"

(64, 65). Blind raters systematically categorizing elements of speech samples according to nonpsychotic thought disorder criteria successfully differentiated patients with somatization disorder and antisocial personality disorder from each other and from controls with neither disorder.

NATURAL HISTORY

As already noted, it is not easy to determine when the illness began. The vague and often inconsistent history makes the chronology of symptoms difficult to establish. The patient may insist that she has always been "sick" and may describe early difficulties that are hard to evaluate. These patients may also suffer from other illnesses, and, therefore, descriptions of childhood or adolescent disorders that allegedly were diagnosed as rheumatic fever, appendicitis, poliomyelitis, or typhoid fever can be most difficult to judge.

The symptoms fluctuate in severity, but the characteristic features persist: recurrent pains, conversion symptoms, nervousness and depression, sexual and marital discord, repeated hospitalization, and repeated surgery (42). Although systematic follow-up until death of a series of patients has not yet been reported, there is no indication that more than a minority of patients experience marked improvement or permanent remission. Twenty to thirty years of symptoms is typical, and patients who have had the illness for more than 40 years are not unusual (68). There is no evidence of excess mortality (26).

In contrast, the long-term course of the patient with conversion symptoms is determined by the underlying illness rather than by the nature of the symptoms themselves. Because conversion symptoms may be seen in a wide variety of medical, neurological, and psychiatric disorders (37, 46, 89), patients with these symptoms have a variable prognosis and course.

COMPLICATIONS

The most frequent and important complications of somatization disorder are repeated surgical procedures, drug dependence, marital separation or divorce, and suicide attempts. The first two are presumably preventable if physicians learn to recognize the disorder and manage patients properly. Knowledge that somatization disorder may be an alternate explanation for various pains and other symptoms can help surgeons withhold or postpone cases when objective indications are equivocal or missing. Habit-forming or addictive drugs should be avoided for recurrent or persistent pain. Whether the physician can modify marital discord through psychotherapy is uncertain, but recognizing the frequency of separation and divorce, the physician can certainly direct attention to these problems. The same may be said about suicide attempts, but there the physician can approach patients with somatization disorder knowing that the risk of completed suicide is low.

FAMILY STUDIES

Studies using the Briquet's syndrome criteria suggest that the disorder runs in families (6, 23, 92). It was found in one study that about 20% of first-degree (siblings, parents, children) female relatives of index cases met the criteria for the same condition, a 10-fold increase over the prevalence in the general population of women, lending strong support to the validity of the concept of hysteria as an illness. A second study, using "blind" examiners, showed lower numbers and only a 3.5-fold increase in first-degree female relatives compared to similar relatives of index women with a range of other psychiatric disorders (41), but it again confirmed the familial aggregation of cases.

Family studies also indicate that a significant association exists between somatization disorder and antisocial personality. First-degree male relatives of women selected by the Briquet's syndrome criteria show an increased prevalence of sociopathy and alcoholism (6, 41, 92). The first-degree female relatives of convicted male felons also show an increased prevalence of Briquet's syndrome (43). The findings, in conjunction with the observation that many female sociopaths present with or develop the full Briquet's syndrome or meet the criteria for somatization disorder (20), have suggested that at least some cases of somatization disorder (Briquet's syndrome) and sociopathy share a common etiology.

The widely recognized observation that somatization disorder is predominantly a disorder of women, whereas antisocial personality is predominantly a disorder of men, raises the interesting possibility that, depending on the sex of the individual, the same etiological and pathogenetic factors may lead to different, although sometimes overlapping, clinical pictures. Future studies may also show a familial aggregation involving borderline and dissociative disorders as well as somatization disorder and antisocial personality. It has been suggested that many individuals with any or all of these four clinical conditions may be suffering from a common syndrome whose overt manifestations vary in accordance with gender and a variety of clinical and social circumstances (63).

Two studies (13, 14, 86) of adopted children whose biological parents showed antisocial behavior revealed greater-than-expected frequency in female offspring of Briquet's syndrome or somatization disorder or other multiple unexplained somatic complaints, further supporting the hypothesis that these are related disorders. One of these studies was carried out in the United States, the other in Sweden.

DIFFERENTIAL DIAGNOSIS

Three psychiatric conditions must, at times, be considered in the differential diagnosis of somatization disorder: panic disorder, major depressive disorder, and schizophrenia. As already noted, the characteristic symptoms of somatization disorder include many that are also seen in panic disorder and depression. If the patient is a young woman with menstrual and sexual difficulties who presents with a full range of anxiety or depressive symptoms, she may nearly meet the diagnostic criteria. Age of onset, details of the symptom picture, course, and mental status will usually help clarify the diagnostic problem. A number of patients with schizophrenia also meet the diagnostic criteria for Briquet's syndrome or somatization disorder. Also, an occasional patient with these latter conditions who does not show definite evidence of schizophrenia when first seen will, in time, develop the typical clinical picture of schizophrenia (94). In contrast to the overlap observed between antisocial personality and somatization disorder in individuals as well as in families, any overlap of schizophrenia with antisocial personality or somatization disorder within individual patients has not been demonstrated to be accompanied by familial associations between schizophrenia and these disorders.

CLINICAL MANAGEMENT

The diagnosis of somatization disorder (based on Briquet's syndrome criteria) provides two advantages. For patients with the full diagnostic picture, the physician can predict in over 90% of cases that the characteristic symptoms will continue through time and that other illnesses, which in retrospect could account for the original clinical picture, will not become evident. For patients who do not present with the full diagnostic picture, especially for those who have conversion symptoms and little else, the physician can expect that in a substantial number of cases other disorders will become evident that may, in retrospect, account for the original clinical picture (67, 89). Many, perhaps most, of the patients whose symptoms resemble somatization disorder but fail to meet the explicit diagnostic criteria will remain undiagnosed at follow-up. Enough of them, however, will turn out to have other serious medical, neurological, or psychiatric disorders to justify the kind of diagnostic open-mindedness that can lead to early recognition of the other illnesses.

Somatoform conditions can be difficult to treat (7, 61, 95, 97). The typical clinical picture of recurrent, multiple, vague symptoms combined with doctor-shopping and frequent requests for time and attention can frustrate many physicians. Few of these patients referred for psychiatric treatment persist with such treatment (42). Thus, the burden of caring for them continues to rest with other physicians. A controlled, randomized study indicates, however, that psychiatric consultation may be helpful in reducing the extent and cost of medical care (80). A review (50) of 31 controlled trials of cognitive-behavioral therapy (CBT) for "somatization or symptom syndromes" (p. 205) (not necessarily somatization disorder/Briquet's syndrome) showed promising results with significant improvements in symptoms. The lasting effectiveness of CBT for somatization, however, has been debated (1). These questions and the cost of treating patients with somatization disorder eventually led to an NIH-funded research project designed to study patients meeting the formal criteria for somatization disorder in a randomized, single-blind efficacy study of CBT (versus care as usual) (2). The results of this formal first study were encouraging because a significant number of patients were rated as "much" to "very much" improved with CBT compared to augmented medical care, and the patients reported an increase in functioning with a corresponding decrease in symptoms and healthcare costs. Replication will be necessary.

Until there is general acceptance of a particular therapeutic intervention, the physician's major goal should be to avoid the complications described earlier. Success will depend on winning the patient's confidence without allowing her symptomatic behavior to exhaust the physician's sympathy. The patient and family can be told that the patient tends to experience symptoms that suggest other disorders, but that they are not medically serious. On this basis, the physician can approach each new complaint circumspectly and conservatively, especially with regard to elaborate or expensive diagnostic studies. As the physician grows familiar with the patient, the physician will become increasingly confident in his or her clinical judgments. Remembering that somatization disorder can "explain" many puzzling symptoms, the physician, always looking for objective evidence of other disorders, can avoid unnecessary hospitalization and surgery.

The physician should strive to substitute discussions of the patient's life problems, personality, and concerns for a quick-triggered response of ordering additional tests and X-rays or yet another medication. At the same time, the physician must recognize the limitations resulting from our lack of knowledge about the causes and mechanisms of the disorder.

REFERENCES

1. Allen, L. A., Escobar, J. I., Lehrer, P. M., Gara, M. A., and Woolfolk, R. L. Psychosocial treatments for multiple unexplained physical symptoms: a review of the literature. Psychosom. Med., *64*:939–950, 2002.
2. Allen, L. A., Woolfolk, R. L., Escobar, J. I., Gara, M. A., and Hamer, R. M. Cognitive-behavioral therapy for somatization disorder: a randomized controlled trial. Arch. Intern. Med., *166*:1512–1518, 2006.
3. American Psychiatric Association. DSM-5 Fact Sheets. Somatic Symptom Disorder. American Psychiatric Association Publishing, 2013. Last accessed 5/26/18. https://www.psychiatry.org/psychiatrists/practice/dsm/educational-resources/dsm-5-fact-sheets.
4. American Psychiatric Association. *Diagnostic and Statistical Manual for Mental Disorders,* 5th edition. Washington, DC: Author, 2013.
5. Andreasen, N. C., and Grove, W. M. Thought, language, and communication in schizophrenia: diagnosis and prognosis. Schizophr. Bull., *12*:348–359, 1986.
6. Arkonac, O., and Guze, S. B. A family study of hysteria. N. Engl. J. Med., *268*:239–242, 1963.
7. Bird, J. The behavioral treatment of hysteria. Br. J. Psychiatry, *134*:129–137, 1979.
8. Blinder, M. G. The hysterical personality. Psychiatry, *29*:227–235, 1966.
9. Bliss, E. L. A symptom profile of patients with multiple personalities, including MMPI results. J. Nerv. Ment. Dis., *172*:197–202, 1984.
10. Boor, M. The multiple personality epidemic. Additional cases and inferences regarding diagnosis, etiology, dynamics, and treatment. J. Nerv. Ment. Dis., *170*:302–304, 1982.
11. Breuer, J., and Freud, S. *Studies in Hysteria,* Brill, A. A. (trans.). New York: Journal of Nervous and Mental Disease Monograph, 1936.
12. Briquet, P. *Traité clinique et thérapeutique à l'hystére.* Paris: J-B Bailliére & Fils, 1859.
13. Cadoret, R. J. Psychopathology in adopted-away offspring of biologic parents with antisocial behavior. Arch. Gen. Psychiatry, *35*:176–184, 1978.
14. Cadoret, R. J., Cunningham, L., Loftus, R., and Edwards, J. Studies of adoptees from psychiatrically disturbed biological parents: III. Medical symptoms and illnesses in childhood and adolescence. Am. J. Psychiatry, *133*:1316–1318, 1976.
15. Carothers, J. C. Hysteria, psychopathy and the magic word. Mankind Q., *16*:93–103, 1975.
16. Chodoff, P. The diagnosis of hysteria: an overview. Am. J. Psychiatry, *131*:1073–1078, 1974.

17. Chodoff, P., and Lyons, H. Hysteria, the hysterical personality and "hysterical" conversion. Am. J. Psychiatry, 114:734–740, 1958.
18. Cloninger, C. R. Somatoform and dissociative disorders. In The Medical Basis of Psychiatry, 2nd edition, Clayton, P., Winokur, G. (eds.). Philadelphia: Saunders, pp. 169–192, 1994.
19. Cloninger, C. R., and Guze, S. B. Female criminals: their personal, familial, and social backgrounds. The relation of these to the diagnoses of sociopathy and hysteria. Arch. Gen. Psychiatry, 23:554–558, 1970.
20. Cloninger, C. R., and Guze, S. B. Psychiatric illness and female criminality: the role of sociopathy and hysteria in the antisocial woman. Am. J. Psychiatry, 127:303–311, 1970.
21. Cloninger, C. R., Martin, R. L., Guze, S. B., and Clayton, P. J. A prospective follow-up and family study of somatization in men and women. Am. J. Psychiatry, 143:873–878, 1986.
22. Cohen, M., Robins, E., Purtell, J., Altmann, M., and Reid, D. Excessive surgery in hysteria. JAMA, 151:977–986, 1953.
23. Coryell, W. A blind family history study of Briquet's syndrome. Arch. Gen. Psychiatry, 37:1266–1269, 1980.
24. Coryell, W., and Norten, S. G. Briquet's syndrome (somatization disorder) and primary depression: comparison of background and outcome. Compr. Psychiatry, 22:249–256, 1981.
25. Creed, F., and Barsky, A. A systematic review of the epidemiology of somatisation disorder and hypochondriasis. J. Psychosom. Res., 56:391–408, 2004.
26. de Figuieredo, J. M., Baiardi, J. J., and Long, D. M. Briquet syndrome in a man with chronic intractable pain. Johns Hopkins Med. J., 147:102–106, 1980.
27. DeSouza, C., and Othmer, E. Somatization disorder and Briquet's syndrome. An assessment of their diagnostic concordance. Arch. Gen. Psychiatry, 41:334–336, 1984.
28. Dimsdale, J. E. DSM-5 proposals for somatic symptom disorders. American Psychiatric Association 165th Annual Meeting, Philadelphia. May, 2012.
29. Dimsdale, J. E., Creed, F., Escobar, J., Sharpe, M., Wulsin, L., Barsky, A., Lee, S., Irwin, M. R., and Levenson, J. Somatic symptom disorder: an important change in DSM. J. Psychosom. Res., 75:223–228, 2013.
30. duGruy, F., Columbia, L., and Dickinson, P. Somatization in a family practice. J. Fam. Pract., 25:45–51, 1987.
31. Edell, W. S. Role of structure in disordered thinking in borderline and schizophrenic disorders. J. Pers. Assess., 51:23–41, 1987.
32. Eysenck, H. The Dynamics of Anxiety and Hysteria. New York: Praeger, 1957.
33. Farley, J., Woodruff, R. A., and Guze, S. B. The prevalence of hysteria and conversion symptoms. Br. J. Psychiatry, 114:1121–1125, 1968.
34. Fink, P., Ewald, H., Jensen, J., Sørensen, L., Engberg, M., Holm, M., and Mink-Jørgensen, P. Screening for somatization and hypochondriasis in primary care and neurological in-patients: a seven-item scale for hypochondriasis and somatization. J. Psychosom. Res., 46:261–273, 1999.
35. Frances, A. DSM-5 somatic symptom disorder. J. Nerv. Ment. Dis., 201:530–531, 2013.
36. Frances, A., and Chapman, S. DSM-5 somatic symptom disorder mislabels medical illness as mental disorder. Aust. N. Z. J. Psychiatry, 47:483–484, 2013.
37. Gatfield, P. D., and Guze, S. B. Prognosis and differential diagnosis of conversion reactions (a follow-up study). Dis. Nerv. Syst., 23:1–8, 1962.

38. Greaves, G. B. Multiple personality. 165 years after Mary Reynolds. J. Nerv. Ment. Dis., *168*:577–596, 1980.

39. Guze, S. B. The diagnosis of hysteria: what are we trying to do? Am. J. Psychiatry, *124*:491–498, 1967.

40. Guze, S. B. The role of follow-up studies: their contribution to diagnostic classification as applied to hysteria. Semin. Psychiatry, 2:392–402, 1970.

41. Guze, S. B., Cloninger, C. R., Martin, R. L., and Clayton, P. J. A follow-up and family study of Briquet's syndrome. Br. J. Psychiatry, *149*:17–23, 1986.

42. Guze, S. B., and Perley, M. J. Observations on the natural history of hysteria. Am. J. Psychiatry, *119*:960–965, 1963.

43. Guze, S. B., Wolfgram, E. D., McKinney, J. K., and Cantwell, D. P. Psychiatric illness in the families of convicted criminals: a study of 519 first-degree relatives. Dis. Nerv. Syst., *28*:651–659, 1967.

44. Guze, S. B., Woodruff, R. A., and Clayton, P. J. A study of conversion symptoms in psychiatric outpatients. Am. J. Psychiatry, *128*:643–646, 1971.

45. Guze, S. B., Woodruff, R. A., and Clayton, P. J. Hysteria and antisocial behavior: further evidence of an association. Am. J. Psychiatry, *127*:957–960, 1971.

46. Hafeiz, H. B. Hysterical conversion: a prognostic study. Br. J. Psychiatry, *136*:548–551, 1980.

47. Hauser, W., and Wolfe, F. The somatic symptom disorder in DSM 5 risks mislabelling people with major medical diseases as mentally ill. J. Psychosom. Res., *75*:586–587, 2013.

48. Hudziak, J. J., Boffelli, T. J., Kreisman, J. J., Battaglia, M. M., Stanger, C., Guze, S. B., and Kriesman, J. J. A clinical study of borderline personality disorder: the significance of Briquet's syndrome (hysteria), somatization disorder, antisocial personality disorder, and substance abuse disorders. Am. J. Psychiatry, *153*:1598–1606, 1996.

49. Kimble, R., Williams, J. G., and Agra, S. A comparison of two methods of diagnosing hysteria. Am. J. Psychiatry, *132*:1197–1199, 1975.

50. Kroenke, K., and Swindle, R. Cognitive-behavioral therapy for somatization and symptom syndromes: a critical review of controlled clinical trials. Psychother. Psychosom., *69*:205–215, 2000.

51. Kroll, P., Chamberlain, K. R., and Halpern, J. The diagnosis of Briquet's syndrome in a male population. J. Nerv. Ment. Dis., *167*:171–174, 1979.

52. Lenze, E. L., Miller, A., Munir, Z., Pornoppadol, C., and North, C. S. Psychiatric symptoms endorsed by somatization disorder patients in a psychiatric clinic. Ann. Clin. Psychiatry, *11*:73–79, 1999.

53. Lewis, D. O., and Shanok, S. S. Medical histories of delinquent and non-delinquent children: an epidemiologic study. Am. J. Psychiatry, *134*:1020–1025, 1977.

54. Lilienfeld, S. O., VanValkenburg, C., Larnitz, K., and Akiskal, H. S. The relationship of histrionic personality disorder to antisocial personality and somatization disorders. Am. J. Psychiatry, *143*:718–722, 1986.

55. Mai, F. M., and Merskey, H. Briquet's Treatise on Hysteria. A synopsis and commentary. Arch. Gen. Psychiatry, *37*:1401–1405, 1980.

56. Mai, F. M., and Merskey, H. Historical review. Briquet's concept of hysteria: an historical perspective. Can. J. Psychiatry, *26*:57–63, 1981.

57. Marsden, C. D. Hysteria: a neurologist's view. Psychol. Med., *16*:277–288, 1986.

58. Martin, R. L. Problems in the diagnosis of somatization disorder: effects on research and clinical practice. Psychiatr. Ann., *18*:357–362, 1988.

59. Mohr, P. D., and Bond, M. J. A chronic epidemic of hysterical blackouts in a comprehensive school. Br. Med. J., *284*:961–962, 1982.

60. Morrison, J. R. Early birth order in Briquet's syndrome. Am. J. Psychiatry, *140*:1596–1598, 1983.

61. Murphy, G. E. The clinical management of hysteria. JAMA, *247*:2559–2564, 1982.

62. Murphy, G. E., Robins, E., Kuhn, N., and Christiansen, R. F. Stress, sickness and psychiatric disorder in a "normal" population: a study of 101 young women. J. Nerv. Ment. Dis., *134*:228–236, 1962.

63. North, C. S. The classification of hysteria and related disorders: historical and phenomenological considerations. Behav. Sci. (Basel), *5*:496–517, 2015.

64. North, C. S., Hansen, K., Wetzel, R. D., Compton, W., Napier, M., and Spitznagel, E. L. Non-psychotic thought disorder: objective clinical identification of somatization and antisocial personality in language patterns. Compr. Psychiatry, *38*:171–178, 1997.

65. North, C. S., Kienstra, D. M., Osborne, V. A., Dokucu, M. E., Vassilenko, M., Hong, B., Wetzel, R. D., and Spitznagel, E. L. Interrater reliability and coding guide for nonpsychotic formal thought disorder. Percept. Mot. Skills, *103*:395–411, 2006.

66. North, C. S., Ryall, J. M., Ricci, D. A., and Wetzel, R. D. *Multiple Personalities, Multiple Disorders: Psychiatric Classification and Media Influence.* New York: Oxford University Press, 1993.

67. Perley, M. J., and Guze, S. B. Hysteria—the stability and usefulness of clinical criteria. N. Engl. J. Med., *266*:421–426, 1962.

68. Pribor, E. F., Smith, D. S., and Yutzy, S. H. Somatization disorder in elderly patients. Am. J. Geriatr. Psychiatry, *2*:109–117, 1994.

69. Purtell, J. J., Robins, E., and Cohen, M. E. Observations on the clinical aspects of hysteria: a quantitative study of 50 patients and 156 control subjects. JAMA, *146*:902–909, 1951.

70. Reis, R. K. Single case study. DSM-III differential diagnosis of Munchausen's syndrome. J. Nerv. Ment. Dis., *168*:629–632, 1980.

71. Robins, E., Murphy, G. E., Wilkinson, R. H., Jr., Gassner, S., and Kayes, J. Some clinical considerations in the prevention of suicide based on a study of 134 successful suicides. Am. J. Publ. Health, *49*:888–899, 1959.

72. Robins, E., Purtell, J. J., and Cohen, M. E. "Hysteria" in men. N. Engl. J. Med., *246*:677–685, 1952.

73. Robins, L. N. *Deviant Children Grown Up: A Sociological and Psychiatric Study of Sociopathic Personality.* Baltimore: Williams & Wilkins, 1966.

74. Rounsaville, B. J., Harding, P. S., and Weissman, M. M. Single case study. Briquet's syndrome in a man. J. Nerv. Ment. Dis., *167*:364–367, 1979.

75. Savill, T. D. *Lectures on Hysteria and Allied Vasomotor Conditions.* London: H.J. Glaisher, 1909.

76. Schmidt, E. H., O'Neal, P., and Robins, E. Evaluation of suicide attempts as guide to therapy. Clinical and follow-up study of 109 patients. JAMA, *155*:547–557, 1954.

77. Simon, G. E., and VonKorff, M. Somatization and psychiatric disorder in the NIMH Epidemiologic Catchment Area study. Am. J. Psychiatry, *148*:1494–1500, 1991.

78. Slater, E. Diagnosis of "hysteria". Br. Med. J., *29*:1395–1399, 1965.

79. Small, G. W., and Nicoli Jr, A. M. Mass hysteria among schoolchildren. Early loss as a predisposing factor. Arch. Gen. Psychiatry, *39*:721–724, 1982.

80. Smith, G. R., Monson, R. A., and Ray, D. C. Psychiatric consultation in somatization disorder. N. Engl. J. Med., *314*:1407–1413, 1986.

81. Spalt, L. Hysteria and antisocial personality. A single disorder? J. Nerv. Ment. Dis., *168*:456–464, 1980.

82. Stefansson, J. G., Messina, J. A., and Meyerwitz, S. Hysterical neurosis, conversion type: clinical and epidemiological considerations. Acta Psychiatr. Scand., *53*:119–138, 1976.

83. Swartz, M., Blazer, D., Woodbury, M., George, L., and Landerman, R. Somatization disorder in a US southern community: use of a new procedure for analysis of medical classification. Psychol. Med., *16*:595–609, 1986.

84. Tomasson, K., Kent, D., and Coryell, W. Somatization and conversion disorders: comorbidity and demographics at presentation. Acta Psychiatr. Scand., *84*:288–293, 1991.

85. Veith, I. *Hysteria: The History of a Disease.* Chicago: University of Chicago Press, 1965.

86. Von Knorring, A.-L. *Adoption Studies on Psychiatric Illness.* Sweden: Umea, 1983.

87. Wakefield, J. C. DSM-5, psychiatric epidemiology and the false positives problem. Epidemiol. Psychiatr. Sci., *24*:188–196, 2015.

88. Wakefield, J. C. Diagnostic issues and controversies in DSM-5: return of the false positives problem. Annu. Rev Clin. Psychol., *12*:105–132, 2016.

89. Watson, C. G., and Buranen, C. The frequency and identification of false positive conversion reactions. J. Nerv. Ment. Dis., *167*:243–247, 1979.

90. Weissman, M. M., Myers, J. K., and Harding, P. S. Psychiatric disorders in a US urban community: 1975–1976. Am. J. Psychiatry, *135*:459–462, 1978.

91. Wetzel, R. D., Guze, S. B., Cloninger, C. R., Martin, R. L., and Clayton, P. J. Briquet's syndrome (hysteria) is both a somatoform and a "psychoform" illness: a Minnesota Multiphasic Personality Inventory study. Psychosomat. Med., *56*:564–569, 1994.

92. Woerner, P. I., and Guze, S. B. A family and marital study of hysteria. Br. J. Psychiatry, *114*:161–168, 1968.

93. Woodruff, R. Hysteria: an evaluation of objective diagnostic criteria by the study of women with chronic medical illness. Br. J. Psychiatry, *114*:1115–1119, 1968.

94. Woodruff, R. A., Clayton, P. J., and Guze, S. B. Hysteria: studies of diagnosis, outcome, and prevalence. JAMA, *215*:425–428, 1971.

95. Yutzy, S. H. Somatization. In *Psychosomatic Medicine in the 21st Century,* Blumenfield, B., Strain, J. J. (eds.). Baltimore: Lippincott, Williams, and Wilkins, pp. 537–543, 2006.

96. Yutzy, S. H., Cloninger, C. R., Guze, S. B., Pribor, E. F., Martin, R. L., Kathol, R. G., Smith, G. R., and Strain, J. J. DSM-IV field trial: testing a new proposal for somatization disorder. Am. J. Psychiatry, *152*:97–101, 1995.

97. Yutzy, S. H., and Parish, B. S. Somatoform disorders. In *The American Psychiatric Press Textbook of Psychiatry,* fifth edition, Hales, R. E., Yudofsky, S. C., Gabbard, G. O. (eds.). Washington, DC: American Psychiatric Press, pp. 609–642, 2008.

98. Yutzy, S. H., Pribor, E. F., Cloninger, C. R., and Guze, S. B. Reconsidering the criteria for somatization disorder. Hosp. Commun. Psychiatry, *43*:1075–1076, 1149, 1992.

99. Zanarini, M. C., Gunderson, J. G., and Frankenburg, F. R. Cognitive features of borderline personality disorder. Am. J. Psychiatry, *147*:57–63, 1990.

100. Ziegler, F. J., Imboden, J. B., and Meyer, E. Contemporary conversion reactions: clinical study. Am. J. Psychiatry, *116*:901–910, 1960.

CHAPTER 9

✧

Antisocial Personality Disorder

"Antisocial personality disorder" refers to a pattern of recurrent antisocial, delinquent, and criminal behavior that begins in childhood or early adolescence and is manifested by disturbances in many areas of life: family relations, education, work, military service, and marriage. The older term, "sociopathy," is occasionally used in the sections that follow, particularly in reference to the older studies, but this term is considered to be synonymous here with antisocial personality disorder.

HISTORICAL BACKGROUND

Prichard's 1835 monograph, *A Treatise on Insanity and Other Disorders Affecting the Mind*, is often cited as furnishing the first description of what is now called "antisocial or sociopathic personality" (72). Under the label "moral insanity" he defined the disorder in this way (p. 15):

> The intellectual faculties appear to have sustained little or no injury, while the disorder is manifested principally or alone in the state of the feelings, temper, or habits. In cases of this description the moral and active principles of the mind are strongly perverted and depraved; the power of self-government is lost or impaired; and the individual is found to be incapable . . . of conducting himself with decency and propriety . . . [having] undergone a morbid change.

As Craft argued (18), Prichard included under this rubric many examples of "temporary mental illness," and most of those cases were probably patients with affective disorder. Craft (p. 10) quoted Clouston's 1883 volume (pp. 347–348) (15): "Prichard . . . vividly described the disease, but I should place most of his cases in my category of simple mania."

Clouston (15) referred also to children "so constituted that they cannot be educated in morality on account of an innate brain deficiency . . . incapable of knowing . . . right and wrong . . . . Such moral idiots I, like others, have met with frequently . . . and persons with this want of development we may label under moral insanity" (pp. 347–348).

Craft pointed out that Prichard used "moral" in three ways: first, in referring to "moral" treatment, meaning psychological treatment; second, in referring to emotional or affective responses in contrast to intellectual ones; and third, in an ethical sense of right or wrong. Most of the time, Prichard used the term in the first two ways and only incidentally in the last way.

As Craft also noted, Benjamin Rush, in 1812, described "derangement of the moral faculties" as follows (pp. 356–357) (80):

The moral faculty, conscience, and sense of deity are sometimes totally deranged. The Duke of Sully has given us a striking instance of this universal moral derangement in the character of a young man who belonged to his suite, of the name of Servin, who, after a life uncommonly distinguished by every possible vice, died, cursing and denying his God. Mr. Haslam has described two cases of it in the Bethlem Hospital, one of whom, a boy of 13 years of age, was perfectly sensible of his depravity, and often asked "why God had not made him like other men." . . . In the course of my life, I have been consulted in three cases of the total perversion of the moral faculties. One of them was in a young man, the second in a young woman, both of Virginia, and the third was in the daughter of a citizen of Philadelphia. The last was addicted to every kind of mischief. Her mischief and wickedness had no intervals while she was awake, except when she was kept busy in some steady and difficult employment. In all of these cases of innate, preternatural moral depravity, there is probably an original defective organization in those parts of the body which are occupied by the moral faculties of the mind.

It was Craft's (18) conclusion that "Rush appears to give the first description of those with sound reason and good intellect who have an innate or lifelong irresponsibility without shame, being unchanged in affect, or by the consequences or by regard for others" (p. 9). Thus, Craft challenged the appropriateness of crediting Prichard with the first description.

Controversy over the concept of "moral insanity" developed partly in regard to the question of whether the "morally insane" should be committed to mental hospitals or should be considered mentally ill in a court of law.

The terms gradually fell into disuse as interest in the whole range of personality disorders grew.

In 1889 Koch (50) introduced the term "psychopathic inferiority" to imply a constitutional predisposition for many deviations of personality, including at least some that are now classified as anxiety disorders. Kraepelin (52), Kahn (47), and Schneider (84) proposed various classifications of personality disorders. Schneider's definition of psychopathic personalities as "all those abnormal personalities who suffer from their abnormalities or cause society to suffer" clearly included much more than "moral imbecility."

The term "psychopathic personality" was used inconsistently, sometimes to refer to the whole spectrum of deviant personalities and sometimes to a subgroup of antisocial or aggressive "psychopaths." Finally, to reduce confusion, the term "sociopathic personality disturbance" was introduced for the latter group and was adopted in 1952 by the American Psychiatric Association's *Diagnostic and Statistical Manual of Mental Disorders*, first edition (*DSM-I*). Nevertheless, many went on using the terms "psychopathy" and "sociopathy" interchangeably, whereas others continued to regard sociopathy as only one form of psychopathy. In a further attempt to reduce confusion, "antisocial personality" was adopted as the official diagnosis for the aggressive or antisocial psychopath or sociopath in later revisions of the *DSM* (*III, III-R, IV, IV-TR*, and *5*) and the International Classification of Disease (ICD). Sir Aubrey Lewis summarized the history of the concept (55). Over time, the antisocial personality disorder diagnosis became widely accepted as the first formally established personality disorder. Unfortunately, because of evidence that psychiatric diagnoses have been applied to political dissenters in other countries, some psychiatrists have been reluctant to use this diagnosis, despite the recognition that individuals with the clinical picture of antisocial personality are found all over the world and that only a few are political dissenters.

EPIDEMIOLOGY

Satisfactory data on the prevalence of antisocial personality disorder are lacking. This partly reflects the failure to reach a general agreement about a definition as well as label evolution. In the Epidemiologic Catchment Area Study, the population prevalence varied between 2.6% and 5.1%, depending on variation in diagnostic criteria (79). (The ratio of males to females in this study varied between 1.62%/1.25% and 9.4%/1.5%.) More recent studies have varied but generally prevalence rates have been between 2% and 3% (16, 66). Higher prevalence rates among men are consistently reported

(22). The prevalence of antisocial personality disorder in forensic settings and correctional settings has been estimated at 50% (43, 79). In general, we do not know what proportion of individuals with antisocial personality disorder come to the attention of physicians. Nevertheless, sociopathy is seen frequently in psychiatric facilities, usually because of associated alcohol and other substance abuse/dependence and depression, and because psychiatric care is made a condition of probation and parole. In one series, 15% of male and 3% of female psychiatric outpatients had antisocial personality disorder (97).

Indirect estimates of population frequency, based on figures for juvenile delinquency and police trouble of all kinds, suggest that antisocial personality is common, probably increasingly so; is much more frequent among males than females; is more common in urban than rural environments; and is most common in low socioeconomic groups (57, 78).

Individuals with antisocial personality usually come from grossly disturbed families. Parental separation or divorce, early death, desertion, alcoholism, and criminality are characteristic. Only a small minority of individuals with antisocial personality disorder, in fact, come from families that are not characterized by one or more of these phenomena (17, 25, 38, 46, 51).

CLINICAL PICTURE

Early antisocial personality (termed "conduct disorder") begins in childhood or early adolescence (3, 65). The first manifestations may be those of the hyperactive child syndrome (25, 59, 67, 82, 83, 96). An adoption study found evidence for a genetic factor associated with some cases of childhood hyperactivity/attention-deficit disorder and adult antisocial personality (9). Other investigators have demonstrated, however, when early hyperactivity is not accompanied by delinquent or antisocial behavior, it much less often leads to antisocial personality patterns. At the same time, delinquency associated with hyperactivity tends to be more severe than delinquency alone, with a worse prognosis for adult adjustment (69, 92). Restlessness, a short attention span, and unresponsiveness to discipline are common. Frequent fighting, often leading to conflicts with adults, and a history of being a general neighborhood nuisance are also common (12, 77).

A disturbed school history is characteristic of early antisocial behavior. In fact, a history of satisfactory school adjustment through high school is so unusual that either the diagnosis or the history should be questioned if it is present. Disruption of classes by talking out of turn, failure to pay attention to the teacher, fighting with classmates, arguing with the teacher, and even fighting with the teacher occur. Academic failures, truancy, and suspension often lead to school dropout or permanent expulsion (12, 40, 77).

Running away from home is also common, though it may be limited to a few one-night episodes. Occasionally, adolescents will disappear for weeks or months. During such absences, they may wander around the country, hitchhiking, doing odd jobs, and bumming around (77).

The job history is characterized by poor performance. Lack of dependability (being late, missing work, quitting without warning), inability to accept criticism and advice, frequent job changes without advancement, and being fired are typical (47, 77). Poor job performance coupled with limited and incomplete education result in low socioeconomic status, low income, and frequent requests for financial assistance from family or society.

Early marriage is typical, especially among women. Very few women with antisocial personality, in fact, fail to marry. Their marriages are marked by infidelity, separation, and divorce. Males have similar marital difficulties. Individuals with the disorder tend to marry those with the disorder (13, 36).

Judges used to handle delinquency by suspending punishment if the offender enlisted in the armed services. Generally, however, individuals with antisocial personality do not do well in military service. Lack of reliability and inability to conform to military discipline results in AWOL absences, difficulties with superiors, court martial, and less-than-honorable discharge. The type of discharge is usually determined by the nature of the offenses, the philosophy of the commanding officer, and general military policy at the time.

Sooner or later, most individuals with the disorder have trouble with the law. Some investigators, in fact, have required police trouble for the diagnosis of antisocial personality disorder (82). Stealing money from the mother's purse or father's wallet or from a schoolmate may be an early sign of a budding criminal career. Shoplifting, peace disturbance (usually associated with drunkenness and fighting), various traffic offenses, auto theft, burglary, larceny, rape, robbery, and homicide may all occur. A sociopathic pattern of behavior is found in many convicted male (37, 42, 82) and female (13) felons.

Many individuals with antisocial personality disorder engage in lying and the use of aliases, usually as understandable responses to social or legal difficulties, but sometimes without any obvious need to avoid punishment or retaliation. Such behavior has been called "pathological lying."

Elaborate stories may be told to confuse or impress relatives. This behavior can take extreme forms, such as masquerading as a physician, military officer, or businessperson. In time, relatives, friends, parole officers, and physicians learn to discount a significant amount of what they are told by the individual.

Conversion symptoms (unexplained neurological symptoms) are common in the disorder; in fact, antisocial personality disorder is second only to somatization disorder (*DSM-IV*) in producing such symptoms (39). Among individuals with antisocial personality, conversion symptoms are characteristically associated with obvious social stresses such as police trouble. The full somatization disorder (*DSM-IV*) may also be seen in association with sociopathy (antisocial personality disorder). Many women with somatization disorder (*DSM-IV*) give a history of previous or concurrent antisocial behavior (13); many young delinquent and antisocial girls develop somatization disorder (*DSM-IV*) as adults (13, 58, 77).

Many studies of delinquents and individuals with antisocial behavior indicate that their average IQ is below normal, but only a minority of these individuals suffer from significant intellectual disability with an IQ less than 70 (18, 57). These studies have not all been adequately controlled for socioeconomic status, sibship size, and other variables correlated with intelligence. Low intelligence probably is not an important factor in the etiology of antisocial personality disorder.

A charming manner, lack of guilt or remorse, absence of anxiety, and failure to learn by experience are said to be characteristic of antisocial personality. The easy-going, open, and winning style, when present, presumably accounts for the success of people with antisocial personality as "confidence men." At best, however, the charm and appeal are superficial; often they are entirely absent.

When seen by psychiatrists, many individuals with antisocial personality report anxiety symptoms, depression, and guilt (10, 97). These frequently occur with alcoholism. The guilt and remorse do not seem to lead to reduction of antisocial behavior, however. This persistence of antisocial behavior, despite repeated failure and punishment, is the basis for the statement that people with antisocial personality "do not learn from experience." Suicide attempts are not rare, but completed suicide, in the absence of alcoholism or drug dependence, is infrequent (26).

Many people occasionally manifest antisocial or delinquent behavior. But only a minority demonstrates a consistent pattern of recurrent and repeated antisocial, delinquent, and criminal behavior beginning in childhood and lasting well into adulthood. The following case provides a vivid example of such persistent and pervasive behavior, justifying the diagnosis of antisocial personality.

A 28-year-old man was seen in a hospital's emergency room because of repeated "spells" or "fits" while in jail; he had been arrested for driving while intoxicated, disturbing the peace, and resisting arrest. The patient's problem behavior had begun at about age 7 or 8 when his parents reported to the local school that they could not handle their son because he was "wild" and "couldn't sit still." Similar behavior had been noted by the school, and a request had been made for the parents to meet with the teacher. From that time forward, a recurrent pattern became evident of fighting in school, other discipline troubles, poor academic performance, several suspensions, and regular truancy.

At the same time, the parents noted that the patient stole money from them and began to stay out late at night, presumably running around with a neighborhood gang. At about age 14, the boy had his first police contact. He and several members of his gang were arrested for stealing from a number of neighborhood stores. Nothing came of this, but at age 17 the patient was arrested for driving a stolen vehicle; he received a suspended sentence. Soon thereafter, he dropped out of school and started to work. His work record was most unsatisfactory, however, because of frequently missing days of work and because he was considered to be a troublemaker by his supervisors. As a result of this pattern, he failed at several jobs. He then enlisted in the army, where his inability to conform to expectations and accept military discipline resulted in a general discharge after 10 months.

Soon after leaving the army, he got married, but as soon as his wife became pregnant, he deserted her. Around that time his parents became aware that he was drinking excessively and experimenting with a variety of illicit street drugs. He and his wife had a stormy marriage with frequent separations and reconciliations. After the birth of three children, they permanently separated. His wife accused him of physical abuse and repeated infidelity, as well as inappropriate physical aggression toward the children (beating).

His work record continued to be erratic, and he was a frequent visitor to local medical clinics and emergency rooms with a variety of physical complaints. On one occasion, he was admitted briefly to a psychiatric unit because of taking an overdose of sleeping pills and illicit drugs.

In summary, this patient's life history is typical for antisocial personality. It includes a panoply of interpersonal and social difficulties, including problems with school, employment, military service, parents, and family, as well as with the police.

BIOLOGICAL FINDINGS

Multitudinous studies have attempted to assess "constitutional" factors in sociopathy over many years (87). One of the earlier organic theories was based on more frequent reports of nonspecifically disordered electroencephalograms (EEGs) among individuals with sociopathy than controls; however, many, if not most, do not have abnormal EEGs (2, 30). Some authors have reported an association between delinquency, learning disability, and neurological impairment, but this has not been a completely consistent finding (91). Many studies have explored psychophysiological response patterns in sociopathy, and a theory of low autonomic and cortical arousal has been formulated to account for a persistent "stimulus hunger" or for the inability to learn socially approved behavior. The theory is thought to explain the impulsive, excitement-seeking, and antisocial behavior of sociopathy (41, 63, 73, 82).

More recent studies have suggested that lowered cerebrospinal fluid 5-hydro-xyindoleacetic acid levels, pointing to some alteration in serotonin metabolism, may predict antisocial behavior, alone or in combination with various measures of autonomic arousal (54). The research findings have not been entirely consistent (63), and some authors (61) have emphasized "a wider degree of variability in arousal levels and reactivity than [in] normal individuals." An association between criminal behavior and chromosomal abnormalities has been reported. In particular, XYY karyotype, unusual height, and impulsive crimes have been associated, but not all studies are consistent (1, 23, 45, 68). On the other hand, more cases of the XXY karyotype (Klinefelter syndrome) than of the XYY karyotype were found in a large Finnish series of male criminals referred for psychiatric evaluation (85). Studies of hormone levels, including androgens and adrenal steroids, have shown inconsistent differences between individuals with and without sociopathy (24, 53, 60).

Extensive neurobiological studies have been undertaken over the past 30 years searching for the etiological basis for sociopathy. While comprehensive review is beyond the scope of this chapter, Cummings (21) has outlined the most relevant noteworthy but nonconvergent investigations. In summary, there is neither an identified organic etiology nor a reliable physiological marker for antisocial personality disorder.

NATURAL HISTORY

Antisocial personality disorder begins early in life (78). In some cases it may begin before the child starts attending school. Few individuals with this disorder get through high school without recurrent difficulties. If the antisocial and delinquent pattern has not begun by age 15 or 16, it is unlikely to occur. The prognosis may be better when the juvenile delinquency is "socialized," that is, when it occurs in a setting of close group involvement or loyalty (44). Lower socioeconomic status, being female, and relative youth may adversely affect the clinical picture, but this is not a consistent finding (48).

The disorder is recurrent and varies in severity. Some individuals with antisocial personality, generally milder cases, may remit during the late teens or early or mid-20s (48). In other instances, antisocial behavior persists into early middle age and then remits (4, 93, 94). Some of these individuals never improve. Attempts to explain remission have been based on hypothetical maturing or burning out.

Remission, when it occurs, usually comes only after years of antisocial behavior, during which education and work achievement have been severely compromised. Individuals with antisocial behavior rarely recover sufficiently to compensate for the "lost years." Thus, "remission" usually means no more than a marginal social adjustment. Even if antisocial behavior subsides, alcohol and drug abuse and dependence persist and influence long-term adjustment (45).

COMPLICATIONS

The complications of antisocial behavior explain why the disorder is legitimately a medical concern. High rates of sexually transmitted disease, extramarital pregnancies, injuries from fights and accidents, alcohol and drug dependence (4, 8, 27, 45, 56), and various medical complications of these conditions mean that individuals with antisocial behavior often come to the attention of physicians. Furthermore, increased mortality from accidents and homicide contributes to a reduced life expectancy, particularly in early adulthood (62, 76). The judicial cost to society is almost incalculable.

FAMILY STUDIES

As noted, individuals with antisocial personality generally come from families with severe social disturbances and disruption. Much of this family pathology consists of antisocial personality and alcoholism (70, 71, 94). In a study of male felons, most of whom had antisocial personality, one-fifth of the first-degree male relatives had antisocial personality disorder and one-third had alcoholism (38). In a study of female felons, half of whom had antisocial personality disorder, one-third of the male relatives had antisocial personality disorder and one-half had alcoholism (14). In a study of children seen in a child guidance clinic (77), one-third of the fathers and one-tenth of the mothers of antisocial children had either antisocial personality disorder or alcohol dependence.

Among the attempts to determine whether this familial pattern reflects genetic factors have been investigations of twins and adoptees. Twin studies generally have focused on antisocial behavior, delinquency, or criminality, without distinguishing between individuals with sociopathy and others who show these behavior patterns. Nevertheless, as most criminals apparently have sociopathy (35), this approach appears somewhat justified. In twin studies, the concordance rates with regard to behavior difficulties, delinquency, and criminality have nearly always been higher for monozygotic than dizygotic twins (63, 88). However, the differences have not been as great as those seen in other psychiatric illnesses where a genetic predisposition is suspected. Furthermore, all of the early series were small and the monozygotic-dizygotic difference in some did not reach statistical significance.

Twin studies of psychiatric illness may involve bias in ascertainment of cases because concordant cases may come to the attention of physicians more often than discordant cases. Population twin registries have been proposed as more suitable for unbiased ascertainment. Christiansen was able to obtain a presumably unselected series of criminal twins through access to a register of all Danish twin births (11). He found that monozygotic twins had a significantly higher concordance rate than dizygotic twins (36% versus 12%). Later efforts have been confounded by multiple factors, including operational issues (examining for different diagnoses [antisocial personality disorder or "psychopathy"] or just variably defined "antisocial" symptoms [aggression or criminality]), assessment methods (self-report, records, or questionnaire), zygosity (usually blood type but occasionally by questionnaire), and age.

Many follow-up studies of children of criminals and "psychopaths" indicate that these children, when adopted early in life by nonrelatives, are more likely to reveal psychopathic and criminal behavior as adults than are adopted children whose biological parents were not criminals or psychopaths (5–7, 19, 20, 86). The association between sociopathy and somatization disorder (*DSM-IV*) within families and in the same individual (discussed in Chapter 8) has been confirmed in other studies (90).

Eventually, meta-analyses (with their own sets of issues) were applied to the twins/adoption studies (estimated at over 100 twins/adoption studies by 2001) (89), and genes were found to account for approximately 40%

of the variance (74). Unfortunately, subsequent molecular genetics studies have not been supportive, with variable and inconsistent findings (81, 95).

DIFFERENTIAL DIAGNOSIS

The differential diagnosis of antisocial personality includes alcohol dependence, drug dependence, somatization disorder, schizophrenia, mania, and organic brain syndrome. Alcohol and drug abuse are frequent complications of antisocial behavior, and they aggravate antisocial and criminal patterns. In addition, however, some alcohol and drug abusers who did not show antisocial behavior in childhood or adolescence before the onset of alcohol or drug dependence do show such behavior as a manifestation of the alcohol or drug dependence. In these cases, the crucial diagnostic feature is the age of onset of antisocial and delinquent behavior; it is usually after age 15 and coincident with or following the onset of the alcohol and drug abuse. When antisocial behavior and alcohol or drug abuse all begin about the same time and before age 15, only follow-up may clarify the diagnosis, and often it is not possible to separate the antisocial behavior from the alcohol or drug dependence.

The familial and clinical associations between antisocial personality disorder and somatization disorder (*DSM-IV*) have already been noted. Many women with antisocial personality and an occasional man with antisocial personality develop the picture of somatization disorder (*DSM-IV*) (40, 58). Moreover, there is an increased frequency of antisocial behavior and delinquency in the past histories and family histories of women with somatization disorder who do not have antisocial personality (40). Finally, somatization disorder (*DSM-IV*) and antisocial personality disorder cluster in the same families. All of these observations suggest that the differential diagnosis between the two conditions may involve the recognition of overlapping manifestations of similar etiological factors (34).

A small minority of men with schizophrenia give a history of antisocial patterns in adolescence, and a small number of young people with antisocial behavior, at follow-up, turn out to have schizophrenia (77), but the prevalence of antisocial personality is not increased in the biological relatives of individuals with schizophrenia compared to the relatives of controls (75). If evidence of schizophrenia has not appeared by the early 20s, however, it is unlikely to develop.

The behavior in early-onset mania may mimic that of antisocial personality, especially in women. Occasionally it will be difficult to distinguish mania from antisocial personality when the latter is complicated by amphetamine or other drug abuse. Follow-up should clarify the issue. Because mania before age 15 remains rare (32), a history of antisocial and delinquent behavior before that age would suggest antisocial personality disorder (conduct disorder) rather than mania. Although antisocial and criminal behavior may accompany delirium or dementia, neither commonly develops in childhood or early adolescence, and follow-up at any age will allow ascertainment of the medical cause.

CLINICAL MANAGEMENT

A major problem in treating antisocial personality disorder is the patient's lack of motivation for change. Few people with antisocial personality disorder volunteer for treatment. They are nearly always brought to the physician's attention by pressure from schools, parents, or judges. Moreover, the commonly disturbed family situation and poor socioeconomic circumstances provide little support for any treatment program. Many therapists believe that early institutional therapy offers the only hope for success, but there is no consensus about this (31). Psychotherapy has not achieved impressive results (98). Broad review of psychological interventional trials has produced inadequate evidence to support any psychological intervention (28). Biological psychiatry proffers no empirically supported treatment intervention (33, 49, 64).

It is particularly difficult to carry out treatment if associated alcoholism or drug dependence cannot be controlled. In many cases, remission of the alcohol or drug abuse is accompanied by a reduction in antisocial and criminal behavior (35). Because antisocial personality disorder begins early and individuals at high risk can be readily recognized (29, 77), early case finding and intervention may ultimately offer hope of intervention with prevention.

REFERENCES

1. Akesson, H. O., Forssman, H., Wahlstrom, J., and Wallin, L. Sex chromosome aneuploidy among men in three Swedish hospitals for the mentally retarded and maladjusted. Br. J. Psychiatry, *125*:386–389, 1974.
2. Arthurs, R., and Cahoon, E. A clinical and electroencephalographic survey of psychopathic personality. Am. J. Psychiatry, *120*:875–877, 1964.
3. Behar, D., and Stewart, M. A. Aggressive conduct disorder: the influence of social class, sex and age on the clinical picture. Psychol. Psychiatry, *25*:119–124, 1984.

4. Bland, R. C., Newman, S. C., and Orn, H. Age and remission of psychiatric disorders. Can. J. Psychiatry, 42:722–729, 1997.
5. Cadoret, R. J. Psychopathology in adopted-away offspring of biologic parents with antisocial behavior. Arch. Gen. Psychiatry, 35:176–184, 1978.
6. Cadoret, R. J., and Cain, C. Sex differences in predictors of antisocial behavior in adoptees. Arch. Gen. Psychiatry, 37:1171–1175, 1980.
7. Cadoret, R. J., Cunningham, L., Loftus, R., and Edwards, J. Studies of adoptees from psychiatrically disturbed biological parents. II. Temperament, hyperactive, antisocial and developmental variables. J. Pediatr., 87:301–306, 1975.
8. Cadoret, R. J., O'Gorman, T. W., Troughton, E., and Heywood, E. Alcoholism and antisocial personality: interrelationships, genetics and environmental factors. Arch. Gen. Psychiatry, 42:161–167, 1985.
9. Cadoret, R. J., Troughton, E., O'Gormon, T. W., and Heywood, E. An adoption study of genetic and environmental factors in drug abuse. Arch. Gen. Psychiatry, 43:1131–1136, 1986.
10. Chiles, J. A., Miller, M. L., and Cox, G. B. Depression in an adolescent delinquent population. Arch. Gen. Psychiatry, 37:1179–1184, 1980.
11. Christiansen, K. O. Crime in a Danish twin population. Acta Genet. Med. Gemellol., 19:323–326, 1970.
12. Cleckley, H. *The Mask of Sanity*. New York: Mosby, 1982.
13. Cloninger, C. R., and Guze, S. B. Psychiatric illness and female criminality: the role of sociopathy and hysteria in the antisocial woman. Am. J. Psychiatry, 127:303–311, 1970.
14. Cloninger, C. R., and Guze, S. B. Psychiatric illness in the families of female criminals: a study of 288 first-degree relatives. Br. J. Psychiatry, 122:697–703, 1973.
15. Clouston, T. S. *Clinical Lectures on Mental Diseases*. London: Churchill, 1883.
16. Coid, J., Yang, M., Tyrer, P., Roberts, A., and Ullrich, S. Prevalence and correlates of personality disorder in Great Britain. Br. J. Psychiatry, 188:423–431, 2006.
17. Cowie, J., Cowie, V., and Slater, E. *Delinquency in Girls*. London: Humanities Press, 1968.
18. Craft, M. *Ten Studies into Psychopathic Personality*. Bristol: John Wright & Sons, 1965.
19. Crowe, R. R. The adopted offspring of women criminal offenders. Arch. Gen. Psychiatry, 27:600–603, 1972.
20. Crowe, R. R. An adoption study of antisocial personality. Arch. Gen. Psychiatry, 31:785–791, 1974.
21. Cummings, M. A. The neurobiology of psychopathy: recent developments and new directions in research and treatment. CNS Spectr., 20:200–206, 2015.
22. Dolan, M., and Vollm, B. Antisocial personality disorder and psychopathy in women: a literature review on the reliability and validity of assessment instruments. Int. J. Law Psychiatry, 32:2–9, 2009.
23. Editorial. What becomes of the XYY male? Lancet, 2:1297–1298, 1974.
24. Ehrenkranz, J., Bliss, E., and Sheard, M. H. Plasma testosterone: correlation with aggressive behavior and social dominance in man. Psychosomat. Med., 36:468–475, 1974.
25. Farrington, D. P. Childhood origins of teenage antisocial behaviour and adult social dysfunction. J. R. Soc. Med., 86:13–17, 1993.
26. Garvey, M. J. Suicide attempts in antisocial personality disorder. Compr. Psychiatry, 21:146–149, 1980.

27. Gerstley, L. J., Alterman, A. I., McLellan, A. T., and Woody, G. E. Antisocial personality disorder in patients with substance abuse disorders: a problematic diagnosis? Am. J. Psychiatry, *147*:173–178, 1990.
28. Gibbon, S., Duggan, C., Stoffers, J., Huband, N., Vollm, B. A., Ferriter, M., and Lieb, K. Psychological interventions for antisocial personality disorder. Cochrane Database Syst. Rev., CD007668, 2010.
29. Glueck, S., and Glueck, E. *Predicting Delinquency and Crime*. Cambridge, MA: Harvard University Press, 1959.
30. Gottlieb, J. S., Ashby, M. C., and Knott, J. R. Primary behavior disorders and psychopathic personality. Arch. Neurol. Psychiatry, *56*:381–400, 1946.
31. Gralnick, A. Management of character disorders in a hospital setting. Am. J. Psychother., *33*:54–66, 1979.
32. Grimmer, Y., Hohmann, S., and Poustka, L. Is bipolar always bipolar? Understanding the controversy on bipolar disorder in children. F1000Prime. Rep., *6*:111, 2014.
33. Gunderson, J. G., and Phillips, K. A. Personality disorders. In *Comprehensive Textbook of Psychiatry, Volume 2*, second edition, Kaplan, H. I., Sadock, B. J. (eds.). Baltimore: Williams & Wilkins, pp. 1425–1444, 1995.
34. Guze, S. B. The role of follow-up studies: their contribution to diagnostic classification as applied to hysteria. Semin. Psychiatry, *2*:392–402, 1970.
35. Guze, S. B., Goodwin, D. W., and Crane, J. B. Criminality and psychiatric disorders. Arch. Gen. Psychiatry, *20*:583–591, 1969.
36. Guze, S. B., Goodwin, D. W., and Crane, J. B. A psychiatric study of the wives of convicted felons: an example of assortative mating. Am. J. Psychiatry, *126*:1773–1776, 1970.
37. Guze, S. B., Goodwin, D. W., and Crane, J. B. Criminal recidivism and psychiatric illness. Am. J. Psychiatry, *127*:832–835, 1970.
38. Guze, S. B., Wolfgram, E. D., McKinney, J. K., and Cantwell, D. P. Psychiatric illness in the families of convicted criminals: a study of 519 first-degree relatives. Dis. Nerv. Syst., *28*:651–659, 1967.
39. Guze, S. B., Woodruff, R. A., and Clayton, P. J. A study of conversion symptoms in psychiatric outpatients. Am. J. Psychiatry, *128*:643–646, 1971.
40. Guze, S. B., Woodruff, R. A., and Clayton, P. J. Hysteria and antisocial behavior: further evidence of an association. Am. J. Psychiatry, *127*:957–960, 1971.
41. Hare, R. D. *Psychopathy: Theory and Research*. New York: John Wiley & Sons, 1970.
42. Hare, R. D. Diagnosis of antisocial personality disorder in two prison populations. Am. J. Psychiatry, *140*:887–890, 1983.
43. Hare, R. D., Hart, S. D., and Harpur, T. J. Psychopathy and the DSM-IV criteria for antisocial personality disorder. J. Abnorm. Psychol., *100*:391–398, 1991.
44. Henn, F. A., Bardwell, R., and Jenkins, R. L. Juvenile delinquents re-visited. Adult criminal activity. Arch. Gen. Psychiatry, *37*:1160–1163, 1980.
45. Hook, E. B. Behavioral implications of the human XYY genotype. Science, *179*:139–150, 1973.
46. Jonsson, G. Delinquent boys, their parents and grandparents. Acta Psychiatr. Scand. Suppl., *195*:1–264, 1967.
47. Kahn, E. *Psychopathic Personalities*. New Haven, CT: Yale University Press, 1931.
48. Kelso, J., and Stewart, M. A. Factors which predict the persistence of aggressive conduct disorder. J. Child Psychol. Psychiatry, *27*:77–86, 1986.
49. Khalifa, N., Duggan, C., Stoffers, J., Huband, N., Vollm, B. A., Ferriter, M., and Lieb, K. Pharmacological interventions for antisocial personality disorder. Cochrane Database Syst. Rev., CD007667, 2010.

50. Koch, J. L. A. *Leitfaden der Psychiatrie*, 2nd edition. Ravensburg, Germany: Dorn, 1889.
51. Koller, K. M., and Castanos, J. N. Family background in prison groups: a comparative study of parental deprivation. Br. J. Psychiatry, *117*:371–380, 1970.
52. Kraepelin, E. *Dementia Praecox and Paraphrenia*, Barclay, R. M., Robertson, G. M. (trans.). Edinburgh: E. & S. Livingstone, 1919.
53. Kreuz, L. E., and Rose, R. M. Assessment of aggressive behavior and plasma testosterone in a young criminal population. Psychosomat. Med., *34*:321–332, 1972.
54. Kruesi, M. J., Hibbs, E. D., Zahn, T. P., Keysor, C. S., Hamburger, S. D., Bartko, J. J., and Rapoport, J. L. A 2-year prospective follow-up study of children and adolescents with disruptive behavior disorders. Arch. Gen. Psychiatry, *49*:429–435, 1992.
55. Lewis, A. Psychopathic personality: a most elusive category. Psychol. Med., *4*:133–140, 1974.
56. Lewis, C. E. Alcoholism, antisocial personality, narcotic addiction: an integrative approach. Psychiatr. Dev., *3*:223–235, 1984.
57. Lundin, W. A. *Statistics on Delinquents and Delinquency*. Springfield, IL: C. C. Thomas, 1964.
58. Maddocks, P. D. A five-year follow-up of untreated psychopaths. Br. J. Psychiatry, *116*:511–515, 1970.
59. Mannuzza, S., Klein, R. G., Bessler, A., Malloy, P., and LaPadula, M. Adult outcome of hyperactive boys. Educational achievement, occupational rank, and psychiatric status. Arch. Gen. Psychiatry, *50*:565–576, 1993.
60. Mattson, A., Schalling, D., Olweus, D. L., Löw, H., and Svensson, J. Plasma testosterone, aggressive behavior, and personality dimensions in young male delinquents. J. Am. Acad. Child Adolesc. Psychiatry, *19*:476–490, 1980.
61. Mawson, A. R., and Mawson, C. D. Psychopathy and arousal: a new interpretation of the psychophysiological literature. Biol. Psychiatry, *12*:49–74, 1977.
62. McFarlane, A. C. Epidemiological evidence about the relationship between PTSD and alcohol abuse: the nature of the association. Addict. Behav., *23*:813–825, 1998.
63. Mednick, S., and Christiansen, K. O. *Biosocial Bases of Criminal Behavior*. New York: Gardner Press, 1977.
64. Meloy, J. R. Antisocial personality disorder. In *Treatment of Psychiatric Disorders, Volume 2*, third edition, Gabbard, G. O. (ed.). Washington, DC: American Psychiatric Press, pp. 2251–2273, 2001.
65. Mitchell, S., and Rosa, P. Boyhood behaviour problems as precursors of criminality: a fifteen-year follow-up study. J. Child Psychol. Psychiatry, *22*:19–33, 1981.
66. Moran, P. The epidemiology of antisocial personality disorder. Soc. Psychiatry Psychiatr. Epidemiol., *34*:231–242, 1999.
67. Morrison, J. Adult psychiatric disorders in parents of hyperactive children. Am. J. Psychiatry, *137*:825–827, 1980.
68. Nielsen, J., and Henrickson, F. Incidence of chromosome aberrations among males in a Danish youth prison. Acta Psychiatr. Scand., *48*:87–102, 1972.
69. Offord, D. R., Sullivan, K., Allen, N., and Abrams, N. Delinquency and hyperactivity. J. Nerv. Ment. Dis., *167*:734–741, 1979.
70. Oliver, J. E. Successive generations of child maltreatment. The children. Br. J. Psychiatry, *153*:543–553, 1988.
71. Oliver, J. E. Intergenerational transmission of child abuse: rates, research, and clinical implications. Am. J. Psychiatry, *150*:1315–1324, 1993.

72. Prichard, J. C. *A Treatise on Insanity and Other Disorders Affecting the Mind.* London: Sherwood, Gilbert, and Piper, 1835.

73. Raine, A., Venables, P. H., and Williams, M. Relationships between central and autonomic measures of arousal at age 15 years and criminality at age 24 years. Arch. Gen. Psychiatry, 47:1003–1007, 1990.

74. Rhee, S. H., and Waldman, I. D. Genetic and environmental influences on antisocial behavior: a meta-analysis of twin and adoption studies. Psychol. Bull., 128:490–529, 2002.

75. Rimmer, J., and Jacobsen, B. Antisocial personality in the biological relatives of schizophrenics. Compr. Psychiatry, 21:258–262, 1980.

76. Robins, L., and O'Neal, P. Mortality, mobility, and crime: problem children thirty years later. Am. Soc. Rev., 23:162–171, 1958.

77. Robins, L. N. *Deviant Children Grown Up: A Sociological and Psychiatric Study of Sociopathic Personality.* Baltimore: Williams & Wilkins, 1966.

78. Robins, L. N. *The Consequences of Conduct Disorder in Girls. Development of Antisocial and Prosocial Behavior.* New York: Academic Press, 1986.

79. Robins, L. N., and Regier, D. A. *Psychiatric Disorders in America: The Epidemiologic Catchment Area Study.* New York: The Free Press, 1991.

80. Rush, B. *Medical Inquiries and Observations Upon the Diseases of the Mind.* Philadelphia: Kimber and Richardson, 1812.

81. Salvatore, J. E., Edwards, A. C., McClintick, J. N., Bigdeli, T. B., Adkins, A., Aliev, F., Edenberg, H. J., Foroud, T., Hesselbrock, V., Kramer, J., Nurnberger, J. I., Schuckit, M., Tischfield, J. A., Xuei, X., and Dick, D. M. Genome-wide association data suggest ABCB1 and immune-related gene sets may be involved in adult antisocial behavior. Transl. Psychiatry, 5:e558, 2015.

82. Satterfield, J. H. The hyperactive child syndrome: a precursor of adult psychopathy. In *Psychopathic Behavior*, Hare, R. D., Schalling, D. (eds.). New York: John Wiley & Sons, pp. 329–346, 1978.

83. Satterfield, J. H., Hoppe, C. M., and Schell, A. M. A prospective study of delinquency in 110 adolescent boys with attention deficit disorder and 88 normal adolescent boys. Am. J. Psychiatry, 139:795–798, 1982.

84. Schneider, K. *Psychopathic Personalities.* London: Cassell, 1958.

85. Schröder, J., de la Chapelle, A., Hakola, P., and Virkkunen, M. The frequency of XYY and XXY men among criminal offenders. Acta Psychiatr. Scand., 63:272–276, 1981.

86. Schulsinger, F. Psychopathy: heredity and environment. Int. J. Ment. Health, 1:190–206, 1972.

87. Shah, S. Z., and Roth, L. H. Biological and psychophysiological factors in criminality. In *Handbook of Criminology*, Glazer, D. (ed.). Chicago: Rand McNally, pp. 101–173, 1974.

88. Slater, E., and Cowie, V. *The Genetics of Mental Disorders.* London: Oxford University Press, 1971.

89. Slutske, W. S. The genetics of antisocial behavior. Curr. Psychiatr. Rep., 3:158–162, 2001.

90. Spalt, L. Hysteria and antisocial personality. A single disorder? J. Nerv. Ment. Dis., 168:456–464, 1980.

91. Spreen, O. The relationship between learning disability, neurological impairment, and delinquency. Results of a follow-up study. J. Nerv. Ment. Dis., 169:791–799, 1981.

92. Stewart, M. A., Cummings, C., Singer, S., and deBlois, C. S. The overlap between hyperactive and unsocialized aggressive children. J. Child Psychol. Psychiatry, 22:35–45, 1981.

93. Stoff, D. M., Breiling, J., and Maser, J. D. (eds.). *Handbook of Antisocial Behavior.* New York: John Wiley, 1997.

94. Sutker, P., and Allain, A. N. Antisocial personality disorder. In *Comprehensive Handbook of Psychopathology*, third edition, Sutker, P. B., Adams, L. J. (eds.). New York: Kluwer Academic/Plenum Publishers, pp. 445–490, 2001.

95. Tielbeek, J. J., Medland, S. E., Benyamin, B., Byrne, E. M., Heath, A. C., Madden, P. A., Martin, N. G., Wray, N. R., and Verweij, K. J. Unraveling the genetic etiology of adult antisocial behavior: a genome-wide association study. PLoS One, 7:e45086, 2012.

96. Weiss, G., Hechtman, L., Milroy, T., and Perlman, T. Psychiatric status of hyperactives as adults: a controlled prospective 15-year follow-up of 63 hyperactive children. J. Am. Acad. Child Adolesc. Psychiatry, 24:211–220, 1985.

97. Woodruff, Jr. R. A., Guze, S. B., and Clayton, P. J. The medical and psychiatric implications of antisocial personality (sociopathy). Dis. Nerv. Syst., 32:712–714, 1971.

98. Woody, G. E., McClellan, A. T., Luborsky, L., and O'Brien, C. P. Sociopathy and psychotherapy outcome. Arch. Gen. Psychiatry, 42:1081–1086, 1985.

CHAPTER 10

✧

Borderline Personality Disorder

Borderline personality disorder (BPD) is a diagnosis in evolution—science continues to accrue evidence in an ongoing manner to demonstrate the validity and reliability of the diagnostic criteria. The cardinal features of BPD, as it is currently conceptualized, are emotional crises, self-mutilation, and chronic suicidality. Patients may present with multiple wrist and forearm scars from self-inflicted lacerations. If permitted, they may call their psychiatrist every day with suicidal threats or multiple times a day with intolerable emotional states. These features are not the only characteristics of BPD, and they are not pathognomonic, but their presence also suggests consideration of the presence of this disorder. Four major areas of psychiatric disturbance are characteristic of BPD: affective instability, cognitive problems, impulsivity, and intense and unstable personal relationships (53).

Borderline personality does not signify borderline schizophrenia. The name "borderline" was originally applied because at the time it was thought to represent a marginal form of schizophrenia.

BPD is one of four disorders currently classified in the Cluster B category of the *DSM-5* personality disorders, with the other three being antisocial, histrionic, and narcissistic personality disorders (5). Cluster B personality disorders are a collection of disorders that share pervasive and long-standing patterns of dramatic, emotional, erratic, and impulsive behaviors. BPD in particular is known for its chronic instability of emotions, self-image, and interpersonal relationships.

The first hint of a "borderline" disorder in the evolving editions of the diagnostic manual of the American Psychiatric Association appeared in 1968 in the second edition, which placed "borderline schizophrenia" within a subcategory of schizophrenia, latent type (97). BPD eventually became an official diagnosis in the manual's third edition in 1980. At that time, BPD was clearly separated from schizophrenia and schizotypal personality disorder. Spitzer and colleagues (97) formally organized the observations of Kernberg (44) and Gunderson and Singer (36) and developed the current diagnostic criteria for BPD.

Despite many years of research characterizing important aspects of this disorder, its conceptualization is still evolving, in the midst of continuing controversy surrounding the categorization and validity of the borderline personality syndrome (11). The disorder's name, signifying the entity as a borderline area of another class of psychopathology, reflects confusion about its validity, dating to its first origins. A recent apt observation by Paris is that "the 'border' on which BPD lies is between multiple trait dimensions and intersecting diagnostic spectra" (p. 468) (69).

Although progress toward validation of the diagnosis has been made (113), the current definition of BPD does not appear to meet the accepted gold standard criteria for diagnostic validity and reliability established nearly 50 years ago (78), especially because of problems of widely inconsistent symptom presentations and phenomenological overlap with other disorders (69). This chapter will identify and discuss the specific areas of diagnostic validity needing further work.

It should be noted that BPD has been a topic of great interest to researchers and clinicians particularly in the last 40 years. The data-based references in this chapter are cited for what they contribute to the developing knowledge base. The reader should not conclude that the amount of research or findings, or even the inclusion of this diagnosis in this text, signifies validity of the current definition of the disorder.

HISTORICAL BACKGROUND

The diagnosis of BPD has relatively recent historical origins in the psychiatric literature. In the early part of the last century, concepts of "borderland neuroses and psychoses" (18) and "borderline" neuroses (98) arose within the context of clinical observations by therapists of patients undergoing psychoanalysis. Descriptions of "borderline" disorders over the next several decades characterized these patients as suffering from narcissism, hypersensitivity, feelings of inferiority and insecurity, delusion-like projection, masochism, personal rigidity, impaired interpersonal and general reality testing, and negative therapeutic response (99). Many of these patients hailed from chaotic and dysfunctional family backgrounds. Three out of four patients reported childhood histories of long-standing and repeated abuse and neglect.

For more than half a century, the classification of this "borderline syndrome" languished in an ill-defined region between neurotic and psychotic illness (33, 99). During this time, many labels were applied to patients sharing these characteristics: ambulatory schizophrenia, simple schizophrenia, latent schizophrenia, subclinical schizophrenia, occult schizophrenia, abortive schizophrenia, preschizophrenia, early schizophrenia, pseudopsychopathic schizophrenia, pseudoneurotic schizophrenia, borderland schizophrenia, atypical psychosis, latent psychosis, borderline psychosis, schizophrenic character, psychotic character, "as-if" personality, infantile personality, and hysteroid dysphoria (36, 45, 99, 100). Research eventually led to the development of nine diagnostic criteria, introduced in *DSM-III* (3). These nine criteria have been demonstrated to differentiate severe borderline personality from schizophrenia (99).

Investigators have long contemplated the relationship of mood dysregulation with BPD (90). Akiskal and colleagues recommended classification of borderline disorders with "subaffective" characterologic syndromes, including cyclothymic, dysthymic, and bipolar II disorders (2). Alternatively, Soloff's group identified mood regulation as a core constitutional and biological feature of borderline personality (92), placing mood features with BPD rather than BPD into a mood disorders category. The rapidly changing affective states inherent in borderline personality prompted characterization of these patients as chronically "stable in their instability" (83). A name briefly proposed, "unstable personality disorder," epitomized this affective instability as a prime feature of the borderline syndrome defined as a personality disorder (97).

Confirming the aforementioned mood, neurotic, and psychotic symptoms in his patients with borderline disorders, Hoch described an even broader array of psychiatric complaints in them. His patients exhibited "panneurosis, pananxiety, and pansexuality together with symptoms of schizophrenia" (p. 1) (36) and "widespread symptoms mimicking the classical neuroses: compulsions, phobias, depressions and so forth, all occurring in a jumble and in such intensity as to cripple the patient's functioning" (p. 349) (99). Tracing the history of the psychiatric classification of these patients, Stone (p. 349) (99) was struck by the range of diagnostic categories of their symptoms. His synopsis of the state of the field reads like the proverbial blind men describing different parts of the elephant:

. . . there is considerable debate, and many psychiatrists see borderline personality as actually a subset of biologic depressive illness. Some see it as a variant of other, better-characterized traditional diagnoses, such as hysteria, sociopathy, or alcoholism since, rarely, patients who appear to be borderlines with alcoholism can become quite normal with sustained sobriety, and sociopaths in tightly closed social systems may become indistinguishable from borderlines. Descriptive subtypes range from the border with the psychoses, in which the patient is chaotic, explosive, or irrational ("schizotypal"), to the border with the neuroses, in which the patient is a depressed, empty clinger with a desperate need for companionship in order just to feel real (the "anaclitic" type). Because some patients lack a sense of their own realness, they adapt like chameleons to the environment of the moment ("as-if personality").

Independently, Guze (37) reported that many patients with BPD also met diagnostic criteria for sociopathy, alcoholism, drug dependence, hysteria, primary or secondary affective illness, or schizophrenic illness. Guze and his colleagues were troubled by the extensive comorbidity observed with borderline personality. This extensive comorbidity has kindled doubt over the ultimate validity of this disorder (29, 37, 40). The critical question is whether these many psychiatric disorders actually coexist with BPD, or whether they merely represent mirages emerging from the plethora of psychiatric symptoms these patients present. The confusing nature of the numerous, varied, and unstable symptom presentations of BPD undoubtedly contribute to the continuing controversy surrounding the unsettled classification of this disorder (114).

EPIDEMIOLOGY

Assorted conceptualizations of BPD have varied widely, yielding vastly differing estimates of the prevalence of the disorder in particular locales (127). Diagnostic imprecision may have contributed to an apparent increase in prevalence of BPD to "epidemic" proportions during the years after its introduction into formal diagnostic criteria in 1980 (61, 127). BPD is presently the most frequently used diagnostic label among the personality disorders. Current estimates, based on meticulous application of established criteria, indicate that as many as 2% of the general population may have BPD, with women representing three-fourths of cases (53).

BPD is found in many settings and populations. Prevalence of the disorder in primary care settings has been estimated at 6% (34). The prevalence is much higher, 15%–20%, in psychiatric inpatient settings (111).

A study of 370 patients treated for substance use disorders diagnosed BPD in 18% of the patients (107). BPD is also reported in association with eating disorders, specifically with bulimia, but not with anorexia nervosa (59, 79). BPD has also been described among patients with anxiety disorders and depression (19, 66). Comorbidity of BPD with other psychiatric disorders may represent a marker for general severity of psychopathology (19, 59, 66).

BPD is not just an American construct. Evidence of this syndrome has been documented in countries around the world, including England (106), France (17), Spain (105), Germany (51), the Netherlands (107), Norway (103), Sweden (49), Switzerland (60), Turkey (85), Brazil (24), New Zealand (16), Japan (19, 59), China (125), India (73), Siberia (84), and Egypt (9).

CLINICAL PICTURE

Patients with BPD can present with many symptoms representing multiple diagnostic categories. They complain of symptoms of psychosis, mania, depression, anxiety, dissociation, sociopathy, substance abuse, eating disorders (especially bulimia), and impulse control disorders. Given the diagnostic complexity of these patients' presentations, the illness can be difficult to understand and to manage. In a study of a psychiatric emergency service, 18 patients with BPD had many more psychiatric complaints and problems than 102 other psychiatric patients visiting the same service. More patients with BPD than those with other psychiatric disorders had suicide attempts, anger and irritability, anhedonia, depression, hypomania, grandiose or omnipotent tendencies, dissociation, sexual promiscuity, destructiveness to property, exploitation of others, alcohol abuse, and transient psychotic episodes without formal thought disorder (72). In a university psychiatry clinic, 9 female patients with Cluster B personality disorders (most representing BPD) described more depressive, manic, anxious, and psychotic symptoms than did 101 other female patients diagnosed with mood, anxiety, and schizophrenic disorders from the same clinic—the same pattern observed among the 32 patients from the same study diagnosed with somatization disorder (52). This pattern of endorsement of many symptoms of diverse psychiatric disorders by patients not suffering from those disorders prompted the emergence of a new term, "psychoform," to describe this classic clinical presentation (52, 63).

The psychoform pattern of reporting many symptoms of multiple psychiatric disorders in BPD is supported by findings of psychological profiles of these patients recorded using the Minnesota Multiphasic Personality Inventory (MMPI). MMPI testing of 26 patients with BPD demonstrated a characteristic "floating" profile in which all the clinical scale scores were in abnormally elevated ranges (defined as T score > 70). The schizophrenia and psychasthenia scales showed the highest elevations (91). The validity scales of most of the MMPI profiles for these patients revealed a style of exaggerated symptom reporting. This study further confirmed that these patients complain vociferously that virtually everything is wrong with their minds.

Not surprisingly, studies have recorded high rates of apparent psychiatric comorbidity in these polysymptomatic patients. Upon finding a 91% diagnostic comorbidity rate in 180 inpatients with BPD, Fyer and colleagues concluded that BPD must represent a heterogeneous category with unclear boundaries, overlapping with many different disorders rather than with any one specific disorder (29). Around the same time, Swartz's group found high rates of current-year psychiatric comorbidity among 21 BPD inpatients and outpatients. Comorbid diagnoses were major depression (81%), generalized anxiety disorder (86%), panic disorder (62%), dysthymia (52%), alcohol abuse/dependence (24%), and drug abuse/dependence (19%) (101). The Swartz et al. study identified a threshold of at least 11 of 24 current-year psychiatric symptoms that predicted the BPD diagnosis with sensitivity and specificity exceeding 85%. These symptoms represent a broad range of psychopathology—panic, anxiety, depression, suicidality, irritability, impulsivity, interpersonal difficulties, brief psychotic phenomena—further illustrating the psychoform character of BPD. This extensive pattern of psychopathology expressed by patients with BPD was well characterized in the title of a recent article authored by Paris: "The Nature of Borderline Personality Disorder: Multiple Dimensions, Multiple Symptoms, But One Category" (69).

Hudziak and his colleagues later found that 100% of 87 patients with BPD in their study met lifetime criteria for one or more additional psychiatric diagnoses. Remarkably, these patients averaged five diagnoses each (40). Around the same time, Zanarini's group described high lifetime comorbidity rates among 379 BPD inpatients: virtually all (98%) had mood disorders, and 73% had "complex" comorbidity (defined as both mood and anxiety disorders with substance abuse and/or an eating disorder) (114). Compared to patients with other personality disorders, the patients with BPD also had significantly higher rates of major depression, bipolar II disorder, panic disorder, generalized anxiety disorder, phobias, posttraumatic stress disorder, obsessive-compulsive disorder, somatization disorder, and eating disorders. Similarly, Zimmerman and Mattia documented current comorbid disorders in 98% of 49 outpatients with BPD, and the average number of comorbid diagnoses was 3.4 (126). Compared to 350 psychiatric outpatients without BPD, the patients with BPD in this study had significantly greater current prevalence of major depression, bipolar I and II disorders, panic disorder, posttraumatic stress disorder, phobic disorders, obsessive-compulsive disorder, eating disorders, and somatoform disorders. Table 10.1 lists the specific comorbidity rates of patients with BPD in these three studies, further demonstrating the uniformly psychoform nature of these patients' complaints.

Symptoms among patients with BPD present not only with a wide range but also with remarkable severity. The Beck Depression Inventory and Hamilton Rating Scale for Anxiety, documenting symptoms of major depression and anxiety disorders, were administered to 283 psychiatric outpatients, and 38 of these patients diagnosed with BPD by structured interview were compared with the others. Only 13 of the 38 patients with BPD were free of major depression, yet this BPD subgroup presented their

TABLE 10.1 STUDIES OF DIAGNOSTIC COMORBIDITY IN PATIENTS
WITH BORDERLINE PERSONALITY DISORDER

Comorbid Disorder Prevalence (%)	Hudziak et al. (Lifetime) (40)	Zanarini et al. (Lifetime) (114)	Zimmerman and Mattia (Current) (126)
Major depression	87	83	61
Dysthymia	44	39	12
Manic episode	19	–	9
Bipolar II disorder	–	10	9
Somatization disorder	45	16	–
Any somatoform disorder	–	39	20
Panic disorder	51	48	31
Generalized anxiety disorder	55	14	14
Simple phobia	31	32	20
Agoraphobia	7	12	2
Social phobia	11	46	42
Alcohol abuse/dependence	49	52	12
Drug abuse/dependence	27	46	3
Antisocial personality disorder	23	–	–
Posttraumatic stress disorder	28	56	36
Obsessive-compulsive disorder	7	16	20
Eating disorder	16	53	17

depression symptoms on these self-rating instruments more severely than did 139 patients without BPD who were diagnosed with major depression, and they also rated their anxiety symptoms more severely than did 134 patients without BPD who were diagnosed with anxiety disorders (19). Zanarini and her colleagues have commented, "It may be that it is their eagerness to confide in others about their dysphoria rather than their actual level of dysphoria which sets borderline patients apart" (p. 164) (122).

The broad psychiatric comorbidity in BPD extends not only to mood, anxiety, and psychotic disorders but also to other personality disorders. A chart review study of 180 inpatients with BPD revealed that 92% met criteria for at least one other personality disorder, and nearly one-half met criteria for two or more other personality disorder diagnoses (29). Similarly, Nurnberg's group found that 82% of BPD outpatients without concurrent major psychiatric disorders had at least one additional personality disorder diagnosis (64). The mean number of additional personality disorder diagnoses was 3.7, although no single accompanying personality disorder predominated. Zanarini's group described sex differences in personality disorder comorbidity among 504 inpatients with personality disorders (115). Comorbid paranoid, passive-aggressive, narcissistic, and antisocial personality disorders were more prevalent among male patients with BPD.

Individual psychological and behavioral features that are considered characteristic of BPD are sometimes also observed in other disorders. It is the occurrence of these features collectively within a single disorder, however, that defines BPD. Patients with BPD struggle with chronic loneliness and emptiness, feelings of inferiority and insecurity, intolerance of anxiety, dependency, helplessness, distrust, poor emotional control, impulsivity, overreactivity to external stressors, projection (e.g., when feeling hostile, accusing others of hostile feelings), "splitting" (i.e., describing self or others as all good or all bad), extreme idealization and devaluation of others, identity disturbance, narcissistic preoccupation with self, special and entitled feelings, lack of empathy for others, extreme attention-seeking, demanding and manipulative behaviors, and wrist-slashing and other self-mutilation (15, 72).

Described as easily bored, stimulation-seeking, and impulsive, patients with BPD are prone to engage in impulsive, potentially self-damaging behaviors such as gambling, excessive spending, binge eating, substance abuse, unsafe sex, or reckless driving. Their self-image may be unstable with dramatic shifts in their goals, values, and roles. Often in the context of emotional storms, they may abruptly change their career plans, friends, or sexual identity. Patients with BPD overreact to interpersonal stresses, erupting into dramatic episodes of despair, panic, or rage. Many patients with BPD have difficulty controlling their anger and may display intense anger outbursts, especially when they feel others are abandoning them. During stressful episodes, they may exhibit dissociative symptoms or brief psychotic-like symptoms (e.g., feelings of unreality of self or the world, body image distortion, visual hallucinations, paranoid feelings, and ideas of reference) (15, 72).

The interpersonal relationships of patients with BPD are characteristically intense and unstable. Their interactions with healthcare professionals are often quite difficult. These patients often demand a great deal of time or special treatment. They may idealize relationships, quickly becoming emotionally involved, then rapidly switching to devalue other persons when their demands are not met, at the same time making accusations of abandonment or lack of concern. Patients with BPD have an uncanny propensity for stimulating conflict and disagreement among their healthcare providers over their care.

Recurrent suicidal behavior is a classic presentation of BPD, particularly during periods of stress. One study found that 73% of inpatients diagnosed with BPD had previously made at least one suicide attempt, and their average number of attempts was 3.4 (95). Suicide attempts in these patients were associated not with comorbid major depression but with antisocial personality disorder. Among the suicide attempters, 20% had antisocial personality, compared to 4% of nonattempters.

One hallmark feature of BPD is self-mutilation, occurring in 90% or more of patients. Although self-mutilation often occurs as part of recurrent suicidal behavior, many patients with BPD engage in self-mutilation during episodes of emotional distress not associated with suicidality (35, 108). Most commonly, patients present with self-inflicted lacerations of the anterior forearms and self-inflicted burns, often in the context of interpersonal stress. Physical examination may reveal multiple superficial scars of the wrists or anterior upper extremities, or a collection of circular burn scars from lighted cigarettes. One patient had hundreds of visible scars from self-inflicted lacerations extending from her wrists to axillae. Self-mutilation is not pathognomonic for BPD, however; it is observed in many other disorders as well.

Clues to the diagnosis of BPD may be detected in speech patterns, collectively termed "nonpsychotic thought disorder" (62), reflecting the cognitive styles of these patients. They exhibit "all-or-nothing" logic and overreactive tendencies, which are expressed in overgeneralized and inappropriately globalized statements. Their verbal expressions are peppered with words and phrases that denote extremes (e.g., "the worst," "never," "always," "nobody," "everybody"). Their speech is characteristically circumstantial and overly inclusive, yet simultaneously vague, impressionistic, imprecise, and lacking important detail. They describe their many symptoms inefficiently and with irrelevancies, apparently unable to provide the specific information requested of them. The history-taking process in these patients can be arduous (26, 47).

BIOLOGICAL FINDINGS

The neurobiology of BPD is poorly understood, but many abnormalities have been reported along several lines of research. Hyperresponsiveness of the hypothalamic-pituitary-adrenal axis has been implicated (76). Another area under investigation is abnormal serotonergic transmission, which may be linked to the disinhibition of aggression that can occur with BPD (53). Structural and functional neuroimaging studies have identified abnormalities in several brain areas mediating serotonergic functions. Findings of reduced volumes in the orbitofrontal and dorsolateral prefrontal cortex, hippocampus, and amygdala; deactivation of anterior cingulate cortex; and hyperactivity in the amygdala in BPD all point to a potential role for serotonin in this disorder (25, 39, 58, 82, 109). In theory, ineffectual prefrontal inhibitory control of amygdala activity may lead to states of emotional overdrive in the amygdala. Collectively, abnormal findings in these systems may represent neurobiological correlates of emotional states in BPD (53).

NATURAL HISTORY

BPD typically manifests during early adulthood with pervasive chronic affective instability and impulsivity. In some patients, behaviors associated with the disorder such as self-mutilation and dramatic suicide gestures begin in adolescence or childhood (113). The clinical course of BPD is frequently described as "stormy" (65), reflecting the chronically turbulent episodes of emotional crises and affective instability characteristic of this disorder. Psychosocial functioning is characteristically significantly impaired in work settings, social relationships, and leisure activities (89).

The association between BPD and patient reports of childhood abuse and neglect histories has long been recognized, and the extent of childhood abuse and neglect in BPD has increasingly been appreciated in the last two decades (124). Zanarini's group found that 91% of 358 patients with BPD reported a history of childhood abuse, and 92% reported childhood neglect (120). A subgroup of 29 BPD inpatients examined by these investigators described particularly severe forms of abuse and neglect, which correlated with severity of their BPD symptoms. The severe abuse reported by these inpatients had typically occurred in both childhood and adolescence on at least a weekly basis, for a minimum of 1 year, by two or more perpetrators, and involving penetration and use of force or violence. Most patients with BPD who describe abuse histories do not report this level of severity of abuse, however. A large longitudinal study controlling for parental psychopathology and level of education found that even verbal abuse and neglect in childhood are associated with the development of borderline and several other personality disorders in adolescence and early adulthood (41, 42). Taken together, however, collective findings from these studies do not demonstrate the association between childhood abuse and BPD to be particularly robust (69).

Although the relationship between reported childhood abuse and BPD has been repeatedly documented, there is insufficient evidence to implicate causality of childhood abuse in the generation of BPD. Zanarini and her colleagues initially assumed such negative early experiences to be instrumental in the generation of borderline psychopathology, but these authors more recently revised their etiological model to account for important contributions of constitutional temperament interacting with early environmental challenges of a range of severity (113).

The validity of memories of childhood abuse reported by patients with BPD has been challenged (67), especially memories claimed to be recovered after having been forgotten or "repressed." Questions have been raised as to whether reported childhood abuse memories may more accurately represent exaggerated reporting behaviors characteristic of many of these patients, distorted perceptions of interpersonal events (67), or even products of therapist suggestion (13, 75). It is likely, however, that patients with BPD actually may have more frequent histories of exposure to adverse environments through their families of origin, in association with the elevated rates of antisocial personality disorder and substance abuse demonstrated among biological relatives of patients with BPD. The clinician is generally not in a position to draw conclusions about the veracity of patient reports of childhood mistreatment, and maintaining an open mind is likely to be in the patient's best interest. Regardless of the validity of the reports of abuse by these patients, the importance to the clinician of the knowledge of these apparent associations is to prompt the clinician to include borderline psychopathology in the differential diagnosis among patients who report childhood abuse and neglect histories.

The long-term course of BPD can be quite variable. The disorder's course is not as bleak as once considered (11, 32, 86, 113, 116). Some patients achieve a stable equilibrium, especially as they develop maturity in the fourth and fifth decades of life. With maturity, some remarkable patients may manage to overcome the grip of the illness on their lives. Social impairment and suicide risk are greatest during the early adult years and tend to diminish with age.

Initial follow-up studies of small samples of patients with BPD collectively pointed to relatively discouraging prospects for recovery (117). Schizophrenia did not develop in these patients. Many, however, had other personality disorder diagnoses in addition to BPD. Two large, more recent systematic outcome studies of patients with BPD with longer follow-up periods suggest more optimistic outcomes. In a study of 100 hospitalized patients with BPD, Paris and colleagues found that 75% no longer met BPD criteria 15 years later (70). These investigators successfully followed 64 of the 100 patients for another 12 years; at an average of 27 years after the index admission, further improvement was evident, and only 5 patients still met BPD criteria (71). A 10-year follow-up study by Zanarini's group of 275 BPD inpatients reported an 88% remission rate with few recurrences (121). Rapid resolution was typical for impulsive symptoms (self-mutilation and manipulative suicide efforts) and interpersonal difficulties (demanding and entitled behaviors and resistance to treatment), but dysphoria (loneliness, emptiness, anger) and abandonment as well as dependency issues tended to be chronic.

The disappearance of BPD in the majority of patients over time has invited questions about the validity of the original BPD diagnosis in these patients, and even about the validity of the diagnostic category in general (69), because personality disorders are defined as being stable and enduring conditions (7). Remission of BPD in these studies, however, was defined as no longer meeting full diagnostic criteria, which is not the same as full remission, which entails the disappearance of all signs and symptoms of the disorder. Closer examination of the findings from the described follow-up studies, however, reveals that while the patients' impulsive and suicidal behaviors tended to improve, their affective instability was chronic and, true to the classic conceptualization of personality disorders, the patients' functional impairment persisted (69).

COMPLICATIONS

Borderline personality disorder is often as severe and functionally disabling as major Axis I psychiatric disorders. A follow-up study of hospitalized patients with BPD determined their outcomes to be worse than those of mania or schizoaffective disorder, approaching the chronicity and severity of schizophrenia (74). Functional impairment in BPD has been described as rivaling that of major depression in domains of work, social relationships, and leisure functioning (89). Nearly two-thirds (64%) of patients previously hospitalized for BPD had not been able to work for at least 1 year (96). A 3- to 10-year follow-up study of 86 borderline patients admitted to a day hospital program documented only 24% employed full-time, full disability in 34%, and only 27% married or cohabitating (80). A 6-year prospective follow-up study of patients with BPD found their social functioning to be even more impaired than among other personality-disordered patients, especially in vocational achievement (117).

Functional impairment in BPD can be quite variable. Some patients work or attend school as well as manage to maintain friendships and leisure activities. At the other end of the spectrum, others cannot maintain stable employment and must rely on disability benefits to support themselves. Some patients with BPD enjoy close, supportive relationships with their families, others have continuously stormy relationships with them, and a few terminate all contact with their families of origin (113).

Suicidal behaviors may represent chronic problems among patients with BPD. Clinicians may be inclined to dismiss frequent suicide gestures as manipulative and posing little risk for suicide. Patients with chronic or repeated suicidality, however, do present significant risk for eventual completed suicide, although compared to the chronic suicide threats and gestures characteristic of these patients, completed suicide is proportionately infrequent (113). A 27-year follow-up study of 64 patients with BPD found that 9% had died by suicide (71). The suicide rate in BPD has been estimated at 400 times the rate of suicide in the general population (65). Early hospital discharge against the patient's wishes or for violating the treatment contract were noted to be associated with completed suicide in two different studies (46, 48). It is unclear from these studies, however, whether the suicides in these patients were specifically associated with psychiatric comorbidities of BPD that are also associated with suicide in other patients, such as major depression and substance use disorders. The frequent suicide gestures in patients with BPD can also result in accidental fatality even when the patient did not intend to die.

Among 84 inpatients with BPD in one study, nearly one-half had made at least one attempt with clear intent to die, and two-thirds of these attempters had made at least one medically serious, potentially lethal, suicide attempt (95). Intent to die was not associated with severity of borderline traits or major depression, but degree of medical lethality was associated with the number of lifetime attempts. Studies have been inconsistent in concluding whether comorbid substance abuse is associated with suicide in BPD (48, 71). Previous suicide attempts by patients with BPD are also found to be associated with completed suicide (48). Therefore, a history of multiple failed suicide attempts among patients with BPD is no guarantee—and no predictor—that subsequent suicide attempts will not be lethal (12).

FAMILY STUDIES

Most studies of psychiatric illness in the families of patients with BPD have relied on patients reporting about family members or chart reviews of recorded family histories. Such "family history" studies are widely considered inferior to direct interviews of the family members themselves (family studies). Family history studies, including those relying on chart review, have identified high prevalence rates of mood disorders among family members of patients with BPD (96) that are similar to those documented among relatives of patients with mood disorders (30, 57), and disputably higher than rates described in relatives of patients with schizophrenia (57, 88). High prevalence rates of BPD (12%) are described in relatives of hospitalized patients with BPD, 10 times higher than in relatives of patients hospitalized for schizophrenia or bipolar disorder (57). Relatives of patients with BPD may also have higher rates of histrionic and antisocial personality disorders than relatives of patients with schizophrenia and bipolar disorders (74), more impulsivity than relatives of patients with other personality disorders or with schizophrenia (88), and two to three times the rates of alcohol disorders compared to relatives of patients with schizophrenia or bipolar disorder (57). Comorbid mood disorders are associated with greater prevalence of alcohol use disorders in family members (30). No excess of schizophrenia or schizotypal personality disorder has been identified in families of patients with BPD (74). Eccentric or peculiar behavior is frequently observed among relatives of BPD inpatients, however (96). Patients with BPD are more likely to be adopted than patients with schizophrenia or bipolar disorder (74), further limiting available family information.

Direct psychiatric interviews of family members in a small study of 11 outpatients with BPD without comorbid mood disorders revealed the prevalence of mood and personality disorders among their 54 relatives to be similar to rates in families of patients with mood disorders, and higher than in relatives of controls with no psychiatric illness (77). This suggests that BPD may run in families with mood disorders.

Genetic contribution to BPD has been most conclusively demonstrated in a single study of twins from a registry that demonstrated a significantly higher rate of BPD concordance among monozygotic (35%) than among dizygotic (7%) twin pairs (104). Multivariate genetic analyses have further shown that a group of traits suggesting emotional dysregulation, including instability of emotions, thinking patterns, sense of self, and interpersonal relationships, has a heritability estimate of 47% (53).

DIFFERENTIAL DIAGNOSIS

The differential diagnosis of BPD encompasses depressive and anxiety disorders, bipolar disorders, schizoaffective disorder, schizophrenia, bulimia, substance use disorders, somatization disorder, and other personality disorders, especially of the Cluster B grouping of personality disorders (65). This is because patients with BPD report many symptoms of other disorders.

Pope and colleagues demonstrated that differences in family histories, treatment response, and outcomes distinguish BPD from schizophrenia and mood disorders (74). Zanarini's group examined 22 borderline personality features identified by the Revised Diagnostic Interview for Borderline Patients and found that while 18 features discriminated BPD from other personality disorders, only 7 were relatively specific to BPD: psychotic-like thought, self-mutilation, manipulative suicide efforts, abandonment issues, demanding and entitlement behaviors, stormy course of treatment, and elicitation of negative therapist responses (122). Several studies have observed that the general psychoform pattern of reporting multiple psychiatric symptoms across many diagnostic classes is a major feature differentiating BPD from other psychiatric disorders (69, 114, 115, 123, 126).

The characteristic pattern in which BPD patients report extensive symptoms of many psychiatric disorders that do not add up to consistent diagnostic entities (i.e., multiple psychoform symptoms) has invited questions about the validity of the diagnosis of BPD. Many patients with somatization disorder, however, similarly describe multiple symptoms of many psychiatric categories (52, 63, 110), but this pattern has not reduced the well-established validity of this diagnosis. The key to distinguishing somatization disorder from BPD is to identify the classic pattern of multiple medically unexplained complaints throughout the body's organ systems in somatization disorder patients that is not a defining characteristic of BPD. Many patients with BPD display somatoform symptoms such as unexplained vomiting (43) and may utilize medical treatment excessively (81), but not to the degree that defines somatization disorder. It is not unusual for patients to meet criteria for both disorders (40, 114).

In the last quarter of a century, scientific investigation has emphasized the relationship between dissociative disorders and BPD. The validity of dissociative disorders, however, has been extensively debated. The defining elements of dissociative disorders are disruption in the usually integrated functions of consciousness, memory, identity, or perception of the environment (4). Dissociative disorders, like somatization and borderline personality disorder, classically present with many symptoms in multiple psychiatric categories (20, 27, 63). Therefore, overlap of these disorders is not unexpected. Most patients with multiple personality disorder (recently renamed as "dissociative identity disorder") also have somatization disorder, BPD, or both (63), complicating attempts to differentiate multiple personality disorder from borderline and somatoform disorders. Patients with multiple personality disorder have been observed to complain of symptoms even more profusely than patients with only borderline or somatization disorder (27, 50, 87). In a study of 60 female BPD inpatients, those with dissociation reported higher rates of self-mutilation, childhood abuse, current depressive symptoms, and psychiatric treatment utilization (14). Lauer and colleagues (50) found no differences between patients with BPD and multiple personality disorder in family history, childhood history, psychiatric comorbidity, and symptom complaints aside from more dissociative symptoms among multiple personality disorder patients. They concluded that multiple personality disorder may simply represent a severe manifestation or variant (an "epiphenomenon") of BPD.

Because the psychoform presentation of BPD can mimic virtually any psychiatric disorder, independent evidence of the characteristic patterns of other disorders should be sought to confirm or rule out these other diagnoses in patients thought to have BPD. Conversely, because patients with other psychiatric disorders may transiently exhibit BPD features during illness episodes, it is advisable to refrain from making the diagnosis of BPD until a history of early onset of the behavior and a long-standing course of BPD independent of other psychiatric illness can be established.

CLINICAL MANAGEMENT

Patients with BPD in treatment have been described as challenging and demanding. Zanarini and colleagues identified specific features of these patients' behavior that frighten or annoy therapists: accusations that the therapist is mean and uncaring, demanding behaviors, and frequent suicide threats and gestures that may appear manipulative (113). Some patients seem to worsen during treatment. Zanarini and colleagues described these patients as having "a toxic reaction to" therapy (p. 522) (113).

General principles of BPD treatment involve exercising flexibility, establishing rules for dealing with crises and suicidality, achieving agreement about patient and therapist roles and responsibilities, mutually setting limits on topics of discussion, carefully maintaining professional boundaries that are often tested by the intense interpersonal styles of patients with BPD, and consulting with colleagues as needed (1, 8, 65). Managing and reducing behavioral dyscontrol, intense dysphoria, and suicidal behaviors are early goals of treatment. Longer-term goals are to improve functioning, productivity, and emotional stability (53).

Few controlled studies of treatment for BPD have been carried out, and these studies have suffered from high dropout rates, potential for placebo effects, and emphasis on less severe and predominantly female populations, limiting interpretation and generalizability of the findings (53, 102).

It is generally agreed at present that psychotherapy should be considered a first-line treatment for BPD (113). Supportive psychotherapy with an active problem-solving emphasis is recommended in conjunction with adjunctive, symptom-targeted pharmacotherapy (6, 53). Assumptions that childhood adversity is the sole source of these patients' distress and disability provide a nonproductive premise for the basis of psychotherapy in these patients (113). Focusing on early maltreatment by others can derail these patients from healthy objectives of gaining insight into and changing their behavior and further alienate these patients from family members who might otherwise provide helpful social support.

Dialectical behavior therapy, a specialized derivative of cognitive therapy developed for patients with chronic suicidality or BPD, teaches problem-solving skills, emotional regulation strategies, distress tolerance, and interpersonal skills in outpatient settings (54). This form of therapy has proved effective in nonrandomized and randomized controlled trials for patients with chronic suicidality or BPD (53, 55, 56). Two other specialized therapies, mentalization-based (10) and schema-focused (31) therapies, have also shown promise in therapeutic trials. These specialized therapies are intensive and potentially useful for the most severe and chronic cases (113).

Even with substantial efforts, systematic review and meta-analysis of randomized controlled trials in 2017 found effect sizes to be small, with substantial risk of bias and reporting bias as well as uneven findings at follow-up (22).

Medications should be considered adjunctive to psychotherapy rather than the mainstay of treatment for BPD (113). Despite this recommendation, however, aggressive pharmacotherapy is too often seen (118, 119) and undoubtedly involves a tendency to mistake the unstable moods of these patients for the sustained mood swings of bipolar disorder and to misconceptualize BPD as representing a form of bipolar disorder (69, 113). Hospitalization and pharmacotherapy have little benefit beyond providing a brief stopgap in the long-term management of emotional crises and suicidality in patients with BPD. Psychiatric hospitalization has not been demonstrated to prevent suicide in patients with BPD, and it sometimes has untoward effects (68). Habitual reliance on hospitalization and pharmacotherapy in the long-term management of BPD can lead to escalation of maladaptive behaviors in these patients (53). Overdose remains a common problem.

Pharmacotherapy may be most beneficial in early phases of psychotherapy by calming intense emotions and allowing the patient to reflect and develop cognitive strategies for coping (53, 69). Although pharmacotherapy aims to reduce unstable moods, impulsive behavior, and distorted thinking and perceptions (1, 65), the benefit from antidepressant, mood stabilizer, and antipsychotic medications commonly prescribed for BPD may represent no more than nonspecific or sedating characteristics of these agents (113).

Although antidepressants and low-dose antipsychotic medications have long been used in treatment of BPD, results have been modest or mixed at best. Patients with BPD sometimes worsen on antidepressants (21, 93, 94). Antidepressant effects appear to be independent of comorbid mood disorders (88), and typically residual symptoms continue (21). Newer antidepressants have more favorable safety profiles than older antidepressants in borderline patients, especially those at risk for impulsive suicide attempts, but the benefit of these medications has not been tested in controlled, randomized studies.

In small placebo-controlled studies, antimanic agents have been shown to reduce interpersonal sensitivity and irritability and anger (28), and antipsychotics to reduce anxiety, paranoia, anger, and hostility (112).

The mechanism of improvement is unclear, likely related in part to non-specific sedative effects. The use of antipsychotic medication for agitation and psychotic-like features, however, is usually reserved for the most severe cases and should be weighed against the risk of significant adverse effects such as neuroleptic malignant syndrome, tardive dyskinesia, sudden death, metabolic syndrome, and other side effects of antipsychotic agents. Newer antipsychotic medications are preferable to the older agents in attempting to manage psychotic-like symptoms for their lower propensity for tardive dyskinesia, but their use may be complicated by metabolic syndrome. Because many patients with BPD complain of profuse anxiety, benzodiazepines are often used (and requested by many of these patients), but their use must be carefully monitored for risk of misuse or addiction (1). No clear medication choice has emerged for long-term management of BPD (21, 38).

A review of 13 studies of electroconvulsive therapy for depression in patients with BPD found that it can be effectively administered in these patients, although outcomes may not be as favorable as in depressed patients without BPD (23). Rigorous randomized treatment studies with follow-up are needed.

Unfortunately, the characteristic extensive, varied, and shifting psychiatric symptoms reported by patients with BPD complicate diagnosis and treatment of this condition (114). Because other psychiatric disorders may complicate BPD and are potentially treatable, clinicians are reminded to complete the psychiatric evaluation for other psychiatric disorders (126). Management of BPD can be expected to be less tumultuous when comorbid disorders are quiescent or absent.

REFERENCES

1. [No authors listed]. Borderline personality: new recommendations. Harv. Ment Health Lett., 18:4–6, 2002.
2. Akiskal, H. S. Subaffective disorders: dysthymic, cyclothymic and bipolar II disorders in the "borderline" realm. Psychiatr. Clin. North Am., 4:25–46, 1981.
3. American Psychiatric Association. Diagnostic and Statistical Manual of Mental Disorders, 3rd edition. Washington, DC: Author, 1980.
4. American Psychiatric Association. Diagnostic and Statistical Manual of Mental Disorders, 4th edition. Washington, DC: Author, 1994.
5. American Psychiatric Association. Diagnostic and Statistical Manual of Mental Disorders, 4th edition, text revision. Washington, DC: Author, 2000.
6. American Psychiatric Association. Practice Guideline for the Treatment of Patients with Borderline Personality Disorder. Washington, DC: American Psychiatric Association Press, 2001.

7. American Psychiatric Association. *Diagnostic and Statistical Manual for Mental Disorders,* 5th edition. Washington, DC: Author, 2013.

8. Aronson, T. A. A critical review of psychotherapeutic treatments of the borderline personality. Historical trends and future directions. J. Nerv. Ment. Dis., 177:511–528, 1989.

9. Asaad, T., Okasha, T., and Okasha, A. Sleep EEG findings in ICD-10 borderline personality disorder in Egypt. J. Affect. Dis., 71:11–18, 2002.

10. Bateman, A. W., and Fonagy, P. Mentalization-based treatment of BPD. J. Pers. Disord., 18:36–51, 2004.

11. Biskin, R. S., and Paris, J. Diagnosing borderline personality disorder. CMAJ., 184:1789–1794, 2012.

12. Black, D. W., Blum, N., Pfohl, B., and Hale, N. Suicidal behavior in borderline personality disorder: prevalence, risk factors, prediction, and prevention. J. Pers. Disord., 18:226–239, 2004.

13. Boakes, J. False complaints of sexual assault: recovered memories of childhood sexual abuse. Med. Sci. Law, 39:112–120, 1999.

14. Brodsky, B. S., Cloitre, M., and Dulit, R. A. Relationship of dissociation to self-mutilation and childhood abuse in borderline personality disorder. Am. J. Psychiatry, 152:1788–1792, 1995.

15. Butler, A. C., Brown, G. K., Beck, A. T., and Grisham, J. R. Assessment of dysfunctional beliefs in borderline personality disorder. Behav Res. Ther., 40:1231–1240, 2002.

16. Carter, J. D., Joyce, P. R., Mulder, R. T., Sullivan, P. F., and Luty, S. E. Gender differences in the frequency of personality disorders in depressed outpatients. J. Pers. Disord., 13:67–74, 1999.

17. Chabrol, H., Chouicha, K., Montovany, A., and Callahan, S. [Symptoms of DSM IV borderline personality disorder in a nonclinical population of adolescents: study of a series of 35 patients]. Encephale, 27:120–127, 2001.

18. Clark, L. P. Some practical remarks upon the use of modified psychoanalysis in the treatment of borderland neuroses and psychoses. Psychoanal. Rev., 6:306–308, 1919.

19. Comtois, K. A., Cowley, D. S., Dunner, D. L., and Roy-Byrne, P. P. Relationship between borderline personality disorder and Axis I diagnosis in severity of depression and anxiety. J. Clin. Psychiatry, 60:752–758, 1999.

20. Coons, P. M. The differential diagnosis of multiple personality: a comprehensive review. Psychiatr. Clin. North Am., 7:51–67, 1984.

21. Cornelius, J. R., Soloff, P. H., Perel, J. M., and Ulrich, R. F. Continuation pharmacotherapy of borderline personality disorder with haloperidol and phenelzine. Am. J. Psychiatry, 150:1843–1848, 1993.

22. Cristea, I. A., Gentili, C., Cotet, C. D., Palomba, D., Barbui, C., and Cuijpers, P. Efficacy of psychotherapies for borderline personality disorder: a systematic review and meta-analysis. JAMA Psychiatry, 74:319–328, 2017.

23. DeBattista, C., and Mueller, K. Is electroconvulsive therapy effective for the depressed patient with comorbid borderline personality disorder? J. ECT, 17:91–98, 2001.

24. Del Ben, C. M., Rodrigues, C. R., and Zuardi, A. W. Reliability of the Portuguese version of the structured clinical interview for DSM-III-R (SCID) in a Brazilian sample of psychiatric outpatients. Braz. J. Med. Biol. Res., 29:1675–1682, 1996.

25. Driessen, M., Herrmann, J., Stahl, K., Zwaan, M., Meier, S., Hill, A., Osterheider, M., and Petersen, D. Magnetic resonance imaging volumes of the hippocampus

and the amygdala in women with borderline personality disorder and early traumatization. Arch. Gen. Psychiatry, 57:1115–1122, 2000.

26. Drob, S., Stewart, S., and Bernard, H. The problem of reinterpretive distortions in group psychotherapy with borderline patients. Group, 6:14–22, 1982.

27. Fink, D., and Golinkoff, M. MPD, borderline personality disorder and schizophrenia: a comparative study of clinical features. Dissociation, 3:127–134, 1990.

28. Frankenburg, F. R., and Zanarini, M. C. Divalproex sodium treatment of women with borderline personality disorder and bipolar II disorder: a double-blind placebo-controlled pilot study. J. Clin. Psychiatry, 63:442–446, 2002.

29. Fyer, M. R., Frances, A. J., Sullivan, T., Hurt, S. W., and Clarkin, J. Comorbidity of borderline personality disorder. Arch. Gen. Psychiatry, 45:348–352, 1988.

30. Gasperini, M., Battaglia, M., Scherillo, P., Sciuto, G., Diaferia, G., and Bellodi, L. Morbidity risk for mood disorders in the families of borderline patients. J. Affect. Disord., 21:265–272, 1991.

31. Giesen-Bloo, J., van Dyck, R., Spinhoven, P., van Tilburg, W., Dirksen, C., van Asselt, T., Kremers, I., Nadort, M., and Arntz, A. Outpatient psychotherapy for borderline personality disorder: randomized trial of schema-focused therapy vs transference-focused psychotherapy. Arch. Gen. Psychiatry, 63:649–658, 2006.

32. Grilo, C. M., Sanislow, C. A., Gunderson, J. G., Pagano, M. E., Yen, S., Zanarini, M. C., Shea, M. T., Skodol, A. E., Stout, R. L., Morey, L. C., and McGlashan, T. H. Two-year stability and change of schizotypal, borderline, avoidant, and obsessive-compulsive personality disorders. J. Consult Clin. Psychol., 72:767–775, 2004.

33. Grinker, R. R. Neurosis, psychosis, and the borderline states. In *Comprehensive Textbook of Psychiatry*, 2nd edition, Friedman, A. M., Kaplan, H. I., Sadock, B. J. (eds.). Baltimore: Williams & Wilkins, pp. 845–850, 1975.

34. Gross, R., Olfson, M., Gameroff, M., Shea, S., Feder, A., Fuentes, M., Lantigua, R., and Weissman, M. M. Borderline personality disorder in primary care. Arch. Intern. Med., 162:53–60, 2002.

35. Gunderson, J. G., and Ridolfi, M. E. Borderline personality disorder. Suicidality and self-mutilation. Ann. N. Y. Acad. Sci., 932:61–73, 2001.

36. Gunderson, J. G., and Singer, M. T. Defining borderline patients: an overview. Am. J. Psychiatry, 132:1–10, 1975.

37. Guze, S. B. Differential diagnosis of the borderline personality syndrome. In *Borderline States in Psychiatry*, Mack, J. E. (ed.). New York: Grune & Stratton, pp. 69–74, 1975.

38. Hancock-Johnson, E., Griffiths, C., and Picchioni, M. A focused systematic review of pharmacological treatment for borderline personality disorder. CNS Drugs, 31:345–356, 2017.

39. Herpertz, S. C., Dietrich, T. M., Wenning, B., Krings, T., Erberich, S. G., Willmes, K., Thron, A., and Sass, H. Evidence of abnormal amygdala functioning in borderline personality disorder: a functional MRI study. Biol. Psychiatry, 50:292–298, 2001.

40. Hudziak, J. J., Boffelli, T. J., Kreisman, J. J., Battaglia, M. M., Stanger, C., Guze, S. B., and Kriesman, J. J. A clinical study of borderline personality disorder: the significance of Briquet's syndrome (hysteria), somatization disorder, antisocial personality disorder, and substance abuse disorders. Am. J. Psychiatry, 153:1598–1606, 1996.

41. Johnson, J. G., Cohen, P., Smailes, E. M., Skodol, A. E., Brown, J., and Oldham, J. M. Childhood verbal abuse and risk for personality disorders during adolescence and early adulthood. Compr. Psychiatry, 42:16–23, 2001.

42. Johnson, J. G., Smailes, E. M., Cohen, P., Brown, J., and Bernstein, D. P. Associations between four types of childhood neglect and personality disorder symptoms during adolescence and early adulthood: findings of a community-based longitudinal study. J. Pers. Disord., 14:171–187, 2000.

43. Johnson, T. M. Vomiting as a manifestation of borderline personality disorder in primary care. J. Am. Board Fam. Pract., 6:385–394, 1993.

44. Kernberg, O. Borderline personality organization. J. Am. Psychoanal. Assoc., 15:641–685, 1967.

45. Khouri, P. J., Haier, R. J., Rieder, R. O., and Rosenthal, D. A symptom schedule for the diagnosis of borderline schizophrenia: a first report. Br. J. Psychiatry, 137:140–147, 1980.

46. Kjelsberg, E., Eikeseth, P. H., and Dahl, A. A. Suicide in borderline patients—predictive factors. Acta Psychiatr. Scand., 84:283–287, 1991.

47. Kroll, J. *The Challenge of the Borderline Patient.* New York: W.W. Norton, 1989.

48. Kullgren, G. Factors associated with completed suicide in borderline personality disorder. J. Nerv. Ment. Dis., 176:40–44, 1988.

49. Larsson, J. O., and Hellzen, M. Patterns of personality disorders in women with chronic eating disorders. Eat. Weight Disord., 9:200–205, 2004.

50. Lauer, J., Black, D. W., and Keen, P. Multiple personality disorder and borderline personality disorder. Distinct entities or variations on a common theme. Ann. Clin. Psychiatry, 5:129–134, 1993.

51. Leichsenring, F. Quality of depressive experiences in borderline personality disorders: differences between patients with borderline personality disorder and patients with higher levels of personality organization. Bull. Menninger Clin., 68:9–22, 2004.

52. Lenze, E. L., Miller, A., Munir, Z., Pornoppadol, C., and North, C. S. Psychiatric symptoms endorsed by somatization disorder patients in a psychiatric clinic. Ann. Clin. Psychiatry, 11:73–79, 1999.

53. Lieb, K., Zanarini, M. C., Schmahl, C., Linehan, M. M., and Bohus, M. Borderline personality disorder. Lancet, 364:453–461, 2004.

54. Linehan, M. M. Dialectical behavior therapy for borderline personality disorder. Theory and method. Bull. Menninger Clin., 51:261–276, 1987.

55. Linehan, M. M., Armstrong, H. E., Suarez, A., Allmon, D., and Heard, H. L. Cognitive-behavioral treatment of chronically parasuicidal borderline patients. Arch. Gen. Psychiatry, 48:1060–1064, 1991.

56. Linehan, M. M., Tutek, D. A., Heard, H. L., and Armstrong, H. E. Interpersonal outcome of cognitive behavioral treatment for chronically suicidal borderline patients. Am. J. Psychiatry, 151:1771–1776, 1994.

57. Loranger, A. W., and Tulis, E. H. Family history of alcoholism in borderline personality disorder. Arch. Gen. Psychiatry, 42:153–157, 1985.

58. Lyoo, I. K., Han, M. H., and Cho, D. Y. A brain MRI study in subjects with borderline personality disorder. J. Affect. Disord., 50:235–243, 1998.

59. Matsunaga, H., Kiriike, N., Nagata, T., and Yamagami, S. Personality disorders in patients with eating disorders in Japan. Int. J. Eat. Disord., 23:399–408, 1998.

60. McQuillan, A., Nicastro, R., Guenot, F., Girard, M., Lissner, C., and Ferrero, F. Intensive dialectical behavior therapy for outpatients with borderline personality disorder who are in crisis. Psychiatr. Serv., 56:193–197, 2005.

61. Millon, T. On the genesis and prevalence of the borderline personality disorder: a social learning thesis. J. Pers. Disord., 1:354–372, 1987.

62. North, C. S., Hansen, K., Wetzel, R. D., Compton, W., Napier, M., and Spitznagel, E. L. Non-psychotic thought disorder: objective clinical identification of

somatization and antisocial personality in language patterns. Compr. Psychiatry, 38:171–178, 1997.

63. North, C. S., Ryall, J. M., Ricci, D. A., and Wetzel, R. D. *Multiple Personalities, Multiple Disorders: Psychiatric Classification and Media Influence*. New York: Oxford University Press, 1993.

64. Nurnberg, H. G., Raskin, M., Levine, P. E., Pollack, S., Siegel, O., and Prince, R. The comorbidity of borderline personality disorder and other DSM-III-R Axis II personality disorders. Am. J. Psychiatry, 148:1371–1377, 1991.

65. Oldham, J. M. A 44-year-old woman with borderline personality disorder. JAMA, 287:1029–1037, 2002.

66. Ozkan, M., and Altindag, A. Comorbid personality disorders in subjects with panic disorder: do personality disorders increase clinical severity? Compr. Psychiatry, 46:20–26, 2005.

67. Paris, J. Memories of abuse in borderline patients: true or false? Harv. Rev. Psychiatry, 3:10–17, 1995.

68. Paris, J. Chronic suicidality among patients with borderline personality disorder. Psychiatr. Serv., 53:738–742, 2002.

69. Paris, J. The nature of borderline personality disorder: multiple dimensions, multiple symptoms, but one category. J. Pers. Disord., 21:457–473, 2007.

70. Paris, J., Brown, R., and Nowlis, D. Long-term follow-up of borderline patients in a general hospital. Compr. Psychiatry, 28:530–535, 1987.

71. Paris, J., and Zweig-Frank, H. A 27-year follow-up of patients with borderline personality disorder. Compr. Psychiatry, 42:482–487, 2001.

72. Perry, J. C., and Klerman, G. L. Clinical features of the borderline personality disorder. Am. J. Psychiatry, 137:165–173, 1980.

73. Pinto, C., Dhavale, H. S., Nair, S., Patil, B., and Dewan, M. Borderline personality disorder exists in India. J. Nerv. Ment. Dis., 188:386–388, 2000.

74. Pope, H. G., Jr., Jonas, J. M., Hudson, J. I., Cohen, B. M., and Gunderson, J. G. The validity of DSM-III borderline personality disorder. A phenomenologic, family history, treatment response, and long-term follow-up study. Arch. Gen. Psychiatry, 40:23–30, 1983.

75. Powell, R. A., and Boer, D. P. Did Freud mislead patients to confabulate memories of abuse? Psychol. Rep., 74:1283–1298, 1994.

76. Rinne, T., de Kloet, E. R., Wouters, L., Goekoop, J. G., DeRijk, R. H., and van den Brink, W. Hyperresponsiveness of hypothalamic-pituitary-adrenal axis to combined dexamethasone/corticotropin-releasing hormone challenge in female borderline personality disorder subjects with a history of sustained childhood abuse. Biol. Psychiatry, 52:1102–1112, 2002.

77. Riso, L. P., Klein, D. N., Anderson, R. L., and Ouimette, P. C. A family study of outpatients with borderline personality disorder and no history of mood disorder. J. Pers. Disord., 14:208–217, 2000.

78. Robins, E., and Guze, S. B. Establishment of diagnostic validity in psychiatric illness: its application to schizophrenia. Am. J. Psychiatry, 126:983–987, 1970.

79. Rosenvinge, J. H., Martinussen, M., and Ostensen, E. The comorbidity of eating disorders and personality disorders: a meta-analytic review of studies published between 1983 and 1998. Eat. Weight Disord., 5:52–61, 2000.

80. Sandell, R., Alfredsson, E., Berg, M., Crafoord, K., Lagerlof, A., Arkel, I., Cohn, T., Rasch, B., and Rugolska, A. Clinical significance of outcome in long-term follow-up of borderline patients at a day hospital. Acta Psychiatr. Scand., 87:405–413, 1993.

81. Sansone, R. A., Wiederman, M. W., and Sansone, L. A. Borderline personality symptomatology, experience of multiple types of trauma, and health care utilization among women in a primary care setting. South. Med. J., *89*:1162–1165, 1996.

82. Schmahl, C. G., Vermetten, E., Elzinga, B. M., and Douglas, B. J. Magnetic resonance imaging of hippocampal and amygdala volume in women with childhood abuse and borderline personality disorder. Psychiatr. Res., *122*:193–198, 2003.

83. Schmideberg, M. The treatment of psychopaths and borderline patients. Am. J. Psychother., *1*:45, 1947.

84. Semke, V. I., Polozhii, B. S., Krasik, E. D., Vasil'eva, O. A., Zalevskii, G. V., and Kornetov, N. A. [Epidemiology, clinical aspects and prevention of borderline conditions in the regions of Siberia and Far East]. Zh. Nevropatol. Psikhiatr. Im S. S. Korsakova, *91*:7–11, 1991.

85. Senol, S., Dereboy, C., and Yuksel, N. Borderline disorder in Turkey: a 2- to 4-year follow-up. Soc. Psychiatry Psychiatr. Epidemiol., *32*:109–112, 1997.

86. Shea, M. T., Stout, R., Gunderson, J., Morey, L. C., Grilo, C. M., McGlashan, T., Skodol, A. E., Dolan-Sewell, R., Dyck, I., Zanarini, M. C., and Keller, M. B. Short-term diagnostic stability of schizotypal, borderline, avoidant, and obsessive-compulsive personality disorders. Am. J. Psychiatry, *159*:2036–2041, 2002.

87. Shearer, S. L. Dissociative phenomena in women with borderline personality disorder. Am. J. Psychiatry, *151*:1324–1328, 1994.

88. Silverman, J. M., Pinkham, L., Horvath, T. B., Coccaro, E. F., Klar, H., Schear, S., Apter, S., Davidson, M., Mohs, R. C., and Siever, L. J. Affective and impulsive personality disorder traits in the relatives of patients with borderline personality disorder. Am. J. Psychiatry, *148*:1378–1385, 1991.

89. Skodol, A. E., Gunderson, J. G., McGlashan, T. H., Dyck, I. R., Stout, R. L., Bender, D. S., Grilo, C. M., Shea, M. T., Zanarini, M. C., Morey, L. C., Sanislow, C. A., and Oldham, J. M. Functional impairment in patients with schizotypal, borderline, avoidant, or obsessive-compulsive personality disorder. Am. J. Psychiatry, *159*:276–283, 2002.

90. Skodol, A. E., Stout, R. L., McGlashan, T. H., Grilo, C. M., Gunderson, J. G., Shea, M. T., Morey, L. C., Zanarini, M. C., Dyck, I. R., and Oldham, J. M. Co-occurrence of mood and personality disorders: a report from the Collaborative Longitudinal Personality Disorders Study (CLPS). Depress. Anxiety, *10*:175–182, 1999.

91. Snyder, S., Pitts, W. M., Goodpaster, W. A., Sajadi, C., and Gustin, Q. MMPI profile of DSM-III borderline personality disorder. Am. J. Psychiatry, *139*:1046–1048, 1982.

92. Soloff, P. H., Cornelius, J., and George, A. The depressed borderline: one disorder or two? Psychopharmacol. Bull., *27*:23–30, 1991.

93. Soloff, P. H., George, A., Nathan, R. S., Schulz, P. M., and Perel, J. M. Paradoxical effects of amitriptyline on borderline patients. Am. J. Psychiatry, *143*:1603–1605, 1986.

94. Soloff, P. H., George, A., Nathan, R. S., Schulz, P. M., Ulrich, R. F., and Perel, J. M. Progress in pharmacotherapy of borderline disorders. A double-blind study of amitriptyline, haloperidol, and placebo. Arch. Gen. Psychiatry, *43*:691–697, 1986.

95. Soloff, P. H., Lis, J. A., Kelly, T., Cornelius, J., and Ulrich, R. Risk factors for suicidal behavior in borderline personality disorder. Am. J. Psychiatry, *151*:1316–1323, 1994.

96. Soloff, P. H., and Millward, J. W. Psychiatric disorders in the families of borderline patients. Arch. Gen. Psychiatry, *40*:37–44, 1983.

97. Spitzer, R. L., Endicott, J., and Gibbon, M. Crossing the border into borderline personality and borderline schizophrenia. The development of criteria. Arch. Gen. Psychiatry, *36*:17–24, 1979.

98. Stern, A. Psychoanalytic investigation of and therapy in the borderline group of neuroses. Psychoanal. Q., 7:467–489, 1938.

99. Stone, M. H. The borderline syndrome: evolution of the term, genetic aspects, and prognosis. Am. J. Psychother., 31:345–365, 1977.

100. Stone, M. H. Toward a psychobiological theory of borderline personality disorder. Dissociation, 1:2–15, 1988.

101. Swartz, M. S., Blazer, D. G., George, L. K., Winfield, I., Zakris, J., and Dye, E. Identification of borderline personality disorder with the NIMH Diagnostic Interview Schedule. Am. J. Psychiatry, 146:200–205, 1989.

102. Tarnopolsky, A., and Berkowitz, M. Borderline personality: a review of recent research. Br. J. Psychiatry, 151:724–734, 1987.

103. Torgersen, S., Kringlen, E., and Cramer, V. The prevalence of personality disorders in a community sample. Arch. Gen. Psychiatry, 58:590–596, 2001.

104. Torgersen, S., Lygren, S., Oien, P. A., Skre, I., Onstad, S., Edvardsen, J., Tambs, K., and Kringlen, E. A twin study of personality disorders. Compr. Psychiatry, 41:416–425, 2000.

105. Torrens, M., Serrano, D., Astals, M., Perez-Dominguez, G., and Martin-Santos, R. Diagnosing comorbid psychiatric disorders in substance abusers: validity of the Spanish versions of the Psychiatric Research Interview for Substance and Mental Disorders and the Structured Clinical Interview for DSM-IV. Am. J. Psychiatry, 161:1231–1237, 2004.

106. van Hanswijck de Jonge, P., Van Furth, E. F., Lacey, J. H., and Waller, G. The prevalence of DSM-IV personality pathology among individuals with bulimia nervosa, binge eating disorder and obesity. Psychol. Med., 33:1311–1317, 2003.

107. Verheul, R., Kranzler, H. R., Poling, J., Tennen, H., Ball, S., and Rounsaville, B. J. Co-occurrence of Axis I and Axis II disorders in substance abusers. Acta Psychiatr. Scand., 101:110–118, 2000.

108. Verheul, R., Van Den Bosch, L. M., Koeter, M. W., De Ridder, M. A., Stijnen, T., and van den Brink, W. Dialectical behaviour therapy for women with borderline personality disorder: 12-month, randomised clinical trial in the Netherlands. Br. J. Psychiatry, 182:135–140, 2003.

109. Westen, D., Ludolph, P., Misle, B., Ruffins, S., and Block, J. Physical and sexual abuse in adolescent girls with borderline personality disorder. Am. J. Orthopsychiatry, 60:55–66, 1990.

110. Wetzel, R. D., Guze, S. B., Cloninger, C. R., Martin, R. L., and Clayton, P. J. Briquet's syndrome (hysteria) is both a somatoform and a "psychoform" illness: a Minnesota Multiphasic Personality Inventory study. Psychosom. Med., 56:564–569, 1994.

111. Widiger, T. A., and Sanderson, C. J. Personality disorders. In *Psychiatry*, Tasman, A., Kay, J., Lieberman, J. A. (eds.). Philadelphia: Saunders, pp. 1291–1317, 1997.

112. Zanarini, M. C., and Frankenburg, F. R. Olanzapine treatment of female borderline personality disorder patients: a double-blind, placebo-controlled pilot study. J. Clin. Psychiatry, 62:849–854, 2001.

113. Zanarini, M. C., and Frankenburg, F. R. The essential nature of borderline psychopathology. J. Pers. Disord., 21:518–535, 2007.

114. Zanarini, M. C., Frankenburg, F. R., Dubo, E. D., Sickel, A. E., Trikha, A., Levin, A., and Reynolds, V. Axis I comorbidity of borderline personality disorder. Am. J. Psychiatry, 155:1733–1739, 1998.

115. Zanarini, M. C., Frankenburg, F. R., Dubo, E. D., Sickel, A. E., Trikha, A., Levin, A., and Reynolds, V. Axis II comorbidity of borderline personality disorder. Compr. Psychiatry, *39*:296–302, 1998.

116. Zanarini, M. C., Frankenburg, F. R., Hennen, J., Reich, D. B., and Silk, K. R. The McLean Study of Adult Development (MSAD): overview and implications of the first six years of prospective follow-up. J. Pers. Disord., *19*:505–523, 2005.

117. Zanarini, M. C., Frankenburg, F. R., Hennen, J., and Silk, K. R. The longitudinal course of borderline psychopathology: 6-year prospective follow-up of the phenomenology of borderline personality disorder. Am. J. Psychiatry, *160*:274–283, 2003.

118. Zanarini, M. C., Frankenburg, F. R., Hennen, J., and Silk, K. R. Mental health service utilization by borderline personality disorder patients and Axis II comparison subjects followed prospectively for 6 years. J. Clin. Psychiatry, *65*:28–36, 2004.

119. Zanarini, M. C., Frankenburg, F. R., Khera, G. S., and Bleichmar, J. Treatment histories of borderline inpatients. Compr. Psychiatry, *42*:144–150, 2001.

120. Zanarini, M. C., Frankenburg, F. R., Reich, D. B., Marino, M. F., Lewis, R. E., Williams, A. A., and Khera, G. S. Biparental failure in the childhood experiences of borderline patients. J. Pers. Disord., *14*:264–273, 2000.

121. Zanarini, M. C., Frankenburg, F. R., Reich, D. B., Silk, K. R., Hudson, J. I., and McSweeney, L. B. The subsyndromal phenomenology of borderline personality disorder: a 10-year follow-up study. Am. J. Psychiatry, *164*:929–935, 2007.

122. Zanarini, M. C., Gunderson, J. G., Frankenburg, F. R., and Chauncey, D. L. Discriminating borderline personality disorder from other Axis II disorders. Am. J. Psychiatry, *147*:161–167, 1990.

123. Zanarini, M. C., Ruser, T., Frankenburg, F. R., and Hennen, J. The dissociative experiences of borderline patients. Compr. Psychiatry, *41*:223–227, 2000.

124. Zanarini, M. C., Yong, L., Frankenburg, F. R., Hennen, J., Reich, D. B., Marino, M. F., and Vujanovic, A. A. Severity of reported childhood sexual abuse and its relationship to severity of borderline psychopathology and psychosocial impairment among borderline inpatients. J. Nerv. Ment. Dis., *190*:381–387, 2002.

125. Zhong, J., and Leung, F. Should borderline personality disorder be included in the fourth edition of the Chinese classification of mental disorders? Chin. Med. J. (Engl.), *120*:77–82, 2007.

126. Zimmerman, M., and Mattia, J. I. Axis I diagnostic comorbidity and borderline personality disorder. Compr. Psychiatry, *40*:245–252, 1999.

127. Zimmerman, M., and Mattia, J. I. Differences between clinical and research practices in diagnosing borderline personality disorder. Am. J. Psychiatry, *156*:1570–1574, 1999.

CHAPTER 11

༄

Alcohol Use Disorder

Disorders of excessive alcohol use have been described under different names across history. Older names for the disorder are "inebriety," "drunkenness," (70) and "dipsomania" (100). "Alcoholism" was first coined by Magnus Huss in Sweden in 1849 to refer to cases of "alcohol addiction" (70). *DSM-I* (3) and *DSM-II* (4) used the term "alcoholism." In 1980, *DSM-III* (5) replaced the diagnosis of "alcoholism" with separate diagnoses of "alcohol abuse" and "alcohol dependence." *DSM-5* subsequently replaced these terms with a single diagnosis of "alcohol use disorder" (6). The evolution in the terminology for disorders of excessive alcohol use has progressed in parallel with evolution from early understanding of these disorders as originating from personality defects and social and moral deficiencies to modern views based on biological and genetic origins (100).

HISTORICAL BACKGROUND

As early as 3500 B.C., people were making and drinking alcohol in the lower Mesopotamian regions of what is now western Iran. Apparently this civilization was already enjoying both wine and beer. Both red wine stains and chemical evidence of beer fermentation in residue were found by group of researchers in the early 1990s in pottery vessels in Sumerian ruins of the Godin Tepe trading outpost and fortress in the Zagros Mountains (93, 94). One of the scientists making the discovery said, "I think a lot of serious drinking was going on there" (141). This civilization was one of the oldest literate places in the world, and it had a complex society of prospering city-states supported by horticulture of domesticated plants and irrigation agriculture (94). The domestication of barley to make bread in the early transition to agriculture by the Mesopotamians around 8000 B.C. provided the technology for beer-making. A long-standing debate in archaeology is the obvious question of which came first after the domestication of barley: beer or bread? (141).

Meanwhile, the Chinese were also fermenting alcoholic beverages from rice, honey, and fruit as early as 7000 B.C. This discovery was made by analysis of residues from pottery jars found in the early Neolithic village of Jiahu in the Hunan province of China (90). The Chinese refined their methods of fermented beverage production over the next 5,000 years, and vessels sealed around 1000 B.C. that were found in 2003 revealed "a delicious aroma and a light flavor" (p. 17597) (90).

The means of making alcohol were undoubtedly available to humans as far back as 200 million years ago, but when exactly humans first imbibed is lost in prehistoric history (114). The likely sources of material for fermentation to alcohol in the Paleolithic and Neolithic eras were fruit juice for wine, grain for beer, and honey for mead. Etymological evidence suggests that honey was the prime source of intoxicating beverage in antiquity: both of the terms from which the word *mead* is derived (*methy* in Sanskrit and *madhu* in Greek) mean both "honey" and "intoxicating drink" (114).

Over thousands of years, alcohol has been used for several purposes: medicinally, in religious ceremonies, and recreationally (114). In the Old Testament, Noah "planted a vineyard. He drank of the wine and was drunken" (Genesis 9:21–22) (2). The Mesopotamian civilization produced some of the earliest descriptions of alcohol intoxication and attempted antidotes (114). During the seventeenth Egyptian Dynasty at about the time of the reign of Hammurabi (circa 2100 B.C.) taverns were prevalent. A hieroglyphic message on a relic from that time, uttered by a female courtier stated, "Give me eighteen bowls of wine! . . . Behold, I love drunkenness!" (p. 847) (114). According to historians, drunkenness was not uncommon in Egypt in that era, occurring in all social categories from the lowest classes to the ruling classes (125). It was customary for both men and women to wind up sick at banquets, as illustrated by a recovered fresco from the second millennium B.C. depicting a woman banqueter turning from the table to vomit into a bowl held by a servant (114).

Pleas for moderation have followed these recorded trails of drunkenness. The first temperance tract appears to have occurred in dynastic Egypt (114). A quote attributed to Genghis Khan is: "A soldier must not get drunk oftener than once a week. It would, of course, be better if he did not get drunk at all, but one should not expect the impossible" (p. 19) (86). The Old Testament is tolerant of alcohol but condemns drunkenness: "Give strong drink unto him that is ready to perish, and wine unto those that be of heavy hearts. Let him drink, and forget his poverty, and remember his misery no more" (Proverbs 31:6-7) (1).

The process of distillation was discovered about 800 A.D. in Arabia (114). The word *alcohol* comes from the Arabic *alkuhl*, referring to the essence or the essential spirit of fermented beverages. For centuries, distilled alcohol was used in medicine, but by the seventeenth century it had also become a drug of abuse on a large scale. By the late seventeenth century, the annual worldwide production of distilled liquors, chiefly gin, was enormous.

Ancient and classical writers used words that are universally translated as "drunkenness." The people who had it were "drunkards." In the four-teenth century, Chaucer used *dronkelewe* to mean addiction to alcohol as a mental illness (22). By the nineteenth century, "inebriety" was the favored descriptor; those who manifested it were not merely inebriated—they were "inebriates." A Swedish public health authority, Magnus Huss, in 1849 coined the term "alcoholism." The word caught on: Danish has *alkoholisme*; Dutch, *alcoholisme*; English, *alcoholism*; Finnish, *alkoholismi*; German, *alkoholismus*; Italian, *alcolismo*; Norwegian, *alkoholisme*; Polish, *alkoholizm*; Portuguese, *alcoolismo*; Russian, *alkogolism*; Serbo-Croatian, *alkoholizam*; Slovene, *alkoholizem*; Spanish, *alcoholismo*; Swedish, *alkoholism* (69).

The "disease concept" of alcoholism originated in the writings of Benjamin Rush and the British physician Thomas Trotter (115), and during the last half of the nineteenth century, the notion that alcoholism was a disease became popular with physicians. Earlier (in the 1830s), Dr. Samuel Woodward, the first superintendent of Worcester State Hospital in Massachusetts, and Dr. Eli Todd of Hartford, Connecticut, suggested the establishment of special institutions for inebriates. The first was opened in Boston in 1841. In 1904, the Medical Temperance Society changed its name to the American Medical Association for the Study of Inebriety and Narcotics. The *Journal of Inebriety*, established in 1876, was founded on the "fact that inebriety is a neurosis and psychosis." (p. 32) (86).

During Prohibition, however, the concept of alcoholism as a disease had lost its vogue (65). The 18th Amendment to the U.S. Constitution prohibiting alcoholic beverages became effective in 1920 and was con-tinued for 13 years before its repeal (76). The disease concept of alco-holism was revived after the repeal of Prohibition. Pioneering studies performed at the Yale School of Alcohol Studies and the writings of E. M. Jellinek were largely responsible for the subsequent popularization of the disease concept of alcoholism in the twentieth century. In the mid-1960s, the US government began supporting alcohol and other drug research on an expanded scale; by the 1980s, the federal government and most state governments were sponsoring substance treatment programs. Proprietary hospitals for alcohol and drug use disorders spread across the continent in large numbers, but for-profit hospitals such as these were stifled with the advent of "managed care." Nonetheless, care continued with development of several different models, including inpatient (shorter stays of 1–4 days versus 28), outpatient, and residential (short stay of 3–6 weeks and long stay of 6–12 months).

EPIDEMIOLOGY

The "intoxicant of choice" in Judeo-Christian culture has historically been alcohol, as described 300 years ago: "To drink is a Christian diversion/ Unknown to the Turk and the Persian," (p. 51) (25). Although the Turks and Persians were not strangers to alcohol, their preference for intoxicants favored the poppy and hemp plants (86).

Societal levels of alcohol consumption have been attributed to the "stresses" of modern living, but such assumptions do not correspond to amounts consumed over time (86). The highest annual per capita amounts of consumption in the United States were in the early 1800s, estimated as the equivalent of six to seven gallons of 200-proof absolute alcohol per person. At that time, the preferred beverages were whiskey and cider, which had the important feature of being portable, a major consideration in times before the development of trains (86). Alcohol consumption after that time decreased with the advent of modern transportation that made it easier to transport less compact forms of alcohol.

After the end of Prohibition, in 1933, consumption of alcohol by Americans gradually increased to a high of 2.76 gallons of pure alcohol per person per year in 1980, with a subsequent decline to just over 2 gallons per person in the late 1990s, which was again followed by a gradual rise to 2.34 gallons per year in 2013 (101). Between 2002 and 2013, the proportion of Americans who drink increased from 65% to 73% (48).

Alcohol consumption varies greatly from country to country. Internationally, the lowest per capita rate of alcohol consumption is in Pakistan (.02 gallons annually), with many Middle Eastern and North African countries sharing similarly low rates. The highest rate is in Moldova (4.81 gallons), and similarly high rates are found in Russia as well as several Eastern European countries (143).

Most adults in the United States are light drinkers. About one-fourth (23%) of men and one-third of women (30%) abstain in any given year (48). According to a 2012 Gallup poll, male drinkers average 6.2 drinks per week, and female drinkers average 2.2 (40). Heavy episodic drinking (also known as "binge drinking" or "daily risk drinking") is defined as consuming at least five alcoholic beverages for men and four for women on at least one occasion in the last month (defining a "daily drinking limit") (29). "Heavy" drinking, which can be deleterious to the individual's health, is defined by the US government as consuming 14 or more drinks per week for men and 7 or more for women (defining a "weekly drinking limit," which, when exceeded, constitutes "weekly risk drinking") (29). Nearly three-fourths of both male and female drinkers are known to exceed one or both of these drinking limits in a given year (33).

Most alcohol is consumed by a small fraction of the population. The top 2.5% of drinkers by volume account for nearly one-fourth of all alcohol consumed, the top 15% consume nearly three-fourths, and the top 20% consume 80% (33).

Drinking patterns vary markedly across different demographic subpopulations. For both men and women, the prevalence of drinking is highest and abstention is lowest in the 25- to 34-year age range (7, 17). Males are two to three times as likely as females to be "heavy" drinkers at all ages (68). However, changing social norms for women in Western culture are bringing more permissive drinking norms and values, and as more women have been pursuing occupational and educational opportunities outside of the home, the gender gap in levels of consumption and in alcohol-related consequences has been closing in younger cohorts (31, 48, 55). Among people ages 65 years and older, abstainers exceed drinkers among both men and women, and only about 10% of men and 2% of women in this age group are heavy drinkers (15). In the United States, the highest and heaviest alcohol consumption are in the Northeast and North Central states and lowest in the South (72).

Although conceptually intertwined, alcohol consumption and alcoholism represent very different constructs. Estimating the prevalence of alcohol use disorders is fraught with methodological hazards. A long-standing lack of consensus on the definition of alcoholism has been further complicated by changing diagnostic criteria for alcohol use disorders over time (54, 77). The methods to assess these disorders have varied from structured diagnostic interviews to clinical assessments to symptom checklists. These different methods have proved to be highly inconsistent in identification of cases and estimation of prevalence (48). Even structured diagnostic interviews, considered to be most effective in precise assessment of diagnostic criteria, are known to have important differences in features, leading to disagreements about diagnosis of alcohol use disorders (49). Other methodological issues, such as sampling complexities, participation bias, and recall bias, represent further threats to valid and consistent findings in prevalence studies of alcohol use disorders.

Recently published research has provided updated estimates of the general population prevalence of alcohol use disorders and findings on recent changes in prevalence. The National Epidemiologic Survey on Alcohol and Related Conditions (NESARC) collected nationally representative surveys of US adults, with a first round of data collected in 2001–2002 and more recent data collected in 2012–2013, using well-tested structured diagnostic interviews (48). The latest findings of the NESARC studies indicate that 17% of men and 9% of American women meet 12-month criteria for a *DSM-IV* alcohol use disorder (48). Males, whites, and young adults are found to have the highest rates of alcohol use disorders (50), consistent with findings that young white males represent the population subgroup with the highest prevalence of alcohol use disorders (50). The NESARC research found that the population prevalence of alcohol use disorders increased by 49% between 2002 and 2013, from 9% to 13% (48). These increases were greatest among women, the elderly, racial/ethnic minorities, and the socioeconomically disadvantaged.

CLINICAL PICTURE

Alcohol use disorders culminate from behavior involving the consumption of large quantities of alcohol on repeated occasions. Motivations underlying such behavior have long been contemplated. When asked why they drink excessively, many individuals with alcohol use disorders attribute their drinking to a particular mood, such as depression or anxiety, or to situational problems. Some describe an overpowering "need" to drink, variously described as a craving or compulsion. Many individuals with alcohol use disorders, however, are unable to offer a plausible explanation of their excessive drinking (81).

The essential feature of alcohol use disorder is a cluster of cognitive, behavioral, and physiological symptoms indicating that the individual continues using alcohol despite significant alcohol-related problems. These problems may include tolerance, withdrawal, and craving of alcohol.

Like other drug dependencies, alcohol use disorder is accompanied by a preoccupation with obtaining and using the drug in quantities sufficient to produce intoxication over long periods. It is especially true early in the course of alcohol use disorders that patients may deny this preoccupation or attempt to rationalize their need by assertions that they drink no more than their friends. Possibly as part of this denial or rationalization, many people who drink to excess spend their time with other heavy drinkers.

A patient named David explained (pp. 27–29) (86):

> My need was easy to hide from myself and others (maybe I'm kidding myself about the others). I only associated with people who drank. I married a woman who drank. There were always reasons to drink. I was low, tense, tired, mad, happy. I probably drank as often because I was happy as for any other reason. And occasions for drinking—when drinking was appropriate, expected—were endless, football games, fishing trips, parties, holidays, birthdays, Christmas, or merely Saturday night. Drinking became interwoven with everything pleasurable—food, sex, social life. When I stopped drinking, these things, for a time, lost all interest for me, they were so tied to drinking.

As the disease progresses and problems from drinking become more serious, the individual may drink alone, sneak drinks, hide the bottle, and take other measures to conceal the seriousness of their condition. This is almost always accompanied by feelings of guilt and remorse, which in turn may produce more drinking, temporarily relieving the feelings. Remorse may be particularly intense in the morning, when the person has not had a drink for a number of hours, and this may provoke morning drinking (p. 28) (86):

> For years [David wrote], I drank and had very little hangover, but now the hangovers were gruesome. I felt physically bad—headachy, nauseous, weak, but the mental part was the hardest. I loathed myself. I was waking early and thinking what a mess I was, how I had hurt so many others and myself. The words "guilty" and "depression" sound superficial in trying to describe how I felt. The loathing was almost physical—a dead weight that could be lifted in only one way, and that was by having a drink, so I drank, morning after morning. After two or three, my hands were steady, I could hold some breakfast down, and the guilt was gone, or almost.

Prolonged drinking, even if initiated to relieve guilt and anxiety, commonly produces anxiety and depression (82). The full range of symptoms associated with depression and anxiety disorders—including terminal insomnia, low mood, irritability, and anxiety attacks with chest pain, palpitations, and dyspnea—often appear. Alcohol temporarily relieves these symptoms, resulting in a vicious cycle of drinking–depression–drinking, which may ultimately result in a classical withdrawal syndrome. Often the patient makes a valiant effort to stop drinking and may succeed for a period of several days or weeks, only to fall off the wagon again (p. 29) (86):

> At some point I was without wife, home, or job. I had nothing to do but drink. The drinking was now steady, days on end. I lost appetite and missed meals (besides money was short). I awoke at night, sweating and shaking, and had a drink. I awoke in the morning vomiting and had a drink. It couldn't last. My ex-wife found me in my apartment shaking and seeing things, and got me in the hospital. I dried out, left, and went back to drinking. I was hospitalized again, and this time stayed dry for 6 months. I was nervous and couldn't sleep, but got some of my confidence back, and found a part-time job. Then my ex-boss offered my job back and I celebrated by having a drink. The next night I had two drinks. In a month I was drinking as much as ever and again unemployed.

Repeated experiences like this easily lead to feelings of despair and hopelessness. By the time patients seek professional help, they have often reached rock bottom. Their situation seems hopeless and, after years of heavy drinking, their problems have become so numerous that they feel nothing can be done about them. At this point, they may be ready to acknowledge their alcohol problem but feel powerless to stop drinking. But many do stop—permanently—as will be discussed later.

Alcohol is one of the few psychoactive drugs that sometimes produce classical amnesia, referred to as "blackouts." Early alcohol research from the 1950s portrayed such blackouts as a hallmark of progressive alcoholism (64). More recent work, however, has shown that most people who experience alcoholic blackouts are not alcohol dependent (75), even though blackouts are strong predictors of drinking-related problems (60). Blackouts are particularly common among younger drinkers and are associated with drinking that results in rapidly rising blood alcohol levels (60, 75). Although blackouts may not be predictive of progressive alcohol dependence, it may be that the individual's behavior after the blackout experience that is influential in determining future drinking behavior (75).

Blackout episodes with drinking can be particularly distressful to individuals with alcohol dependence because they may fear that they have unknowingly harmed someone or behaved imprudently while intoxicated (p. 37) (86):

> A thirty-nine-year-old salesman awoke in a strange hotel room. He had a mild hangover but otherwise felt normal. His clothes were hanging in the closet: he was clean-shaven. He dressed and went down to the lobby. He learned from the

clerk that he was in Las Vegas and that he had checked in two days previously. It had been obvious that he had been drinking, the clerk said, but he hadn't seemed very drunk. The date was Saturday the fourteenth. His last recollection was of sitting in a St. Louis bar on Monday the ninth. He had been drinking all day and was drunk, but could remember everything perfectly until about three p.m., when "like a curtain dropping," his memory went blank. It remained blank for approximately five days. Three years later, those five days were still a blank. He was so frightened by the experience that he abstained from alcohol for two years.

Alcoholic blackouts represent an impairment of memory encoding, which is the initial recognition and interpretation of stimuli. Encoding provides a critical context for the formation and recall of episodic memories. The amnesia of alcoholic blackouts is typically anterograde, for memories of ongoing events. Retrograde amnesia can also occur, however, if a large amount of alcohol is consumed after memories are established in a completely sober state (75). During a blackout, remote and immediate memory may be intact, but the individual may experience a specific short-term memory deficit with inability to recall events that happened 5 or 10 minutes before. Because motor and other intellectual faculties are relatively well preserved, during blackouts individuals can perform complicated acts and appear normal to the casual observer.

Most alcoholic amnesia episodes represent partial or fragmentary loss of memory rather than complete memory loss. Thus, cueing the individual to events during the blackout can sometimes elicit forgotten memories (75). Theoretically, returning to an intoxicated state might prompt the return of memories blacked out by intoxication, but this has not been shown to regularly aid recall of these memories (74). Once in a while, a curious thing may happen: a person may recall things that happened during a previous drinking period that had been forgotten when sober, such as hiding money or alcohol, forgetting about it when sober, and remembering it again during the next drinking episode. One remarkable example of drinking-related recovery of memory is as follows (p. 38) (86):

A forty-seven-year-old housewife often wrote letters when she was drinking. Sometimes she would jot down notes for a letter and start writing it but not finish it. The next day, sober, she would be unable to decipher the notes. Then she would start drinking again, and after a few drinks the meaning of the notes would become clear and she would resume writing the letter. "It was like picking up the pencil where I had left off."

Anecdotal reports suggest that benzodiazepine medication combined with alcohol increases the likelihood of a blackout occurring with smaller amounts of alcohol than is usually required (98, 122). Benzodiazepines may also by themselves lead to short-term anterograde memory impairment in a dose-dependent fashion, but benzodiazepines do not typically produce the dense blackouts associated with heavy alcohol use (12, 83, 104).

Before an alcohol use disorder can be treated, it first must be recognized. Physicians are in a particularly good position to identify a drinking problem early through three main approaches: they can take a history, perform a physical examination, and order laboratory tests.

The alcohol inquiry must be designed by the examiner using the physician's own style to elicit the history and, eventually, the diagnostic criteria. After rapport is developed and the examiner is ready to turn to this section, the clinical approach may be direct ("Tell me about your current and past use of alcohol") or indirect ("Has alcohol ever interfered with your social, work, interpersonal or legal affairs?") The examiner should avoid a staccato firing of questions, judgmental approach, or aggressive style, all of which will likely inhibit open disclosure by the patient. Over the last 50 years, brief screening surveys have been developed for various settings, including the Michigan Alcoholism Screening Test (MAST) (124), CAGE questionnaire (37), and Alcohol Use Disorders Identification Test (AUDIT) (116). Even though the screening parts of these instruments may be helpful to the clinician in developing a set of questions and even perhaps a style of approach, the reader is reminded that brief surveys neither capture all cases nor diagnose illness. The clinician must take the time to develop rapport and talk with the patient to obtain a specific history of alcohol consumption patterns and sufficient information for diagnostic assessment of problem drinking.

Following are some potential medical indications of a drinking problem:

1. Arcus senilis—a ringlike opacity of the cornea—occurs commonly with age, causes no visual disturbance, and is considered an innocent condition. The ring forms from fatty material in the blood. Alcohol increases fat in the blood and more patients with alcohol addiction have the ring than others their age (9, 38).
2. A red nose (acne rosacea) suggests the owner has a weakness for alcoholic beverages. Often, however, people with red noses are teetotalers or even rabid prohibitionists, and they resent the insinuation.

3. Red palms (palmer erythema) are also suggestive, but not diagnostic, of alcoholism.
4. Cigarette burns between the index and middle fingers or on the chest and contusions and bruises should raise suspicions of alcoholic stupor.
5. Painless enlargement of the liver may suggest a larger alcohol intake than the liver can process. Severe, constant upper abdominal pain and tenderness radiating to the back indicates pancreatic inflammation, and alcohol sometimes is the cause.
6. Reduced sensation and weakness in the feet and legs may occur from excessive drinking.
7. Laboratory tests provide other clues. The major alcohol biomarkers are gamma-glutamyl transpeptidase (GGT), alanine amino-transferase (ALT), aspartate aminotransferase (AST), and mean corpuscular volume (MCV) (63). Historically, the test used most commonly in clinical practice is GGT. Although more than half of alcohol-dependent patients have increased amounts of this protein, it is nonspecific for alcoholism because it can also be elevated in nonalcoholic liver disease, biliary disease, obesity, and certain medications. These tests are hampered by low sensitivity and specificity and variable performance in different populations. The carbohydrate-deficient transferrin (CDT) test, approved by the U.S. Food and Drug Administration (FDA) in 2001, has high specificity but it is expensive and not widely available (63).

In their search for signs of excessive alcohol use, physicians sometimes slip into a moralistic attitude that alienates the patient. For personal reasons, physicians may believe any drinking is wrong, but they still should be aware of research suggesting that moderate drinking may actually confer specific health benefits and even contribute to longevity (96, 99). The lowest mortality from all causes is associated with consumption of one (for women) to two (for men) alcoholic beverages per day. Specifically, "beneficial" effects of alcohol include increased high-density lipoprotein (HDL) cholesterol, thought to contribute to lower likelihood of cardiovascular illness (i.e., myocardial infarction, heart failure, and ischemic stroke) and reduced risk for diabetes mellitus, dementia, and osteoporosis among moderate drinkers (99). Heavier drinking substantially increases the risk for all of these conditions. The risk of cancer, however, increases with any amount of alcohol consumed, even at the lowest levels. Greater amounts of alcohol consumption are especially associated with risk for breast, liver, esophageal, colon, and head and neck cancers (79, 99).

The weight of evidence does not suggest that nondrinkers should be encouraged to start an alcohol habit and there is no evidence to support immoderate use of alcohol (99, 130). The potential benefits of moderate drinking must be weighed against potential for development of alcohol use disorders and data demonstrating that alcohol contributes to automobile accidents, high blood pressure, breast cancer, adverse outcomes for patients with hepatitis C, and birth defects associated with drinking during pregnancy (128, 130). For healthy individuals who demonstrate ability to enjoy alcohol safely, however, recommendation of abstinence is not indicated, although continued monitoring is (130).

BIOLOGICAL FINDINGS

Current understanding of the biology of alcohol addiction is yet rudimentary. Unlike opioids and nicotine, alcohol has no known receptor in the human brain (35). Alcohol affects a number of neurotransmitter systems in various brain regions that are known to play a role in reward and reinforcement processes considered fundamental to addictions. Administration of alcohol enhances gamma-aminobutyric acid (GABA, the brain's main inhibitory neurotransmitter), inhibits glutamate (an excitatory neurotransmitter), and increases dopamine, serotonin, and opioid peptides (59, 87).

The dopamine system is considered to be central in the development and maintenance of alcohol dependence. During the development of an alcohol use disorder, the brain's sensitivity increases to the positive and negative reinforcing properties of ethanol. The brain's drug reward apparatus involves the mesolimbic dopamine pathway projecting from the ventral tegmental area into the nucleus accumbens. Alcohol increases the amount of dopamine in this pathway, and the amount of dopamine increase is associated with the level of high or euphoria reported from alcohol ingestion. With alcohol addiction, alcohol-conditioned cues by themselves prompt increases in striatal dopamine, even more than with actual alcohol ingestion. Once addiction to alcohol has developed, the dopamine response to alcohol ingestion is blunted. During protracted withdrawal in people with alcohol use disorders, dopamine receptors decrease in the striatum, and this is further associated with decreased function of the salience attribution areas of the orbitofrontal cortex and also of inhibitory controls in the anterior cingulate gyrus. The dopamine circuits involved in reward and conditioning thus become imbalanced with brain circuits involved in executive functions (emotional control and decision-making). This imbalance is postulated to contribute to the compulsion to drink and loss of control that are the clinical hallmarks of alcohol use disorder (140).

There is also considerable evidence for the involvement of serotonergic systems in all stages of alcohol dependence, from initiation of drinking to withdrawal and relapse. The brain's serotonergic circuitry is highly complex, with large numbers of receptor subtypes. Dysregulation of serotonin pathways has been demonstrated to be associated with impulsive alcohol consumption and with drinking for the purposes of self-medication of anxiety, contributing to excessive and compulsive drinking, sensitivity to the negative reinforcing effects of alcohol, and relapse behavior. Genotypic differences in brain serotonin circuitry may well contribute to many different pathways to the development of alcohol use disorders (87).

NATURAL HISTORY

Symptoms of alcohol use disorder do not commonly occur for the first time after age 45 (8). If they do, the physician should be alerted to the possibility of a primary mood disorder or brain disease. Alcohol use disorders have been studied less extensively in women than in men, but the evidence suggests that the course of the disorder is more variable in women. In women, the onset often occurs later (23, 61) and spontaneous remission apparently is less frequent (30). Women with the disorder are more likely than their male counterparts to have a history of depressive and anxiety disorders (55).

Historically, consideration has been given to types or patterns of drinking. The patterns are quite variable, and no particular pattern is associated exclusively with alcohol use disorder. Overall, alcohol dependence is a chronic remitting and relapsing disorder with periods of remission lasting for variable lengths of time.

Alcohol use disorder has a higher "spontaneous" remission rate than is often recognized. The incidence of first admissions to psychiatric hospitals for alcohol problems drops markedly in the sixth and seventh decades, as do first arrests for alcohol-related offenses. Although the mortality rate among people with alcohol use disorder is perhaps two to three times that of moderate drinkers, attrition through death is probably insufficient to account for the apparent decrease in problem drinking in middle and late middle life (51, 137).

Based on questionnaire data obtained from patients with alcohol use disorders, Jellinek promulgated earlier views that manifestations of the disorder follow a natural chronological order, with blackouts being one of the early "prodromal" symptoms of the illness (64). Later studies (75, 103) have challenged these ideas, and it is now believed that problems from drinking may occur in various sequences and that blackouts have no special significance as a sign of incipient alcohol problems. Frequently, after years of heavy problem-free drinking, a person may experience a large number of problems in a brief period. Table 11.1 shows the mean age of

TABLE 11.1 ONSET OF ALCOHOLIC MANIFESTATIONS AMONG ALL MEN IN THE SAMPLE (N = 100)

Manifestation	Present (%)	Mean Age at Onset	Percentage Reporting Manifestation (by Age at First Occurrence)*										
			<20	20–24	25–29	30–34	35–39	40–44	45–49	50–54	55–59	60–64	65–70
1. Frequent drunken episodes	98	27	18	17	21	18	13	7	3		1	1	
2. Weekend drunken episodes	82	28	11	18	21	32		6	8	2		1	
3. Morning drinking	84	31	2	17	15	25	17	9	11	1	1	1	
4. Benders	76	31	7	14	18	21	13	9	12	5	1		
5. Neglecting meals	86	32	2	11	14	29	15	10	10	6	1		1
6. "Shakes"	88	33	1	11	15	24	17	9	16	3	2		1
7. Job loss from drinking	69	34	3	7	19	19	26	7	9	6	3	1	
8. Separation or divorce from drinking	44	34		16	7	23	14	20	14	7			
9. Blackouts	64	35	2	6	16	28	25	8	10	3			
10. Joined Alcoholics Anonymous	39	36		8	8	28	20	15	8	10	3		
11. Hospitalization for drinking	100	37	1	3	14	18	20	13	14	9	6		
12. Alcohol withdrawal syndrome	45	38		2	11	11	40	16	7	11	2	1	1

* Figures rounded to nearest whole number for ease of perusal. Sums may therefore not equal 100%. Adapted from Goodwin et al. (44).

onset of alcohol problems in an unselected series of men hospitalized for alcoholism.

In 1960, Jellinek (65) developed a typology subdividing alcoholism along observable drinking patterns. Subsequent research by Edwards and Gross in 1976 (34) moved the field toward establishing a reliable basis for diagnosis of alcohol dependence syndrome by using criteria. Their "provisional description" of certain observable behaviors (e.g., 1. Narrowing of drinking behaviors, 2. Salience of drink-seeking behavior, 3. Increased tolerance to alcohol, 4. Repeated withdrawal symptoms, 5. Avoidance of withdrawal by further alcohol intake, 6. Awareness of compulsion to drink, and 7. Relapse after abstinence) became the bases for the formalized criteria for alcohol dependence found in *DSM-III-R, DSM-IV, DSM-IV-TR*, and *DSM-5* (see Table 11.1) and the international diagnostic criteria (*ICD-10*).

COMPLICATIONS

Because alcohol use disorder is defined by the problems it creates, symptoms and complications inevitably overlap. By the time people with alcohol problems consult a physician, many have developed medical and social complications from drinking. For present purposes, we will consider social and medical complications separately.

High rates of marital separation and divorce accompany alcohol use disorders (27). People with alcohol use disorder often have job troubles, including frequent absenteeism and job loss. They also have a high frequency of accidents—in the home, on the job, and while driving automobiles. More than one-third of highway fatalities in the United States involve a driver who has been drinking, but with national programs implemented to address this problem, the rates have dropped substantially over the last three decades (102). Nearly half of convicted felons have an alcohol use disorder (45), and about half of police activities in large cities are associated with alcohol-related offenses. According to a report by the Federal Aviation Administration (FAA), 6% of pilots killed in private plane crashes were found to have ethanol in excess of FAA regulations (20).

Medical complications fall into three categories: 1) acute effects of heavy drinking, 2) chronic effects of heavy drinking, and 3) withdrawal effects. Consumption of very large amounts of alcohol can lead directly to death by depressing the respiratory center in the medulla. Acute hemorrhagic pancreatitis occasionally occurs from a single heavy drinking episode.

Nearly every organ system can be affected, directly or indirectly, by chronic, heavy use of alcohol. General medical complications of excessive alcohol use include cancer, cardiovascular illness (i.e., cardiomyopathy, my-ocardial infarction, heart failure, and ischemic stroke), diabetes mellitus, os-teoporosis, thrombocytopenia and anemia, myopathy, and dementia (99).

The gastrointestinal system is especially vulnerable to damaging effects of alcohol. Chronic gastritis may occur, although chronic *Helicobacter pylori* infection has been found to be causal in most alcoholic gastritis and not the direct effects of alcohol itself. A thorough review of related research has concluded that the available evidence does not show increased risk of gas-tric or duodenal ulcer disease in association with acute or chronic alcohol consumption (85).

The most damaging effect of alcohol on the gastrointestinal tract is to the liver. Exactly how alcohol damages the liver is still not fully under-stood, despite decades of study. Alcohol induces tissue injury through known pathways involving acetaldehyde production, oxidant injury, and proinflammatory cytokines and chemokines. The underlying mechanisms in these processes, however, are complex, involving alcohol-induced alter-ation in cellular pathways of signal transduction, activation of tumor ne-crosis factor, suppression of natural killer cell functions, and generation of free radicals promoting lipid peroxidation, ultimately resulting in oxidant injury in mitochondria (41, 80, 97).

The first stage of alcoholic liver disease is fatty liver, a rapid response to excessive alcohol consumption. Although high-fat diets alone can cause fatty liver, alcohol can produce fatty liver even without dietary fat intake. High-fat diets increase the likelihood of fatty liver and liver disease asso-ciated with chronic excessive alcohol intake (74, 78). Although fatty liver is reversible, hepatocytes in this condition are vulnerable to adversity and their survival is reduced. Continued alcohol ingestion leads to a progres-sion of inflammatory responses and fibrosis and ultimately cirrhosis of the liver in some individuals. Although most patients with Laennec cirrhosis in Western countries are excessive drinkers, most people with severe al-coholism do not develop cirrhosis (probably less than 10%). This finding leaves unresolved the question of the direct role of alcohol in producing cir-rhosis. It appears that cirrhosis results from the combined effect of alcohol and diet plus other factors, likely including heredity (109).

Because, on average, half of all daily calories consumed by individuals with alcohol use disorders are from alcohol, insufficient intake of vital nutrients can result in serious malnutrition. Gastrointestinal complications of prolonged heavy alcohol use such as pancreatitis can further cause malnutrition through malabsorption. Alcohol also promotes degrada-tion of nutrients, such as vitamin A. Although experimental studies have demonstrated that nutritional deficiencies alone may damage the liver, adequate nutrition does not protect the liver against the toxic effects of chronic excessive alcohol consumption (78).

Alcohol use disorder is associated with pathology of the nervous system. It has long been debated whether peripheral neuropathy, the most common neurological complication, results from multiple vitamin B deficiencies or direct toxic effects of alcohol (67). Recent evidence that thiamine does not reverse the neuropathy, coupled with findings of biological differences between neuropathies of nutritional and alcoholic origins, has prompted the conclusion that it is alcohol itself that is responsible (91). Retrobulbar neuropathy may result in a rare complication of alcoholism and may lead to amblyopia (also called "tobacco-alcohol amblyopia" because of its historic association with both heavy tobacco and alcohol use among World War II veterans), a painless bilateral loss of vision that is usually reversible with adequate dietary and vitamin intake (107).

Other neurological complications involve anterior lobe cerebellar degenerative disease (118) and the Wernicke-Korsakoff syndrome (135). The latter involves thiamine deficiency. The acute Wernicke stage consists of ocular disturbances (nystagmus or sixth-nerve palsy), ataxia, and confusion. It usually clears in a few days but may progress to a chronic brain syndrome (Korsakoff psychosis). Short-term memory loss (anterograde amnesia) is the most characteristic feature of Korsakoff psychosis. "Confabulation" (narration of fanciful tales) may also occur. The Wernicke-Korsakoff syndrome is associated with necrotic lesions of the mammillary bodies, thalamus, and other brainstem areas. Thiamine corrects early Wernicke signs rapidly and *may* prevent development of an irreversible Korsakoff dementia. Once the dementia is established, thiamine does not usually help (see also Chapter 13).

Whether excessive use of alcohol produces cortical atrophy has been debated for decades. A confluence of radiological and pathological evidence has reached a consensus that brain shrinkage, especially in white matter but also in gray matter, occurs with chronic alcohol excess. The frontal cortex appears most sensitive to chronic alcohol-induced damage (123, 129, 132). The motor cortex, cerebellum, pons, mammillary bodies, thalamus, and hypothalamus are also affected. Ventricular and cortical sulci are enlarged. Some of these brain matter changes may reverse within a month of abstinence from alcohol, although permanent and irreversible damage may persist, presumably due to neuronal loss (123, 132).

In chronic alcohol use disorder, cognitive impairments are well described in domains of executive functioning (involving judgment, appropriateness of affect, insight, social functioning, motivation, and attention, learning and memory, and abstract problem- solving). Long-standing excessive alcohol consumption is particularly disruptive to visuospatial abilities (39) and to functions of gait, balance, and postural stability of the lower extremities (53, 132, 133). Cognitive deficits in chronic alcoholism have long been considered to represent "frontal" brain abnormalities (73), but other work has also implicated damage to the pontocerebellar and cerebellothallamocortical systems (53, 133). Although the amount of alcohol consumed has not consistently been found to parallel the severity of cognitive deficits in alcoholic patients, lifetime alcohol consumption is related to problems with gait and balance (133). Continued abstinence may permit partial recovery of brain function, but deficits based on neuronal loss may be permanent and irreversible (73, 110, 132).

Teratogenic effects of alcohol have been suspected for centuries, but only in the half-century has research demonstrated a distinct pattern of birth defects associated with maternal alcoholism during pregnancy. It is called "fetal alcohol syndrome." Affected babies are small and exhibit various combinations of developmental delays, craniofacial abnormalities (short palpebral fissures, epicanthal folds, and maxillary hypoplasia), and microcephaly. Associated behavioral and cognitive problems observed in these children are impaired information processing and memory, intellectual deficiencies, hyperactivity, impulsivity, and social and communication skills deficits. Brain abnormalities documented in the hippocampus, corpus callosum, cerebellum (especially anterior vermis), and basal ganglia (especially caudate nucleus) in fetal alcohol syndrome may explain some of the behavioral and cognitive problems (88, 112, 129). Animal studies have demonstrated specific teratogenic properties of ethyl alcohol in a variety of species, many of the abnormalities being similar to those described in humans (28, 71).

Fetal alcohol syndrome is the leading known cause of intellectual developmental disorder (36). A comprehensive review of research on the prevalence of fetal alcohol syndrome estimated its occurrence in approximately 0.5 to 2.0 per 1,000 births. The prevalence of all alcohol-related neurodevelopmental disorders is far higher, at least 10 per 1,000 births (89). Far more women drink during pregnancy than have fetal alcohol syndrome babies. Not all children prenatally exposed to heavy alcohol intake develop the full syndrome, many experiencing milder forms of brain abnormalities and associated cognitive and behavioral effects. Moderate drinking during pregnancy in amounts below those known to be associated with fetal alcohol syndrome may also have negative behavioral and neurocognitive consequences; the data on risk for fetal malformations or other gestational problems, however, are inconclusive (52). The amount of alcohol needed to harm a fetus is not established. No threshold has been determined for safe levels of drinking in pregnancy; therefore, general recommendations established by the US Surgeon General in 1981 for abstinence during pregnancy still prevail (52).

Grand mal convulsions ("rum fits") occur occasionally, sometimes as long as 2 or 3 days after drinking stops. As a rule, convulsions in alcohol use disorder do not represent epilepsy; electroencephalograms (EEGs) are normal when the individual is not drinking and convulsions occur only during withdrawal (58).

Alcoholic hallucinosis is a rare complication of chronic alcohol use disorder characterized by predominantly auditory hallucinations occurring during or after a period of heavy alcohol use (10). Chronic alcoholic hallucinosis can occur after cessation of heavy drinking and disappearance of other abstinence symptoms (113).

Approximately half of people with an alcohol use disorder will experience an alcohol withdrawal syndrome (6). Alcohol withdrawal syndromes typically manifest within several hours or days of reduction or cessation of heavy and prolonged alcohol consumption and typically last 4–5 days. Common withdrawal symptoms include autonomic hyperactivity (e.g., tachycardia, sweating), tremor, anxiety, sleeplessness, and nausea or vomiting. These symptoms may persist at lower levels of intensity for months beyond the culmination of acute withdrawal. Sometimes transient hallucinations or illusions and even grand mal seizures can occur in alcohol withdrawal.

The term "delirium tremens" (DTs) refers to an alcohol withdrawal syndrome that results in delirium (a rapid-onset fluctuating disturbance of attention and cognition, sometimes with hallucinations) (121). This syndrome usually begins within about 3 days of the onset of the alcohol withdrawal syndrome and typically lasts 2 to 3 days. The condition is fatal in 1–4% of patients hospitalized for the condition (121). One must always suspect intercurrent medical illness when delirium occurs during withdrawal. The physician should be particularly alert to hepatic decompensation, pneumonia, subdural hematoma, pancreatitis, and fractures.

The hallucinations and confusion sometimes associated alcohol withdrawal states may precipitate fear and associated behaviors, such as jumping out of hospital windows and other forms of disorganized self-harm that represent attempts to escape misperceived terrors. These patients require close monitoring to prevent misadventure (pp. 245–246) (47):

After a week of heavy drinking and little food, a 30-year-old newspaper reporter tried to drink a morning cup of coffee and found that his hands were shaking so violently he could not get the cup to his mouth. He managed to pour some whisky into a glass and drank as much as he could. His hands became less shaky but now he was nauseated and began having "dry heaves." He tried repeatedly to drink but could not keep the alcohol down. He felt ill and intensely anxious and decided to call a doctor friend. The doctor recommended hospitalization.

On admission, the patient had a marked resting and exertional tremor of the hands, and his tongue and eyelids were tremulous. He also had feelings of "internal" tremulousness. Lying in the hospital bed, he found the noises outside his window unbearably loud and began seeing "visions" of animals and, on one occasion, a dead relative. He was terrified and called a nurse, who gave him a tranquilizer. He became quieter and his tremor was less pronounced. At all times he realized that the visual phenomena were "imaginary." He always knew where he was and was oriented otherwise. After a few days the tremor disappeared and he no longer hallucinated. He still had trouble sleeping but otherwise felt back to normal and vowed never to drink again.

Suicide is an important complication of alcoholism. About one-quarter of suicides occur in the context of alcoholism, predominantly among white men over age 35. Apparently patients with alcohol use disorders are more likely than patients with major depression to commit suicide after loss of a wife, close relative, or other serious interpersonal disruption, and to have experienced recent financial difficulty (26, 117). They are also more likely to be divorced or separated, recently unemployed, younger, lacking recent somatic illness, and intoxicated at the time of the suicide (117).

FAMILY AND GENETIC STUDIES

Every family study of alcoholism, regardless of country of origin, has shown much higher rates of alcoholism among the relatives of alcoholic patients than in the general population (62, 131, 136). A person with alcohol use disorder in a parent has a five-fold increased risk for the disorder, and alcohol use disorder in a sibling increases one's chance of developing the disorder at some time in life to about one in three (130). Not everything that runs in families is inherited, however (62, 131, 136). Speaking French, for example, runs in families and is not inherited. How does one separate nature from nurture in familial illnesses? Both twin and adoption studies have been used to address this question for many of the conditions described in this book, and this is no less true for alcoholism. Here, briefly, are the results.

Several twin studies demonstrated significantly greater concordance for alcoholism in identical twins than in fraternal twins—the more severe the alcoholism, the greater the difference (35, 108, 131, 138). Early twin studies in northern Europe, dating to the 1960s to 1980s, described these effects in male twins, but the situation was not so clear in women. In those days the studies did not include enough women to provide sufficient statistical power to test for genetic heritability. Later studies, however, included enough women to demonstrate the same level of genetic heritability in liability for alcoholism as in men—in the range of 50%–60% (16, 108, 138).

Beginning in the early 1970s, results of several adoption studies in northern Europe and the United States indicated that alcoholism appears to be inherited through biological fathers, with adoptive fathers providing no measurable contribution (13, 18, 19, 46). Male biological offspring of alcoholic fathers also had elevated rates of childhood conduct disorder compared to offspring of nonalcoholic biological fathers.

Despite overwhelming evidence of genetic liability to risk for alcoholism, it is easy to overlook reports that alcoholism also occurs in families with no other alcoholic members. In most studies, about half of patients hospitalized for alcohol use disorder give a family history of the disorder and about half do not. A number of investigators have compared the groups with and without a family history of alcoholism, and two consistent conclusions have emerged. Individuals with familial alcoholism who develop alcohol dependence 1) show the first signs of dependence at a younger age than do those without familial alcoholism, and 2) have a more severe form of dependence with a more rapid, fulminating course (43). Individuals with nonfamilial alcoholism appear to have a greater likelihood of returning to controlled drinking after treatment than do those with familial alcoholism (95).

The psychiatric disorders known to accompany alcoholism in individuals also aggregate in families with alcoholism (especially depressive, anxiety, somatization, and eating disorders in women and hyperactivity and other substance use disorders and antisocial personality disorder in men) (35, 105). There is also evidence that familial alcoholism is less likely than nonfamilial alcoholism to have psychiatric comorbidity, consistent with conceptualization of familial alcoholism as the "primary" disorder (18, 43). The type of alcoholism that runs in families, however, may be specifically associated with antisocial personality disorder and childhood conduct disorder and hyperactivity (57, 106). Cloninger defined two subtypes of alcoholism with distinct course and relationship to antisocial personality disorder. Type I alcoholism has adult onset and rapid progression to dependence without criminality, and type II is characterized by male predominance, early onset, and sociopathy, and is more heritable than type I (24, 126).

Despite substantial comorbidity (in individuals) and coaggregation (in families) of other psychiatric disorders with alcohol use disorder, available evidence suggests that about 75% of the genetic liability to alcoholism is disease specific (35). Two major studies have demonstrated the familial transmission of opiate, cocaine, and cannabis dependency to be independent of alcohol (11, 92). Nicotine, however, may share its familial transmission of addiction liability with alcohol (35).

Genetic variations in the neurotransmitter systems mediating reward, reinforcement, tolerance, and withdrawal may predispose some individuals to the craving and loss of control that characterize addiction and have been targets for genetic studies of alcoholism. No candidate genes have emerged, but the genes for alcohol dehydrogenase (ADH) and aldehyde dehydrogenase (ALDH) involving alcohol metabolism may well be protective against the development of alcohol use disorders (131, 136).

DIFFERENTIAL DIAGNOSIS

Chronic excessive use of alcohol produces a wide range of psychiatric symptoms that, in various combinations, can mimic other psychiatric disorders. Therefore, while a person is drinking heavily and during the withdrawal period, it is difficult to determine whether he or she suffers from a psychiatric condition other than alcoholism.

Other drug use often accompanies alcohol use disorder. It may be difficult to determine which symptoms are produced by alcohol and which by cocaine, amphetamines, opiates, and so on. Patients who have been drinking heavily and not eating may become hypoglycemic (139), and this condition may produce symptoms resembling those seen in alcohol withdrawal.

A psychiatric condition commonly associated with alcohol use disorder is major depressive disorder (14). Women with alcohol use disorder apparently suffer more often from major depressive disorder than do their male counterparts (16, 144). The diagnosis of major depressive disorder usually can be made by past history or by observing the patient during long periods of abstinence (14). Comorbid major depressive disorder is more likely to be the primary diagnosis in women than in men (144); furthermore, family history of major depressive disorder and initial onset of the depression before the onset of the alcohol problem suggest that major depressive disorder is the primary disorder (14).

A focused search for an "alcoholic personality" type has been ongoing for nearly a century. Efforts continue (142), but the only personality type found to have some predisposition toward alcohol use disorder has been antisocial personality disorder, with a prevalence of about 15% in men and 5% in women with alcohol use disorder (56, 111, 119).

CLINICAL MANAGEMENT

The treatment of alcohol use disorder and the management of alcohol withdrawal symptoms present separate problems. In the absence of serious medical complications, the alcohol withdrawal syndrome is usually transient and self-limited; the patient recovers within several days regardless of treatment (21). Insomnia and irritability may persist for longer periods.

Treatment for alcohol withdrawal is symptomatic and prophylactic. Relief of agitation and tremulousness can be achieved with a variety of medications (e.g., including alcohol, paraldehyde, chloral hydrate, clonidine, beta-adrenergic antagonists, and carbamazepine), but currently, benzodiazepines (e.g., lorazepam, diazepam, oxazepam, and chlordiazepoxide) are widely considered the drugs of choice for withdrawal. As a class they are considered superior because of efficacy (reduction in withdrawal symptomatology), safety (dosing), possible reduction in seizure risk, and limited side-effect profile (particularly compared to the other agents). Several can be administered parenterally to intoxicated patients without apparent significant risk and continued orally during the withdrawal period. Use of antipsychotic agents should be avoided if possible because these medications lower seizure threshold, especially in the early stages, and are associated with increased mortality, reportedly from hypotension or hepatic encephalopathy. Antipsychotics can be considered for adjunctive use late in withdrawal if benzodiazepines alone do not control agitation, delirium, and hallucinations (66).

Clinicians generally manage alcohol withdrawal with scheduled benzodiazepines monitored by frequent vital signs checks (every 4 to 6 hours but sometimes up to hourly) and assessment of symptom severity to prompt supplemental medication as needed. The Clinical Institute Withdrawal Assessment for Alcohol revised (CIWA-Ar) (134), a rapidly administered scale, can assist in assessment of severity and progression of alcohol withdrawal. Because this scale does not differentiate between alcohol withdrawal delirium and delirium of other origins, its utility is limited to monitoring of the course of delirium as part of an alcohol withdrawal syndrome that has already been clinically established (21, 66).

Administration of large doses of vitamins—particularly the B vitamins—is obligatory, given the role of these vitamins in preventing peripheral neuropathy and the Wernicke-Korsakoff syndrome. The B vitamins are water soluble, and there is no apparent danger in administering them in large doses.

Grand mal seizures may occur in up to one-third of patients hospitalized for alcohol withdrawal syndrome, and they typically occur within 24 to 48 hours of onset of alcohol withdrawal (21). Alcohol withdrawal seizures are more common in patients with a seizure disorder history, but phenytoin (Dilantin) is not consistently effective at preventing them. Fortunately, benzodiazepines such as lorazepam or chlordiazepoxide may be helpful in preventing alcohol withdrawal seizures (21, 66).

Patients who develop delirium should be considered dangerous to themselves and others, and protective measures should be taken. Ordinarily, sedatives will calm the patient sufficiently to control agitation, and restraints will not be necessary. Administration of intravenous benzodiazepines in escalating doses may be necessary for severe agitation. Most important, if delirium occurs, further exploration should be conducted to rule out serious medical illness missed in the original examination. When delirium occurs, as previously noted, an attendant should always be present. It is sometimes helpful to have a friend or relative present.

Uncomplicated outpatient alcohol detoxification has been found to be effective and safe for a significant subset of patients with alcohol use disorder (21). Although the approach varies, nonpharmacological detoxification is best suited for patients with mild symptoms, only mild to moderate dependence, and no significant withdrawal history. Patients may reside for 3 or 4 days in therapeutic housing that provides support and ensures safety, rest, and proper nutrition. Observation in this setting also allows for medical intervention in case a complication arises.

The treatment of alcohol use disorder should not begin until withdrawal symptoms subside. Treatment has two goals: 1) sobriety and 2) amelioration of psychiatric conditions associated with alcohol use disorders. A small minority of people recovering from alcohol use disorder can eventually drink in moderation, but for several months after a heavy drinking bout, total abstinence is desirable for three reasons. First, it will allow time for assessment of the patient's level of motivation and selection of what may be the optimal approach for achieving the best outcome for the patient. Second, the physician must follow the patient, sober, for a considerable period to potentially diagnose a coexistent psychiatric problem. Third, it is important for the patient to learn that he or she can cope with ordinary life problems without alcohol. Most relapses occur within the first 3 months of completing specialty treatment, and relapse after 1 year of sobriety is relatively low (42). Over the long term, about one-third of patients treated for alcohol use disorder have a good outcome (abstinence or moderate drinking), one-third show partial improvement, and one-third have continuing alcohol problems (42).

Disulfiram (Antabuse) has a long history of use in maintenance of alcohol abstinence. In the nineteenth century it was discovered that individuals industrially exposed to disulfiram used in the vulcanization of rubber developed intolerance to alcohol. This finding suggested that properties of disulfiram might have potential utility for treatment of alcoholism (128). Disulfiram inhibits aldehyde dehydrogenase, leading to an accumulation of acetaldehyde if alcohol is consumed. In 1949, disulfiram was the first drug approved by the FDA for the treatment of alcoholism. When consumed with alcohol, acetaldehyde is highly toxic and produces severe anxiety, vomiting, flushing, and headache. These reactions are sufficiently aversive that most patients who take disulfiram avoid alcohol altogether. A recent meta-analysis of randomized controlled trials demonstrated significant effectiveness for disulfiram (127). Side effects (bad taste, headaches, sedation, rash, impotence, and hepatotoxicity), potentially dangerous reactions with alcohol, and adherence problems with this drug have relegated it to second-line treatment for alcohol relapse prevention (42, 120, 128). Earlier complications involving rare cases of severe hypotension and even fatalities have curtailed the use of this drug to lower doses (e.g., 200–250 mg/day).

In 1995, the FDA approved naltrexone (ReVia) for the treatment of alcoholism. It is prescribed in doses of 50–100 mg/day or 150 mg three times a week (120). This drug has been found to diminish craving for alcohol and reduce feelings of reward and pleasure from drinking (119). Results of recent reviews including meta-analyses have indicated that naltrexone significantly reduces the rate of relapse, by about 20% overall (32, 84, 120, 128). Unfortunately, the beneficial effects of this drug appear to decrease over the first 2 weeks of its administration (128).

In 2004, the FDA approved acamprosate (calcium homotaurinate) for treatment of alcoholism. Acamprosate modulates the glutaminergic and GABA-ergic systems and exerts its therapeutic effects through modulation of dopamine-mediated alcohol reinforcement (128). In studies of more than 5,000 patients in 40 countries, acamprosate has been found to reduce relapse and improve maintenance of abstinence from alcohol, with small-to-moderate effect sizes (128). Acamprosate is contraindicated for patients with severe renal impairment (128).

Psychosocial treatments are the most widely used interventions for alcohol use disorders. Historically, these include cognitive-behavioral therapies, 12-step programs such as those used in Alcoholic Anonymous, and family and social therapies. There is little evidence to support psychodynamically oriented treatments (128). Although abstinence has been a primary goal of alcohol treatment in the past, more recent approaches have focused on harm reduction strategies to reduce the overall amount of drinking (128). A recent advance in alcohol treatment interventions is motivational interviewing (MI). MI is an evidence-based counseling method that promotes patient motivation to change in a harm-reduction model that involves exploration and resolution of patient ambivalence toward change. MI interventions can be accomplished in sessions of 15–30 minutes (120, 128).

In conclusion, it should be emphasized that relapses are characteristic of alcohol use disorders. Therefore, physicians treating this disease should avoid anger or excessive pessimism when such relapses occur. Patients with alcohol use disorders have contact with nonpsychiatric physicians at least as often as they do with psychiatrists. Therefore, general practitioners and internists can be at least as helpful as psychiatrists for these patients.

REFERENCES

1. King Jame Bible, Proverbs 31:6-7. Bible Hub, 2012. Last accessed 11/4/2017. http://biblehub.com/kjv/proverbs/31.htm.
2. The Holy Bible, English Standard Version, Genesis 9:21-22. Bible Hub, 2016. Last accessed 11/4/2017. https://www.biblegateway.com/passage/?search=Genesis+9%3A21-25&version=KJV.
3. American Psychiatric Association. *Diagnostic and Statistical Manual: Mental Disorders*, 1st edition. Washington, DC: Author, 1952.
4. American Psychiatric Association. *Diagnostic and Statistical Manual of Mental Disorders*, 2nd edition. Washington, DC: Author, 1968.
5. American Psychiatric Association. *Diagnostic and Statistical Manual of Mental Disorders*, 3rd edition. Washington, DC: Author, 1980.
6. American Psychiatric Association. *Diagnostic and Statistical Manual for Mental Disorders*, 5th edition. Washington, DC: Author, 2013.
7. Anthony, J. C., and Echeagaray-Wagner, F. Epidemiologic analysis of alcohol and tobacco use. Alcohol Res. Health, 24:201–208, 2000.
8. Atkinson, R. M., Tolson, R. L., and Turner, J. A. Late versus early onset problem drinking in older men. Alcohol. Clin. Exp. Res., 14:574–579, 1990.
9. Barchiesi, B. J., Eckel, R. H., and Ellis, P. P. The cornea and disorders of lipid metabolism. Surv. Ophthalmol., 36:1–22, 1991.
10. Bhat, P. S., Ryali, V., Srivastava, K., Kumar, S. R., Prakash, J., and Singal, A. Alcoholic hallucinosis. Ind. Psychiatry J., 21:155–157, 2012.
11. Bierut, L. J., Dinwiddie, S. H., Begleiter, H., Crowe, R. R., Hesselbrock, V., Nurnberger, J. I., Jr., Porjesz, B., Schuckit, M. A., and Reich, T. Familial transmission of substance dependence: alcohol, marijuana, cocaine, and habitual smoking: a report from the Collaborative Study on the Genetics of Alcoholism. Arch. Gen. Psychiatry, 55:982–988, 1998.
12. Blin, O., Simon, N., Jouve, E., Habib, M., Gayraud, D., Durand, A., Bruguerolle, B., and Pisano, P. Pharmacokinetic and pharmacodynamic analysis of sedative

and amnesic effects of lorazepam in healthy volunteers. Clin. Neuropharmacol., 24:71–81, 2001.

13. Bohman, M. Some genetic aspects of alcoholism and criminality. Arch. Gen. Psychiatry, 35:259–276, 1978.

14. Brady, K. T., and Verduin, M. L. Pharmacotherapy of comorbid mood, anxiety, and substance use disorders. Subst. Use Misuse, 40:2021–2028, 2005.

15. Breslow, R. A., Faden, V. B., and Smothers, B. Alcohol consumption by elderly Americans. J. Stud. Alcohol, 64:884–892, 2003.

16. Brienza, R. S., and Stein, M. D. Alcohol use disorders in primary care: do gender-specific differences exist? J. Gen. Intern. Med., 17:387–397, 2002.

17. Britton, A., Ben-Shlomo, Y., Benzeval, M., Kuh, D., and Bell, S. Life course trajectories of alcohol consumption in the United Kingdom using longitudinal data from nine cohort studies. BMC Med., 13:47, 2015.

18. Cadoret, R. J., Cain, C. A., and Grove, W. M. Development of alcoholism in adoptees raised apart from alcoholic biologic relatives. Arch. Gen. Psychiatry, 37:561–563, 1980.

19. Cadoret, R. J., and Gath, A. Inheritance of alcoholism in adoptees. Br. J. Psychiatry, 132:252–258, 1978.

20. Canfield, D. V., Dubowski, K. M., Chaturvedi, A. V., and Whinnery, J. E. (2011). Drugs and alcohol in civil aviation accident pilot fatalities from 2004–2008. Report no. DOT/FAA/AM-11/13. Washington, DC: Office of Aerospace Medicine, Federal Aviation Administration.

21. Carlson, R. W., Kumar, N. N., Wong-Mckinstry, E., Ayyagari, S., Puri, N., Jackson, F. K., and Shashikumar, S. Alcohol withdrawal syndrome. Crit. Care Clin., 28:549–585, 2012.

22. Chaucer, G. The Canterbury Tales: The Pardoner's Tale. In The Student's Chaucer, Skeats, W. W. (ed.). New York: Oxford University Press, 1900.

23. Chung, N., Langenbucher, J., McCrady, B., Epstein, E., and Cook, S. Use of survival analyses to examine onset and staging of DSM-IV alcohol symptoms in women. Psychol. Addict. Behav., 16:236–242, 2002.

24. Cloninger, C. R., Sigvardsson, S., Gilligan, S. B., von Knorring, A. L., Reich, T., and Bohman, M. Genetic heterogeneity and the classification of alcoholism. Adv. Alcohol Subst. Abuse, 7:3–16, 1988.

25. Congreve, W. The Way of the World: A Comedy. As it Is Acted at the Theatre in Lincolns-Inn-Fields, by His Majesty's Servants. London: Jacob Tonson, 1706.

26. Conner, K. R., and Duberstein, P. R. Predisposing and precipitating factors for suicide among alcoholics: empirical review and conceptual integration. Alcohol. Clin. Exp. Res., 28:6S–17S, 2004.

27. Cranford, J. A. DSM-IV alcohol dependence and marital dissolution: evidence from the National Epidemiologic Survey on Alcohol and Related Conditions. J. Stud. Alcohol Drugs, 75:520–529, 2014.

28. Cudd, T. A. Animal model systems for the study of alcohol teratology. Exp. Biol. Med. (Maywood), 230:389–393, 2005.

29. Dawson, D. A., Grant, B. F., and Li, T. K. Quantifying the risks associated with exceeding recommended drinking limits. Alcohol. Clin. Exp. Res., 29:902–908, 2005.

30. Dawson, D. A., Grant, B. F., Stinson, F. S., Chou, P. S., Huang, B., and Ruan, W. J. Recovery from DSM-IV alcohol dependence: United States, 2001-2002. Addiction, 100:281–292, 2005.

31. Delker, E., Brown, Q., and Hasin, D. S. Alcohol consumption in demographic subpopulations: an epidemiologic overview. Alcohol Res., 38:7–15, 2016.

32. Donoghue, K., Elzerbi, C., Saunders, R., Whittington, C., Pilling, S., and Drummond, C. The efficacy of acamprosate and naltrexone in the treatment of alcohol dependence, Europe versus the rest of the world: a meta-analysis. Addiction, *110*:920–930, 2015.

33. Dufour, M. C. If you drink alcoholic beverages do so in moderation: what does this mean? J. Nutr., *131*:552S–561S, 2001.

34. Edwards, G., and Gross, M. M. Alcohol dependence: provisional description of a clinical syndrome. Br. Med. J., *1*:1058–1061, 1976.

35. Enoch, M. A., and Goldman, D. The genetics of alcoholism and alcohol abuse. Curr. Psychiatr. Rep., *3*:144–151, 2001.

36. Eustace, L. W., Kang, D. H., and Coombs, D. Fetal alcohol syndrome: a growing concern for health care professionals. J. Obstet. Gynecol. Neonatal Nurs., *32*:215–221, 2003.

37. Ewing, J. A. Detecting alcoholism. The CAGE questionnaire. JAMA, *252*:1905–1907, 1984.

38. Ewing, J. A., and Rouse, B. A. Corneal arcus as a sign of possible alcoholism. Alcohol. Clin. Exp. Res., *4*:104–106, 1980.

39. Fama, R., Pfefferbaum, A., and Sullivan, E. V. Perceptual learning in detoxified alcoholic men: contributions from explicit memory, executive function, and age. Alcohol. Clin. Exp. Res., *28*:1657–1665, 2004.

40. Gannon, M. US alcohol drinkers average 4 beverages per week. New York: Live Science, Purch, 2017. Last accessed 11/5/2017. https://www.livescience.com/22492-alcohol-drinkers-four-beverages-week.html.

41. Gao, B., and Bataller, R. Alcoholic liver disease: pathogenesis and new therapeutic targets. Gastroenterology, *141*:1572–1585, 2011.

42. Goh, E. T., and Morgan, M. Y. Review article: pharmacotherapy for alcohol dependence—the why, the what and the wherefore. Aliment. Pharmacol. Ther., *45*:865–882, 2017.

43. Goodwin, D. W. Familial alcoholism: a separate entity? Subst. Alcohol Actions Misuse, *4*:129–136, 1983.

44. Goodwin, D. W., Crane, J. B., and Guze, S. B. Alcoholic "blackouts": a review and clinical study of 100 alcoholics. Am. J. Psychiatry, *126*:191–198, 1969.

45. Goodwin, D. W., Crane, J. B., and Guze, S. B. Felons who drink: an 8-year follow-up. Q. J. Stud. Alcohol, *32*:136–147, 1971.

46. Goodwin, D. W., Schulsinger, F., Hermansen, L., Guze, S. B., and Winokur, G. Alcohol problems in adoptees raised apart from alcoholic biological parents. Arch. Gen. Psychiatry, *28*:238–243, 1973.

47. Goodwin, D. W., Skodol, A. E., Gibbon, M., and Williams, J. B. W. The reporter. In *DSM-III Case Book*, Spitzer, R. L. (ed.). Washington, DC: American Psychiatric Association, pp. 245–246, 1981.

48. Grant, B. F., Chou, S. P., Saha, T. D., Pickering, R. P., Kerridge, B. T., Ruan, W. J., Huang, B., Jung, J., Zhang, H., Fan, A., and Hasin, D. S. Prevalence of 12-month alcohol use, high-risk drinking, and DSM-IV alcohol use disorder in the United States, 2001-2002 to 2012-2013: results from the National Epidemiologic Survey on Alcohol and Related Conditions. JAMA Psychiatry, 74:911–923, 2017.

49. Grant, B. F., Dawson, D. A., Stinson, F. S., Chou, P. S., Kay, W., and Pickering, R. The Alcohol Use Disorder and Associated Disabilities Interview Schedule-IV (AUDADIS-IV): reliability of alcohol consumption, tobacco use, family history of depression and psychiatric diagnostic modules in a general population sample. Drug Alcohol Depend., *71*:7–16, 2003.

50. Grant, B. F., Dawson, D. A., Stinson, F. S., Chou, S. P., Dufour, M. C., and Pickering, R. P. The 12-month prevalence and trends in DSM-IV alcohol abuse and dependence: United States, 1991-1992 and 2001-2002. Drug Alcohol Depend., 74:223–234, 2004.

51. Greenfield, T. K., and Kerr, W. C. Tracking alcohol consumption over time. Alcohol Res. Health, 27:30–38, 2003.

52. Gunzerath, L., Faden, V., Zakhari, S., and Warren, K. National Institute on Alcohol Abuse and Alcoholism report on moderate drinking. Alcohol. Clin. Exp. Res., 28:829–847, 2004.

53. Harper, C., and Matsumoto, I. Ethanol and brain damage. Curr. Opin. Pharmacol., 5:73–78, 2005.

54. Hasin, D. Classification of alcohol use disorders. Alcohol Res. Health, 27:5–17, 2003.

55. Hasin, D. S., and Grant, B. F. The National Epidemiologic Survey on Alcohol and Related Conditions (NESARC) Waves 1 and 2: review and summary of findings. Soc. Psychiatry Psychiatr. Epidemiol., 50:1609–1640, 2015.

56. Hesselbrock, M. N. Childhood behavior problems and adult antisocial personality disorder in alcoholism. In *Psychopathology and Addictive Disorders*, Meyer, R. E. (ed.). New York: Guilford Press, pp. 78–94, 1986.

57. Hesselbrock, V. M., Stabenau, J. R., Hesselbrock, M. N., Meyer, R. E., and Babor, T. F. The nature of alcoholism in patients with different family histories for alcoholism. Prog. Neuropsychopharmacol. Biol. Psychiatry, 6:607–614, 1982.

58. Hillbom, M., Pieninkeroinen, I., and Leone, M. Seizures in alcohol-dependent patients: epidemiology, pathophysiology and management. CNS Drugs, 17:1013–1030, 2003.

59. Hillmer, A. T., Mason, G. F., Fucito, L. M., O'Malley, S. S., and Cosgrove, K. P. How imaging glutamate, gamma-aminobutyric acid, and dopamine can inform the clinical treatment of alcohol dependence and withdrawal. Alcohol. Clin. Exp. Res., 39:2268–2282, 2015.

60. Hingson, R., Zha, W., Simons-Morton, B., and White, A. Alcohol-Induced blackouts as predictors of other drinking related harms among emerging young adults. Alcohol. Clin. Exp. Res., 40:776–784, 2016.

61. Holdcraft, L. C., and Iacono, W. G. Cohort effects on gender differences in alcohol dependence. Addiction, 97:1025–1036, 2002.

62. Iyer-Eimerbrink, P. A. and Nurnberger, J. I., Jr. Genetics of alcoholism. Curr. Psychiatry Rep., 16:518, 2014.

63. Jastrzebska, Zwolak, A., Szczyrek, M., Wawryniuk, A., Skrzydlo-Radomanska, B., and Daniluk, J. Biomarkers of alcohol misuse: recent advances and future prospects. Prz. Gastroenterol., 11:78–89, 2016.

64. Jellinek, E. M. Phases of alcohol addiction. Q. J. Stud. Alcohol, 13:673–684, 1952.

65. Jellinek, E. M. *The Disease Concept of Alcoholism*. New Haven, CT: College & University Press, 1960.

66. Jesse, S., Brathen, G., Ferrara, M., Keindl, M., Ben-Menachem, E., Tanasescu, R., Brodtkorb, E., Hillbom, M., Leone, M. A., and Ludolph, A. C. Alcohol withdrawal syndrome: mechanisms, manifestations, and management. Acta Neurol. Scand., 135:4–16, 2017.

67. Kahana, R. J. A remission through crisis in ulcerative colitis. Psychosomat. Med., 24:499–506, 1962.

68. Karlamangla, A., Zhou, K., Reuben, D., Greendale, G., and Moore, A. Longitudinal trajectories of heavy drinking in adults in the United States of America. Addiction, 101:91–99, 2006.

69. Keller, M. On defining alcoholism: with comment on some other relevant words. In *Alcohol, Science and Society Revisited*, Gomberg, L., White, H. R., Carpenter, J. A. (eds.). Ann Arbor: University of Michigan Press, 1982.

70. Kelly, J. F. Toward an addiction-ary: a proposal for more precise terminology. Alcohol. Treat. Q., *22*:79–87, 2004.

71. Kelly, S. J., Day, N., and Streissguth, A. P. Effects of prenatal alcohol exposure on social behavior in humans and other species. Neurotoxicol. Teratol., *22*:143–149, 2000.

72. Kerr, W. C. Categorizing US state drinking practices and consumption trends. Int. J. Environ. Res. Public Health, 7:269–283, 2010.

73. Kril, J. J., and Halliday, G. M. Brain shrinkage in alcoholics: a decade on and what have we learned? Prog. Neurobiol., *58*:381–387, 1999.

74. Lakshman, M. R. Some novel insights into the pathogenesis of alcoholic steatosis. Alcohol, *34*:45–48, 2004.

75. Lee, H., Roh, S., and Kim, D. J. Alcohol-induced blackout. Int. J. Environ. Res. Public Health, *6*:2783–2792, 2009.

76. Lewis, C. National prohibition in the United States: a cognitive-behavioral perspective: part 2: 20th century national prohibition. J. Addict. Med. Ther., *1*:1–8, 2013.

77. Li, T. K., Hewitt, B. G., and Grant, B. F. The alcohol dependence syndrome, 30 years later: a commentary. The 2006 H. David Archibald lecture. Addiction, *102*:1522–1530, 2007.

78. Lieber, C. S. Alcoholic fatty liver: its pathogenesis and mechanism of progression to inflammation and fibrosis. Alcohol, *34*:9–19, 2004.

79. LoConte, N. K., Brewster, A. M., Kaur, J. S., Merrill, J. K., and Alberg, A. J. Alcohol and cancer: a statement of the American Society of Clinical Oncology. J. Clin. Oncol., *36*:83–93, 2018.

80. Louvet, A., and Mathurin, P. Alcoholic liver disease: mechanisms of injury and targeted treatment. Nat. Rev. Gastroenterol. Hepatol., *12*:231–242, 2015.

81. Ludwig, A. M. On and off the wagon. Reasons for drinking and abstaining by alcoholics. Q. J. Stud. Alcohol, *33*:91–96, 1972.

82. Mackenzie, A., Funderburk, F. R., and Allen, R. P. Sleep, anxiety, and depression in abstinent and drinking alcoholics. Subst. Use Misuse, *34*:347–361, 1999.

83. Maczaj, M. Pharmacological treatment of insomnia. Drugs, *45*:44–55, 1993.

84. Maisel, N. C., Blodgett, J. C., Wilbourne, P. L., Humphreys, K., and Finney, J. W. Meta-analysis of naltrexone and acamprosate for treating alcohol use disorders: when are these medications most helpful? Addiction, *108*:275–293, 2013.

85. Malfertheiner, P., Chan, F. K., and McColl, K. E. Peptic ulcer disease. Lancet, *374*:1449–1461, 2009.

86. Manzardo, A. M., Goodwin, D. W., Campbell, J. L., Penick, E. C., and Gabrielli, Jr. W. F. *Alcoholism: The Facts*, 4th edition. New York: Oxford University Press, 2008.

87. Marcinkiewcz, C. A. Serotonergic systems in the pathophysiology of ethanol dependence: relevance to clinical alcoholism. ACS Chem. Neurosci., *6*:1026–1039, 2015.

88. Mattson, S. N., Schoenfeld, A. M., and Riley, E. P. Teratogenic effects of alcohol on brain and behavior. Alcohol Res. Health, *25*:185–191, 2001.

89. May, P. A., and Gossage, J. P. Estimating the prevalence of fetal alcohol syndrome. A summary. Alcohol Res. Health, *25*:159–167, 2001.

90. McGovern, P. E., Zhang, J., Tang, J., Zhang, Z., Hall, G. R., Moreau, R. A., Nunez, A., Butrym, E. D., Richards, M. P., Wang, C. S., Cheng, G., Zhao, Z., and Wang, C.

Fermented beverages of pre- and proto-historic China. Proc. Natl. Acad. Sci. USA, 101:17593–17598, 2004.

91. Mellion, M., Gilchrist, J. M., and de la Monte, S. Alcohol-related peripheral neuropathy: nutritional, toxic, or both? Muscle Nerve, 43:309–316, 2011.

92. Merikangas, K. R., Stolar, M., Stevens, D. E., Goulet, J., Preisig, M. A., Fenton, B., Zhang, H., O'Malley, S. S., and Rounsaville, B. J. Familial transmission of substance use disorders. Arch. Gen. Psychiatry, 55:973–979, 1998.

93. Michel, R. H., McGovern, P. E., and Badler, V. R. Chemical evidence for ancient beer. Nature, 360:24, 1992.

94. Michel, R. H., McGovern, P. E., and Badler, V. R. Chemical detection of ancient fermented beverages. Analyt. Chem., 65:408–413, 1993.

95. Miller, W. R., and Joyce, M. A. Prediction of abstinence, controlled drinking, and heavy drinking outcomes following behavioral self-control training. J. Consult. Clin. Psychiatry, 47:773–775, 1979.

96. Mintz, J., Mintz, L. I., Arruda, M. J., and Hwang, S. S. Treatments of depression and the functional capacity to work. Arch. Gen. Psychiatry, 49:761–768, 1992.

97. Molina, P. E., McClain, C., Valla, D., Guidot, D., Diehl, A. M., Lang, C. H., and Neuman, M. Molecular pathology and clinical aspects of alcohol-induced tissue injury. Alcohol. Clin. Exp. Res., 26:120–128, 2002.

98. Morris, H. H., III, and Estes, M. L. Traveler's amnesia. Transient global amnesia secondary to triazolam. JAMA, 258:945–946, 1987.

99. Mostofsky, E., Mukamal, K. J., Giovannucci, E. L., Stampfer, M. J., and Rimm, E. B. Key findings on alcohol consumption and a variety of health outcomes from the Nurses' Health Study. Am. J. Public Health, 106:1586–1591, 2016.

100. Nathan, P. E., Conrad, M., and Skinstad, A. H. History of the concept of addiction. Annu. Rev. Clin. Psychol., 12:29–51, 2016.

101. National Institute on Alcohol Abuse and Alcoholism. Apparent per capita ethanol consumption, United States, 1850-2013 (Surveillance Report #102). Bethesda, MD: National Institutes of Health, US Department of Health and Human Services, 2015. Last accessed 11/5/2017. https://pubs.niaaa.nih.gov/publications/surveillance102/tab1_13.htm.

102. National Transportation Safety Board. Reaching zero: actions to eliminate alcohol-impaired driving. Safety Report NTSB/SR-13/01 PB2013-106566. Washington, DC: National Transportation Safety Board, 2013. Last accessed 11/8/2017. https://www.ntsb.gov/safety/safety-studies/documents/sr1301.pdf.

103. Nelson, E. C., Heath, A. C., Bucholz, K. K., Madden, P. A., Fu, Q., Knopik, V., Lynskey, M. T., Lynskey, M. T., Whitfield, J. B., Statham, D. J., and Martin, N. G. Genetic epidemiology of alcohol-induced blackouts. Arch. Gen. Psychiatry, 61:257–263, 2004.

104. Nichols, J. M., and Martin, F. The effect of heavy social drinking on recall and event-related potentials. J. Stud. Alcohol, 57:125–135, 1996.

105. Nurnberger, J. I., Jr., Wiegand, R., Bucholz, K., O'Connor, S., Meyer, E. T., Reich, T., Rice, J., Schuckit, M., King, L., Petti, T., Bierut, L., Hinrichs, A. L., Kuperman, S., Hesselbrock, V., and Porjesz, B. A family study of alcohol dependence: coaggregation of multiple disorders in relatives of alcohol-dependent probands. Arch. Gen. Psychiatry, 61:1246–1256, 2004.

106. Penick, E. C., Read, M. R., Crowley, P. A., and Powell, B. J. Differentiation of alcoholics by family history. J. Stud. Alcohol, 39:1944–1948, 1978.

107. Prakash, J., Ryali, V., Srivastava, K., Bhat, P. S., Shashikumar, R., and Singal, A. Tobacco-alcohol amblyopia: a rare complication of prolonged alcohol abuse. Ind. Psychiatry J., *20*:66–68, 2011.

108. Prescott, C. A., Caldwell, C. B., Carey, G., Vogler, G. P., Trumbetta, S. L., and Gottesman, I. I. The Washington University Twin Study of alcoholism. Am. J. Med. Genet. B Neuropsychiatr. Genet., *134*:48–55, 2005.

109. Ramaiah, S., Rivera, C., and Arteel, G. Early-phase alcoholic liver disease: an update on animal models, pathology, and pathogenesis. Int. J. Toxicol., *23*:217–231, 2004.

110. Reed, R. J., Grant, I., and Rourke, S. B. Long-term abstinent alcoholics have normal memory. Alcohol. Clin. Exp. Res., *16*:677–683, 1992.

111. Robins, L. N., Tipp, J., and Przybeck, T. Antisocial personality. In *Psychiatric Disorders in America: The Epidemiologic Catchment Area Study*, Robins, L. N., Regier, D. A. (eds.). New York: The Free Press, 1991.

112. Roebuck, T. M., Mattson, S. N., and Riley, E. P. A review of the neuroanatomical findings in children with fetal alcohol syndrome or prenatal exposure to alcohol. Alcohol. Clin. Exp. Res., *22*:339–344, 1998.

113. Ropper, A. H., Brown, R. H., and Brown, R. J. Alcohol and alcoholism. In *Adams and Victor's Principles of Neurology*, 7th edition. New York: McGraw-Hill, pp. 1004–1015, 2001.

114. Roueche, B. Cultural factors and drinking patterns. Ann. N. Y. Acad. Sci., *133*:846–855, 1966.

115. Rush, B. *An Inquiry into the Effects of Ardent Spirits upon the Human Body and Mind*, 6th edition. New York: Cornelius Davis, 1811.

116. Saunders, J. B., Aasland, O. G., Babor, T. F., de la Fuente, Jr., and Grant, M. Development of the Alcohol Use Disorders Identification Test (AUDIT): WHO collaborative project on early detection of persons with harmful alcohol consumption—II. Addiction, *88*:791–804, 1993.

117. Schneider, B. Substance use disorders and risk for completed suicide. Arch. Suicide Res., *13*:303–316, 2009.

118. Scholz, E., Diener, H. C., Dichgans, J., Langohr, H. D., Schied, W., and Schupmann, A. Incidence of peripheral neuropathy and cerebellar ataxia in chronic alcoholics. J. Neurol., *233*:212–217, 1986.

119. Schuckit, M. A. The clinical implications of primary diagnostic groups among alcoholics. Arch. Gen. Psychiatry, *42*:1043–1049, 1985.

120. Schuckit, M. A. Alcohol-use disorders. Lancet, *373*:492–501, 2009.

121. Schuckit, M. A. Recognition and management of withdrawal delirium (delirium tremens). N. Engl. J. Med., *371*:2109–2113, 2014.

122. Schwartz, R. H., Milteer, R., and LeBeau, M. A. Drug-facilitated sexual assault ('date rape'). South. Med. J., *93*:558–561, 2000.

123. Scroop, R., Sage, M. R., Voyvodic, F., and Kat, E. Radiographic imaging procedures in the diagnosis of the major central neuropathological consequences of alcohol abuse. Australas. Radiol., *46*:146–153, 2002.

124. Selzer, M. L. The Michigan Alcoholism Screening Test: the quest for a new diagnostic instrument. Am. J. Psychiatry, *127*:1653–1658, 1971.

125. Sigerist, H. E. *The History of Medicine*. New York: M.D. Publications, 1960.

126. Sigvardsson, S., Bohman, M., and Cloninger, C. R. Replication of the Stockholm Adoption Study of alcoholism. Confirmatory cross-fostering analysis. Arch. Gen. Psychiatry, *53*:681–687, 1996.

127. Skinner, M. D., Lahmek, P., Pham, H., and Aubin, H. J. Disulfiram efficacy in the treatment of alcohol dependence: a meta-analysis. PLoS One, *9*:e87366, 2014.

128. Soyka, M., Kranzler, H. R., Hesselbrock, V., Kasper, S., Mutschler, J., and Moller, H. J. Guidelines for biological treatment of substance use and related disorders, part 1: alcoholism, first revision. World J. Biol. Psychiatry, *18*:86–119, 2017.

129. Spampinato, M. V., Castillo, M., Rojas, R., Palacios, E., Frascheri, L., and Descartes, F. Magnetic resonance imaging findings in substance abuse: alcohol and alcoholism and syndromes associated with alcohol abuse. Top. Magn. Reson. Imaging, *16*:223–230, 2005.

130. Standridge, J. B., Zylstra, R. G., and Adams, S. M. Alcohol consumption: an overview of benefits and risks. South. Med. J., *97*:664–672, 2004.

131. Stickel, F., Moreno, C., Hampe, J., and Morgan, M. Y. The genetics of alcohol dependence and alcohol-related liver disease. J. Hepatol., *66*:195–211, 2017.

132. Sullivan, E. V., and Pfefferbaum, A. Neurocircuitry in alcoholism: a substrate of disruption and repair. Psychopharmacology (Berl)., *180*:583–594, 2005.

133. Sullivan, E. V., Rosenbloom, M. J., and Pfefferbaum, A. Pattern of motor and cognitive deficits in detoxified alcoholic men. Alcohol. Clin. Exp. Res., *24*:611–621, 2000.

134. Sullivan, J. T., Sykora, K., Schneiderman, J., Naranjo, C. A., and Sellers, E. M. Assessment of alcohol withdrawal: the revised clinical institute withdrawal assessment for alcohol scale (CIWA-Ar). Br. J. Addict., *84*:1353–1357, 1989.

135. Svanberg, J., Withall, A., Draper B., and Bowden, S. (eds.). *Alcohol and the Adult Brain*. New York: Psychology Press, 2015.

136. Tawa, E. A., Hall, S. D., and Lohoff, F. W. Overview of the genetics of alcohol use disorder. Alcohol Alcohol., *51*:507–514, 2016.

137. Thun, M. J., Peto, R., Lopez, A. D., Monaco, J. H., Henley, S. J., Heath, C. W., Jr., and Doll, R. Alcohol consumption and mortality among middle-aged and elderly U.S. adults. N. Engl. J. Med., *337*:1705–1714, 1997.

138. Tyndale, R. F. Genetics of alcohol and tobacco use in humans. Ann. Med., *35*:94–121, 2003.

139. van de Wiel, A. Diabetes mellitus and alcohol. Diabetes Metab. Res. Rev., *20*:263–267, 2004.

140. Volkow, N. D., Wang, G. J., Fowler, J. S., Tomasi, D., and Telang, F. Addiction: beyond dopamine reward circuitry. Proc. Natl. Acad. Sci. USA, *108*:15037–15042, 2011.

141. Wilford, J. N. Jar in Iranian ruins betrays beer drinkers of 3500 B.C. *New York Times*, November 11, 1992. Last accessed 11/3/2017. http://www.nytimes.com/1992/11/05/world/jar-in-iranian-ruins-betrays-beer-drinkers-of-3500-bc.html?pagewanted=print.

142. Windle, M., and Scheidt, D. M. Alcoholic subtypes: are two sufficient? Addiction, *99*:1508–1519, 2004.

143. World Health Organization. Global status report on alcohol and health. Geneva: WHO Press, 2011. Last accessed 11/12/2017. http://www.who.int/substance_abuse/publications/global_alcohol_report/msbgsruprofiles.pdf.

144. Zilberman, M. L., Tavares, H., Blume, S. B., and el Guebaly, N. Substance use disorders: sex differences and psychiatric comorbidities. Can. J. Psychiatry, *48*:5–13, 2003.

CHAPTER 12

❧

Drug Use Disorder

"Drug use disorder" refers to the presence of any of a collection of drug-specific diagnoses that are characterized by cognitive, behavioral, and physiological symptoms accompanying repeated use of a drug despite significant substance-related problems causing harm to the user or to others. A multitude of terms have been variously applied to this diagnosis, although they are not a part of the current diagnostic nomenclature. The term "addiction" has commonly been used to refer to severe physical and psychological problems related to compulsive and habitual use of substances.

The term "physical addiction" has been used to refer to a drug-induced condition characterized by *physical tolerance* (the need for larger doses of a drug to obtain its original effects) and *physical dependence* (the need to continue administration of a drug to prevent its characteristic withdrawal symptoms). Among drugs, only opiates and barbiturates (and, to a lesser degree, benzodiazepines) produce both physical tolerance and physical dependence. *Psychological addiction/dependence* implies compulsive drug use behavior and excessive involvement in drug use and procurement. The term "habituation" has been used almost synonymously with psychological addiction, specifically referring to a need to use a drug to maintain an optimal state of well-being (45). Physical and psychological addiction may overlap but do not necessarily occur together. For example, a person physically addicted to morphine administered medically for severe chronic pain may have none of the characteristics of psychological addiction. Conversely, an individual may be psychologically addicted to drugs with little or no tolerance or physical dependence.

DSM-IV differentiated substance dependence and substance abuse diagnostically (5). It defined substance *dependence* as "a cluster of cognitive, behavioral, and physiological symptoms indicating that the individual continues use of the substance despite significant substance-related problems" (p. 192) and substance *abuse* as "a maladaptive pattern of substance use manifested by recurrent and significant adverse consequences related to the repeated use of substances" (p. 198). The updated criteria in *DSM-5* combined substance dependence and substance abuse into a single construct and conceptualized all substance use disorders on a continuum of severity defined by the number of symptoms of the disorder (6, 56).

The establishment of uniform criteria across specific drugs represents a substantial movement forward from earlier individualized approaches to the various agents. Further, this simplified and streamlined approach facilitates diagnosis of drug use disorders, which drives treatment planning for this very significant medical problem that affects so many aspects of society. One unsatisfactory consequence of this approach is that the criteria for some types of drug use disorders conform poorly to these rigidly organized definitions; for example, certain substances, such as hallucinogens and phencyclidine, have no established withdrawal syndromes.

HISTORICAL BACKGROUND

The basic needs of the human race . . . are food, clothing, and shelter. To that fundamental trinity most modern authorities would add, as equally compelling, security and love. There are, however, many other needs whose satisfaction, though somewhat less essential, can seldom be comfortably denied. One of these, and perhaps the most insistent, is an occasional release from the intolerable clutch of reality. All men throughout recorded history have known this tyranny of memory and mind, and all have sought . . . some reliable means of briefly loosening its grip.

Berton Roueché (p. 3) (82)

Regardless of whether this fully explains the motivation behind the use of intoxicating substances, it is true they have been used by humankind for thousands of years in nearly every part of the world. Except in a few primitive cultures, humans have discovered plants whose juices and powders that on being properly prepared and consumed have caused desirable alterations of consciousness. In ancient times, these substances were widely used in religious ceremonies (as wine is still used in the Catholic mass and peyote by the North American Church), but they also have been used for recreational purposes. As the sciences of medicine and chemistry progressed, the variety of drugs increased, and for many years, drugs have been diverted from medical use into "illicit" channels as they are today.

Historically, opium has been known for millennia for its ability to relieve pain and was suggested for surgical use more than 2,000 years ago (30). Oral analgesia was achieved in the 1600s by using tincture of opium, commonly known as "laudanum" (in various "recipes"). Opium consists of about 10% morphine. Morphine was first isolated in 1805 by Friedrich Sertürner (90) and named after the Greek god of dreams, Morpheus (44).

The analgesic drugs derived from the opium poppy plant were particularly susceptible to abuse because they produced euphoria as well as analgesia. The spread of opium into England, commercially promoted as part of the Chinese opium trade, led to widespread abuse of the drug in the nineteenth century. The introduction of the hypodermic needle during the American Civil War period facilitated both analgesia and addiction. The use of morphine for nonmedicinal purposes became widespread, and by the turn of the next century, large numbers of people were apparently dependent on the drug, taken intravenously or more often as an ingredient of patent medicines, most notably laudanum (tincture of opium prescribed for severe diarrhea) (70). Heroin, the diethylated form of morphine, was introduced around the turn of the century as a "heroic" solution for the opiate problem (a form of substitution therapy, just as methadone is used today).

Another development of the mid-nineteenth century was the introduction of bromides as sedatives. There was an enormous demand for these compounds and a steady increase in their use. Along with use came misuse, which often resulted in intoxication and psychotic reactions. The bromide problem began to abate in the 1930s as barbiturates and other sedatives became available. The first barbiturate, Veronal, was introduced in 1903, and others appeared in quick succession. The short-acting barbiturates such as pentobarbital and amobarbital became popular in the 1930s and 1940s; their dependence-producing qualities were not immediately recognized (4).

During the late nineteenth century, individuals in the West discovered botanicals used for mind-altering purposes elsewhere, such as cocaine and hashish (the most potent form of cannabis). Cocaine was found to be useful medically (by Sigmund Freud, among others), and a number of well-known physicians and surgeons became "cocaine addicts."

Ether, also discovered in the nineteenth century, was used recreationally, again often by medical professionals, as were nitrous oxide and other volatile solvents. Doctors and nurses, presumably because of their access to these drugs and their familiarity with them, were particularly prone to taking them, although reliable data regarding drug abuse by physicians at any time in history, including today, are not available (25). Meperidine, introduced in the 1940s as a "nonaddictive" synthetic narcotic, led to a mild outbreak of abuse among physicians before its addictive potential was appreciated.

In post–World War II in Japan, thousands of young people turned to amphetamines. Drastic measures were required to control the problem, including the establishment of special psychiatric facilities and stringent legal controls.

Further surges of illicit drug use ensued elsewhere in the decades to follow. This development originated with Hofmann's discovery in 1953 that lysergic acid diethylamide-25 (LSD) produced perceptual distortions and other aberrant mental phenomena. Again, physicians were involved in the introduction of the drug for medical use (65). It was first used in re-search on the US East and West Coasts experimentally because it produced symptoms resembling those seen in psychosis. It was also used therapeu-tically, usually by psychoanalysts who believed the drug would dissolve "repressions." Because LSD is easy to synthesize, it became widely available and has been used, at least experimentally, by several million people, the majority of them of young age and from the middle or upper-middle class.

As mind-altering drugs became widely publicized in the 1960s, increasing numbers of young people experimented with them. An explo-sion of illicit hallucinogen use occurred in the 1960s during the rise of an American "counterculture" involving opposition to the Vietnam War and a "sexual revolution." In the early adolescent group, glue sniffing and in-halation of other volatile solvents were apparently widely practiced then, as they have been in recent decades. Individuals in late adolescence and their early 20s, particularly on college campuses in the 1960s and early 1970s, experimented with LSD and other synthetic hallucinogens such as dimethyltryptamine (DMT) as well as other derivatives of the indole and catecholamines that produced psychedelic effects. Beginning in the mid-1970s, the use of LSD and other psychedelics began to decline and has continued to decline since then (89). Injected amphetamines became pop-ular in the late 1960s. Popularity of this class of drugs waned in the 1980s and early 1990s. However, the mid-1990s saw a rise in the use of smoked or injected methamphetamine. "Downers" such as barbiturates and other sedative-hypnotics became popular among young people in the late 1960s through the mid-1970s.

Cocaine, the psychoactive component from the coca leaves, first became widely available in the United States in the late nineteenth century (107). It was available in drug stores, grocery stores, and bars, and by mail order. Many different preparations added the substance, including wine and Coca-Cola. Problems mounted, and cocaine became Public Enemy Number One with the *Harrison Act* that was passed in 1914 to tightly control distribution and sale. Cocaine, sniffed in powdered form, enjoyed resurgence in popularity in the late 1960s and 1970s on college campuses and in suburbia. As in the case of other street drugs, the "cocaine" that people thought they were obtaining was often either adulterated or completely absent. During the late 1980s and early 1990s, however, changes in the delivery of available compounds (e.g., "freebase" and "crack" forms) of cocaine contributed to a significant upsurge in use. The introduction of the inexpensive crack form of cocaine has been attributed to an increase in homelessness in America and specifically the influx of women and children into the homeless population at that time (71, 72).

In the 1960s and 1970s, marijuana emerged as the most widely used illicit drug in America, not only for its enhancement of sensory processes (92) but also for its other psychotomimetic properties (61). Marijuana is the "tobacco" of the hemp plant. It has grown wild in America since colonial times or before. Widely condemned in the 1930s as a dangerous drug, marijuana was used recreationally only by small population subgroups such as jazz musicians and Mexican immigrant workers (13) until the 1960s. Subsequently, use of cannabis became more widely accepted in Western countries as an ostensibly benign if not completely innocuous substance.

Marijuana has been recognized for its potential in the treatment of medical conditions that are unresponsive to traditional treatment, such as nausea and vomiting side effects of chemotherapy, seizure disorders, disorders of spasticity, multiple sclerosis, and even certain psychiatric disorders. Clear empirical evidence for this benefit is limited, and experts have identified the need for more definitive research to inform considerations of legalization of marijuana for medical use (7, 12, 53, 109).

In 2012, the states of Washington and Colorado proceeded to legalize cannabis for recreational use, and Oregon and Alaska soon followed (43, 53, 64). Epidemiological surveillance data on accidents, presentations of emergency medical care and addiction treatment, and use by minors are being monitored to determine the public health effects of this legislation, but it is yet too early to make conclusions about the public health consequences of this legislation (43). Marijuana and its potent relative, hashish, are still illegal in most countries (7), many of which are signatories to a United Nations treaty prohibiting its sale.

During the 1960s when marijuana and hallucinogens were coming into wide use in the United States, heroin—the fast-acting, potent form of morphine—became a serious medical and legal problem, involving mainly lower-income African American urban men. By the early 1990s it was estimated that New York City alone had more than 100,000 opiate-addicted citizens. Also in the early 1990s there was a change in the demographics of opiate use, with an increase among Hispanic males who were between the ages of 18 and 25 and living in the West (48). The expense of supporting a heroin habit among the growing population of users led to widespread criminal activities, including corruption of police authorities. Deaths resulted from heroin overdose, allergic responses, or medical complications following unsterile intravenous injection (bacterial endocarditis, hepatitis B and C, and human immunodeficiency virus [HIV]). Heroin "epidemics" have paralleled the price of the drug and its relative availability.

The mid-1990s saw a substantial increase in the number of prescribed opioids in the United States, especially oxycodone (OxyContin) (16, 17), which is particularly attractive to illicit users seeking to convert this drug to injectable forms. OxyContin has not been adulterated with acetaminophen or nonsteroidal anti-inflammatory drugs, facilitating the diversion of prescription medication for nontherapeutic purposes (17). In the next decade, the recognition of increasing diversion of prescription opiates prompted pharmaceutical and federal agencies to institute measures to address this growing problem, through development of abuse-deterrent drug formulations, statewide prescription monitoring programs, and targeted physician education (16, 22).

As these efforts reduced available supplies of illicit opiates, individuals already dependent on prescription opioids switched to heroin as a cheaper and more available substance to satisfy their addictions (16). This newly emerging population of heroin users included increasing numbers of older, primarily white, suburban women as well as men, a demographic markedly different from previous cohorts (16). New opiate users began to turn to heroin as prescription opiates became unavailable, generating new waves of heroin overdoses and fatalities among opiate-naïve individuals who are more susceptible (16). The emergence of fentanyl-laced heroin about the same time caused more deaths. Together, these trends propelled a nationwide surge of heroin overdoses and fatalities. Emergency department visits nearly tripled in numbers between 2004 and 2011, and opioid deaths more than quadrupled between 2000 and 2014 (22). Emergency services in many communities were overwhelmed by the deluge of opiate overdoses. Many communities responded by distributing the opiate antagonist agent naloxone to emergency and law enforcement personnel and to trained, registered members of the public to reverse acute opiate overdoses and save lives. This dire opioid situation in America continues at the time of the publication of this book, with no signs of abatement.

Evidence has emerged that nicotine is among the most addictive substances used by humans (9, 46). The notion that nicotine was highly addictive did not achieve official sanction until the last few decades (97). The

US government maintains that hundreds of thousands of Americans die every year of nicotine-related illnesses, particularly heart disease and lung cancer. Even secondhand smoke is dangerous, according to the Surgeon General and the Environmental Protection Agency (3, 69). A brief history of tobacco use therefore seems justified here.

In 1492, Columbus recorded in his diary the gift of "strange dry leaves" (p. 72) from a native of San Salvador (75). Within a few years, tobacco had crossed the Atlantic to Europe and become popular for recreational and medicinal uses. In 1560, Jean Nicot, French ambassador to Portugal, touted tobacco's curative powers. The first commercial tobacco crop was grown in Jamestown in 1612. Within a short time, tobacco cultivation spread throughout the colonies. Britain wanted control of tobacco exports, increasing anti-British sentiment in America. Large plantations sprang up, an impetus for the use of slaves to work the plantations.

In 1881, a cigarette-making machine was invented that was capable of making 120,000 cigarettes a day. Cigarettes became immensely popular. This trend was countered by an enthusiastic antismoking movement and establishment of laws prohibiting smoking, which largely died out by World War I. In 1918, the United States War Department provided tobacco in soldiers' rations. By war's end, cigarettes sales had reached one billion a year. American cigarettes became accepted as currency around the world.

In 1964, the U.S. Surgeon General linked tobacco to cancer, heart disease, and other serious ailments. Warning labels were required on cigarette packs. A ban on radio and television advertising of cigarettes took effect. The 1988 Surgeon General's report (24) concluded the following: 1) cigarettes and other forms of tobacco are addictive; 2) nicotine is the drug in tobacco that causes addiction; and 3) the pharmacological and behavioral processes that determine addiction are similar to those that determine addiction to drugs such as heroin and cocaine (78). This report set the stage for the Food and Drug Administration (FDA) to consider regulation of tobacco in the United States in 1994 and then for the World Health Organization (WHO) to consider the international impact and potential control (108).

Decades ago, half of the adult population in the United States smoked nicotine cigarettes. The figure has now fallen to 15% and will probably drop even more as antismoking sentiments further increase (49). In this political climate, most US workplaces have become smoke-free over recent decades. Nonsmokers became increasingly intolerant of cigarette smoke in their environment, and many smokers tried to stop but had difficulty. Regardless, new smokers continue to emerge in the population, as most initiation of smoking occurs during adolescence (59). Today, smoking prevalence remains highest among young adults, males, less educated and lower-income groups, Midwesterners and Southerners, people with mental illness, disabled individuals, and gay, lesbian, and bisexual members of the population (49).

Against this backdrop, the resource-rich tobacco industry has been unrelenting in its marketing of tobacco, especially to the most vulnerable members of society, and in political and legal efforts (69) to promote continuation of its "scourge of tobacco upon society" (p. 409) (3). New products and devices to deliver nicotine, such as through "vaping" of electronic cigarettes ("e-cigarettes"), have provided fresh consumer markets for the tobacco industry. Arguments have been made that vaping may be less harmful than cigarette smoking and may also assist smoking cessation, but these will likely pale in comparison to the potential for this practice to provide a gateway to nicotine habit formation, increasing smoking prevalence and overall harm (23, 87).

EPIDEMIOLOGY

Epidemiological surveys focusing on prevalence of drug use and abuse involve the usual methodological challenges to reliability (e.g., inconsistent population samples, inaccessibility of drug users, self-report data, instrument selection, retrospective design, nondisclosure of substance use and of criminal activity) encountered in prevalence studies. Epidemiological issues of particular relevance to drug studies are the rapidly changing patterns of drug use as well as varying levels of its social acceptability (41). Despite these challenges, certain broad trends in general drug use and abuse have been identified by epidemiological studies. Distinct waves of drug use in the United States began with an overall increase in the 1970s followed by a decline in the 1980s, with another upswing beginning in 1992 that lasted about a decade (51). The National Epidemiologic Survey on Alcohol and Related Conditions (NESARC) found the 12-month prevalence of drug use disorder to be only 2% in the general US population in 2001–2002, increasing to 4% in 2012–2013 (40). Substance abuse is known to be strongly associated with anxiety, personality, and mood disorders (38, 39, 54, 79, 102).

The statistics on the prevalence of drug use indicate that many people have been exposed to a variety of illicit drugs. Billions of dollars are spent on illicit drugs annually, and tens of billions are lost every year in drug-related crime, health problems, and lowered productivity. Intravenous drug use is second only to men having sex with men (MSM) as a risk factor for acquired immune deficiency syndrome (AIDS) (106).

Popular images of drug abusers have evolved over time. Increasing numbers of socialites, athletes, and Hollywood celebrities have experienced legal difficulties related to their use of drugs such as cocaine and opiates. The 1970s popularity of LSD and psilocybin use as part of the "drug culture" of the time has declined greatly. The recent decriminalization of marijuana in some states reflects changing societal attitudes toward use of this substance.

IDENTIFYING THE DRUG USER

Formal assessment of substance use is part of every patient evaluation. Although each evaluator develops a personal style of approach to assessment, several major issues need consideration. First, on the whole, a matter-of-fact inquiry embedded in the intake is usually most effective, including new assessments in outpatient, inpatient, emergency department, and consultation settings. Second, careful attention to the answers provided is necessary to ascertain whether the patient appears to be carefully avoiding disclosure of the whole truth about the patient's substance use. If so, focused follow-up may be necessary and should be preceded by identification of the reasons why it is important that the physician be provided the complete history ("My role here is to fully assess the situation, which is in your best interest. What I need to complete this evaluation is your assistance in providing the full picture.") Should such attempts meet with failure, approaching collateral informants (e.g., spouse, family, friends, workplace informants), within the rules of confidentiality, may yield valuable information. Third, interviewing an intoxicated individual for anything other than the basics may be fruitless or may produce incorrect or misleading information. Fourth, because the examiner will be asking about behaviors that are counter to cultural norms or even illegal, avoiding a judgmental stance or attitude will facilitate the interview. Finally, inquiry should almost always be made with patients (particularly new patients or those with unknown prior history) into the possibility of pending withdrawal from any agent that may produce significant morbidity (or mortality). Obtaining the history, physical examination, and laboratory testing will complete the assessment of these patients. Although assessing use of each single drug for status of substance use disorder may prove tedious, establishing the proper diagnosis (or diagnoses) is the first step toward initiating appropriate treatment.

DRUG CATEGORIES

Opioids

Opioids are derivatives of naturally occurring plant substances (opiates) from which morphine-like effects or opiate-like substances are synthesized or semi-synthesized in the laboratory. Opiates include opium, heroin, fentanyl, hydromorphone (Dilaudid), codeine, oxycodone (OxyContin), hydrocodone, and paregoric. Meperidine (Demerol) is a synthetic analgesic structurally dissimilar to morphine but pharmacologically similar. Opium and heroin are not available for medical use in the United States.

Heroin can be snorted (insufflation), smoked, or skin-popped (injected subcutaneously). Most people who are addicted to heroin and morphine eventually take opiates intravenously, which produces flushing and a sensation described as similar to orgasm, known as a "rush." Psychomotor activity initially increases, followed by a period of drowsiness and inactivity, a state that has been called "being on the nod" or "nodding out."

In usual therapeutic doses, opioids produce analgesia, drowsiness, and a change in mood described as a sense of well-being. Opioids produce constriction of the pupils, constipation, and occasionally nausea and vomiting; they are also respiratory depressants. Variable potencies of different forms of heroin often result in respiratory distress. Many people with heroin addiction come to the attention of medical authorities after presenting to an emergency department in overdose status.

A drug screen is obviously procured when a somnolent patient presents to the emergency department. In outpatient settings, an evaluator may notice small, poorly reactive pupils, variable mentation at different visits, needle tracks, lower weight than the ideal, and pain complaints that are out of proportion to the physical exam. The evaluator may then request a drug screen and may be surprised when the patient volunteers a history of using a particular narcotic. It is important to ask whether that is the only substance that may be found. Routine drug screens may also be part of treatment programs.

Tolerance develops to most opioid effects, including euphoria. Libido declines; menstruation may cease. Some people with opioid addiction who manage to obtain adequate supplies of opiates are able to dress properly, maintain nutrition, and discharge social and occupational obligations without gross impairment. Others become socially disabled, and the expense of drugs leads to theft, forgery, prostitution, and the sale of drugs to other users.

The first symptoms of opioid withdrawal usually appear 8–12 hours after the last dose once a habit has been established (Table 12.1). These include lacrimation, rhinorrhea, sweating, and yawning. Thereafter, the person may fall into a fitful sleep known as "the yen" and then awaken after several hours, restless and miserable. Additional signs and symptoms peak 48–72 hours after drug discontinuation. These include dilated pupils, anorexia, restlessness, insomnia, irritability, gooseflesh, nausea, vomiting, diarrhea, chills, and abdominal cramps. These manifestations subside gradually and disappear after 7–10 days, although the individual may continue to experience insomnia, weakness, and nervousness.

In addition to acute withdrawal symptoms, opioids may produce a protracted abstinence syndrome lasting several months (15). Body temperature and respiratory rate may be below normal. The person may have trouble sleeping. More important, the craving for opiates may persist for several months after the last dose. This probably contributes to the high recidivism rate in opiate users. Recidivism has also been attributed to a phenomenon called the "conditioned abstinent syndrome" (15). After detoxification, patients returning to the environment in which they used drugs may experience craving for the drug as well as physical manifestations of abstinence because of conditioned stimuli (e.g., seeing old friends and familiar places).

The course of opiate addiction varies depending on the population studied. In Vaillant's 12-year follow-up of people addicted to opiates originally treated at the federal addiction treatment center at Lexington, KY, 98% had returned to the use of opiates within 12 months after release (98). In contrast, a study of Vietnam veterans who used opium and its products extensively during their tour in Vietnam revealed that fewer than 10% continued using the drug in the year after their return to the United States (81). This suggests that circumstances of exposure and availability are important factors in maintaining use. There is some evidence that heroin users who do not die as a result of drugs or criminal activities may spontaneously stop using the drug after their mid-30s. School problems such as delinquency and truancy frequently antedate heroin use (98).

The mortality from opiate withdrawal is negligible despite the unpleasantness of the withdrawal syndrome. Deaths from medical causes occurring among opiate-dependent individuals are mainly attributable to infection, overdose, and hypersensitivity reactions, possibly from diluents such as quinine. Unsterile injections may facilitate septicemia, hepatitis B and C, subacute bacterial endocarditis, tetanus, and HIV infection. Illicitly obtained opiates are highly variable in potency. Accustomed to the normal successive dilutions of the drug passing through distribution channels, opiate users may unexpectedly encounter relatively pure heroin

TABLE 12.1 ABSTINENCE SIGNS IN SEQUENTIAL APPEARANCE AFTER LAST DOSE OF OPIATE IN PATIENTS WITH WELL-ESTABLISHED PARENTERAL HABITS*

Grades of Abstinence	Signs (Observed in Cool Room, Patient Uncovered or under Only a Sheet)	Hours after Last Dose				
		Morphine	Heroin	Meperidine	Dihydromorphinone	Codeine
Grade 0	Craving for drug Anxiety	6	4	2–3	2–3	8
Grade 1	Yawning Perspiration Lacrimation Rhinorrhea Yen sleep	14	8	4–6	4–5	24
Grade 2	Increase in Grade 0–1 signs plus: Mydriasis Gooseflesh (piloerection) Tremors (muscle twitches) Hot and cold flashes Aching bones and muscles Anorexia	16	12	8–12	7	48
Grade 3	Increased intensity of Grade 0–2 signs plus: Insomnia Increased blood pressure Increased temperature (1–2) Increased respiratory rate and depth Increased pulse rate Restlessness Nausea	24–36	18–24	16	12	—

TABLE 12.1 CONTINUED

Grades of Abstinence	Signs (Observed in Cool Room, Patient Uncovered or under Only a Sheet)	Hours after Last Dose				
		Morphine	Heroin	Meperidine	Dihydromorphinone	Codeine
Grade 4	Increased intensity of Grade 0–3 signs plus: Febrile facies Position—curled up on hard surface Vomiting Diarrhea Weight loss (5 lbs. daily) Spontaneous ejaculation or orgasm Hemoconcentration leukocytosis, eosinopenia, increased blood sugar	36–48	24–36	—	16	—

*Not all signs are necessary to diagnose any particular grade. Racemorphan (Dromoran) and levorphanol (Levodromoran), although three times and six times as strong as morphine sulfate, show the same time curve as morphine sulfate. This characteristic is similar for paregoric, laudanum, and hydrochlorides of opium alkaloids (Pantopon), depending on their relative content of morphine.
Adapted from Blachly (11).

or powerful contaminants such as fentanyl, both of which present risk of overdose. Overdoses may be fatal because of respiratory depression and may require ventilatory assistance in a hospital. Naloxone, an opioid antagonist, reverses opiate respiratory depression.

The mainstay of treatment for opioid use disorders is medication-assisted treatment. Three main μ-opioid receptor pharmacological agents have been demonstrated to be effective for treating opioid use disorders and preventing relapse (22, 101).

Developed for treatment of opioid use disorders about a half century ago, methadone is a full μ-opioid receptor agonist that activates opioid receptors (22). It is prescribed in gradually increasing doses over a period of weeks until a high degree of cross-tolerance to all opiates is established, blocking the euphoric effects of intravenous narcotics. Methadone must be taken orally once daily, dispensed from specialty outpatient treatment programs that patients must visit daily to receive the medication.

Buprenorphine (Suboxone) is a nonselective partial μ-opioid receptor agonist that activates opiate receptors but produces a diminished response. It is taken orally or sublingually once daily and has been shown to be as effective as methadone. Its advantages include reduced addictive properties, low overdose potential, and fewer withdrawal symptoms. Prescription by certified physicians makes it more widely available by eliminating the need for patients to visit specialized treatment clinics. To diminish abuse liability, the Suboxone formulation incorporates the antagonist naloxone that induces withdrawal if the drug is injected.

Naltrexone is a μ-opioid receptor antagonist that blocks opioid receptors, interfering with the pleasurable and analgesic effects of opioids. Naltrexone is administered orally or by injection to diminish the reinforcing effects of opioids. It is nonaddictive and not sedating and it appears to be somewhat useful in highly motivated opioid-dependent patients. A long-acting injectable form (Vivitrol) is available as an alternative to daily oral dosing (101).

Acute withdrawal from opiates is most effectively treated with a long-acting oral opioid (usually methadone or buprenorphine) to relieve symptoms followed by a gradual dose reduction to allow the patient to adjust to the absence of an opioid (88). All three medications acting at the μ-opioid receptor (methadone, buprenorphine, and naltrexone) that are used for the treatment of opioid use disorders have been found to prevent the emergence of withdrawal (22). Clonidine, an alpha-adrenergic agonist used for treatment of hypertension, also alleviates the opiate withdrawal syndrome, but its use in the treatment of opiate withdrawal has been supplanted by the opioid agonists (91).

Medications alone apparently are not enough for successful treatment outcomes; a complete program of rehabilitation is typically necessary. Various psychosocial treatment models have been put forward for treatment of opiate abuse, although with only moderate results (26, 29). Self-help groups inspired by people who have recovered from addiction have stimulated enthusiastic responses from some participants, but their efficacy in general remains unknown.

Sedative-Hypnotics

Sedatives produce calmness; hypnotics produce sleep. Both share similar pharmacological actions, hence the term "sedative-hypnotics." In higher doses, drugs marketed as sedatives also produce sleep. Hypnotics prescribed in lower doses produce calmness. The most popular class of sedative-hypnotics is the benzodiazepines. Benzodiazepines are distinguishable from barbiturates and older sedative-hypnotics such as choral hydrate in that animals and people can easily be aroused from benzodiazepine-produced sleep, whereas this is more difficult with the older drugs. The benzodiazepines will be discussed in the next section, and this section will confine itself to the barbiturates.

In contrast to opioids, barbiturates are usually taken orally. The short- and intermediate-acting barbiturates are most frequently used for nonmedical purposes. In both acute and chronic intoxication as well as the withdrawal syndrome, the clinical picture resembles that produced by alcohol. An intoxicated patient may show lethargy, difficulty in thinking, poor memory, irritability, and self-neglect. Nystagmus, ataxia, and a positive Romberg sign are often present.

Generally lessened use of the barbiturates as a class in recent years makes the possibility of encountering a patient in withdrawal rather uncommon, but knowledge of the potentially serious nature of the withdrawal (and treatment) is exceedingly important. Withdrawal symptoms may occur when patients take more than 400 mg of barbiturates per day. The patient becomes anxious, restless, and weak during the first 12 to 16 hours after the usual dose has not been supplied. Tremors of the hands are prominent; deep tendon reflexes are hyperactive. During the second or third day, grand mal seizures may occur, sometimes followed by delirium and rarely even death. The syndrome usually clears in about a week. Long-acting barbiturates such as phenobarbital rarely, if ever, produce major withdrawal symptoms.

Withdrawal manifestations may be prevented or treated by administering a large dose of a short-acting barbiturate such as secobarbital (800–1,000 mg per 24 hours in divided doses) and then gradually reducing the doses over a period of 7–10 days. Phenobarbital, a long-acting drug, is useful in detoxifying sedative-hypnotic dependence by producing a gradual cessation of withdrawal symptoms: 30 mg of phenobarbital is roughly equivalent to 100 mg of the short-acting barbiturates.

The older synthetic hypnotics (e.g., glutethimide [Doriden], methyprylon [Noludar], and ethchlorvynol [Placidyl]) are rarely encountered now.

Benzodiazepines

Benzodiazepines are the most widely prescribed class of medication in the Western world. At least a dozen benzodiazepine drugs are marketed in the

United States and more than 20 have been approved internationally (93). Benzodiazepines are also called "tranquilizers" or "minor" tranquilizers, in contradistinction to "major" tranquilizers such as the antipsychotic drugs. The term "tranquilizer" originated from the observation that benzodiazepines would "tranquilize" wild animals—make them tamer and more manageable—without rendering them unconscious (37).

Compared to the sedative-hypnotic drugs described in the previous section, benzodiazepines have the following advantages: 1) they relieve anxiety without necessarily reducing alertness, impairing coordination, or interfering with normal thinking processes; 2) regularly prescribed doses provide little or no euphoria; 3) they are good muscle relaxants; and 4) they are the safest, most effective drugs for treating alcohol withdrawal and other agitated states produced by many street drugs. Benzodiazepines can be given to intoxicated patients in an emergency room without fear of lethal reactions, although caution should always be exercised. The favorable pharmacokinetic and pharmacodynamic properties of benzodiazepines that make them preferred choices for clinical use include their rapid onset of action, lower propensity for respiratory depression, higher lethal-to-effective dose ratio, and ability to provide anxiolysis without excessive sedation (94).

Benzodiazepines are the most effective drugs available for insomnia. Unlike barbiturates, they lose little of their effectiveness over even long periods of use, and short-acting benzodiazepine hypnotics such as triazolam (Halcion) and temazepam (Restoril) and the non-benzodiazepine gamma aminobutryic acid (GABA)-A alpha-1 selective agent zolpidem (Ambien) leave few after-effects the next morning. These drugs have one great advantage over the barbiturates and other hypnotics routinely used for sleep and relaxation in the past: It is almost impossible to commit suicide by taking an overdose. Very rarely, deaths are reported from overdose, but these almost always involve concomitant use of other sedative agents or alcohol (93).

Abrupt discontinuation of benzodiazepines after long-term use at relatively high dosages can result in severe withdrawal syndromes, manifesting with hallucinations, disorientation, and grand mal seizures (93). Even low-dose use of benzodiazepines over protracted periods can result in milder, short-lived abstinence syndromes with rebound symptoms, anxiety, muscle tension, tremor, restlessness, agitation, and disordered perceptions (77, 93). Thus caution is indicated in prescribing these drugs for long periods, even in low dosage. Geriatric patients are particularly sensitive to benzodiazepines and should be given smaller doses than younger patients.

The onset of withdrawal symptoms occurs more rapidly with the shorter-acting benzodiazepines (2–3 days) than with the longer-acting agents (5–10 days) (93). Gradual withdrawal of these medications, especially with long-term use at higher doses, is thus prudent, and tapering over a period of 4–6 (or even 8) weeks may be needed. Alprazolam (Xanax), a very effective anti-anxiety agent, has the particular disadvantage of producing physical dependence even at moderate, recommended dosages (77, 84). The strategy for withdrawing patients from alprazolam is to taper the medication very slowly, reducing the dosage by as little as 10% every 1–2 weeks (66). Other benzodiazepines may be ineffective for alprazolam withdrawal, because of incomplete cross-tolerance between them, attributed to the far greater affinity of alprazolam's triazole ring for benzodiazepine receptors (84).

While in-depth review of receptor physiology is beyond the scope of this book, it does seem to be a settled issue that GABA is the major inhibitory neurotransmitter in mammalian brains and its effects are mediated through two receptors: GABA-A and GABA-B (77). The presence of a benzodiazepine at the benzodiazepine-binding site on the GABA-A receptor causes the receptor to be more responsive to synaptic GABA. Activation of the GABA-A receptor facilitates the influx of chloride ions hyperpolarizing the neuron and inhibiting depolarization and, therefore, transmission (77). This inhibitory action on neurons is thought to produce the major pharmacological actions of benzodiazepines, including reduced arousal, sedation, and muscle relaxation (77).

Marijuana

Cannabis sativa (hemp) contains psychoactive chemicals known as cannabinoids. One of these, Δ-9-tetrahydrocannabinol (THC), is believed to be the most psychoactive constituent of marijuana. The effects of THC depend on dosage, and they range from mild euphoria with small doses to sedation with high doses. Most of the marijuana that grows wild in the United States contains insufficient amounts of THC to produce measurable psychological effects. Cannabis imported from Mexico, South America, and India, however, contains sufficient THC to produce marked euphoria and, depending on the plant preparation used, paranoid delusions and other psychotomimetic effects. Because THC deteriorates at the rate of 5% per month at room temperature, even the imported cannabis eventually loses its potency. The cannabis in use today tends to have a much higher THC content than that available in the mid-1970s (7).

There are two generally available cannabis preparations: marijuana and hashish. The former consists of a mixture of dried plant products (upper leaves, tops, stems, flowers and seeds). The latter consists of the resins of the plant and is more potent.

Cannabis can be either smoked or eaten. Cannabinoids are lipophilic and rapidly distributed throughout the body, stored in the adipose tissue, and distributed to the body slowly over time. Blood testing can reveal presence of THC more than 30 days after heavy use.

In parts of the world where concentrated cannabis preparations have been used by millions of people for hundreds of years, constant use is said to be associated with serious medical and psychiatric illnesses. Early studies conducted in Jamaica, Costa Rica, and Greece—countries where cannabis has been used regularly for many years—failed to reveal any serious pathology associated with the use of the drug (83). However, subsequent evidence accumulated over several decades suggests that regular use of marijuana is associated with the following hazards (52):

1. Bronchial and pulmonary irritation. Marijuana, because of its relatively poor combustibility, has up to 50% more polyaromatic hydrocarbons in its smoke than tobacco does (47). Cigarette for cigarette, the difference between tobacco and marijuana may be even more significant because of the way marijuana typically is smoked—down to a minuscule butt— and because users retain the smoke in the lungs for a longer period than with tobacco smoking. Studies have found habitual marijuana use to be associated with inflammation of large airways, airway resistance, and lung hyperinflation, promoting persistent respiratory symptoms, including acute and chronic bronchitis, wheezing, and exertional dyspnea (100).

2. Cardiovascular effects. Temporal associations have been established between marijuana use and myocardial infarction, sudden cardiac death, cardiomyopathy, stroke, and transient ischemic attack (96).

3. THC is a potent immune modulator with significant immunosuppressive effects on various immune cells, including T lymphocytes, macrophages, and natural killer cells (55).

4. Studies consistently show short-term adverse effects of marijuana on cognition and immediate memory. These impairments may last for many weeks, months, or years after use (100).

5. Marijuana intoxication impairs reaction time, motor coordination, and visual perception. Studies under simulated conditions and in street traffic have confirmed that the ability to operate a motor vehicle is adversely affected by marijuana use (7, 100).

There is accumulating evidence that the use of cannabis, especially with the far more potent forms of the drug circulating today, is associated with the development of psychotic illness, including schizophrenia (100). This relationship has been found to occur in a dose-dependent relationship, with a four-fold increase in risk among the heaviest users. A causal link between cannabis and psychosis has not, however, been unequivocally established.

Marijuana has well-known abuse potential. Approximately 9% of people who experiment with the drug will become addicted to it (100). Cannabis use is also associated with the use of other illicit substances and with other substance use disorders (12).

Trends in marijuana use have varied during the time that epidemiological data have been collected. By the mid-to-late 1970s, the numbers of high school seniors in the United States using marijuana daily peaked at 10%; these numbers dropped to 5% in 1984 and 2% in 1991 (50). Between 1992 and 2002, the prevalence of marijuana use in the population was steady at 4%, but during this same decade the prevalence of marijuana abuse or dependence increased from 1.2% to 1.5% (21). By 2013, the population prevalence of marijuana use had increased to approximately 12%, although without further increase in the prevalence of abuse or dependence (20, 41, 100).

Cocaine

The United States has experienced two major surges of cocaine abuse. The first occurred in the last decades of the nineteenth century when physicians in particular became reliant on the drug (thinking, as did Freud at first, that it was relatively benign and nonaddictive). The second surge began in the mid-1970s. Cocaine remains a major drug of abuse throughout the United States.

In the 1970s, cocaine was still widely held to be a relatively benign drug. This aided the substantial replacement of amphetamines by cocaine as the preferred illicit stimulant drug. The trade-off—for society and for individuals—did not work (35). Experience since the 1980s has indicated that cocaine (particularly the newer "crack" form of the drug) may be more dependence-producing and dangerous than the amphetamines.

In the early 1980s, increasing numbers of white, employed, middle-class people in their late 20s and 30s who had never before sought psychological help entered treatment for cocaine dependence. A cocaine hotline in Washington, DC, received more than 14,000 calls daily (35, 103). Many of the callers were college graduates, professionals, and business executives.

Half had cocaine habits costing more than their annual salaries. Focus on the drug was intense. Nearly all callers said they could not turn the drug down when it was available. Most said cocaine had become more important to them than either food or sex. They had physical complaints: headaches, sinus infections, and sexual dysfunction. Some had seizures or became paranoid.

Until the late 1980s, the cocaine most often used and most widely available on the street was cocaine hypochloride, a powdered form that was ingested by snorting (36). However, in the mid-1970s some Americans adopted methods similar to South American practices of smoking cocoa paste—a potent alkaline extract from cocoa leaves. It was found that street cocaine can be "freed" from its salts and cutting agents by a chemical process to create "freebased" cocaine, which is potentially hazardous because it involves heating flammable solvents. Another process to deliver cocaine to a form that can be smoked involves dissolving the cocaine in water and mixing it with sodium bicarbonate to yield a base that when dried creates a rock-like substance, called "crack" cocaine. The name "crack" derives from the cracking or popping sound when the drug is lit for smoking (36).

The demographics of cocaine users shifted in the second half of the 1980s with the advent of the inexpensive and hence more accessible "crack" preparation of the drug. Cocaine use among women, minority groups, lower-income groups, and adolescents skyrocketed. Cocaine problems infiltrated the small towns of the Midwest and even invaded suburbia. By 1996, the number of occasional users (less than 12 days per year) had decreased to 2.5 million, compared to 7 million in 1985 (26).

By the mid-1980s, cocaine was universally considered a dangerous drug (1). Because smoked cocaine is inhaled and enters the brain rapidly, it is highly habit forming. The smoked forms of cocaine were considered by many authorities to be the most dangerous of all cocaine preparations. Smoking cocaine increases heart rate and blood pressure; produce tremors, anorexia, and insomnia; sometimes precipitates hallucinations, paranoia, and depression; and may even result in cardiac arrest and lung damage (36). Cocaine has accounted for a number of deaths among celebrities, and it is associated with drug-related crimes and murders.

Cocaine resembles amphetamines in many ways, but in contrast to amphetamines, which are synthetic drugs, cocaine is of botanical origin, originating from shrubs grown in the Andes. Its effects last for a shorter period than those of amphetamines. Like amphetamines, cocaine is a powerful stimulant of the nervous system, producing euphoria, increasing alertness, and suppressing fatigue and boredom (36). Cocaine intoxication may be accompanied by anxiety, agitation, suspiciousness that may extend to paranoia, tremor, mydriasis, diaphoresis, tachycardia, hypertension, and hyperpyrexia. After regular, heavy use of the drug, a withdrawal syndrome of sorts may occur, in which formication (a sensation of bugs crawling under the skin) frequent occurs, together with depression and lassitude (105).

Heavy use of cocaine may produce a schizophreniform psychosis resembling paranoid schizophrenia. Occasional users sometimes report a profound dysphoria, persisting for several days after they have used the drug. Cocaine may have a deleterious effect on the health of pregnant women and on fetal development. Used during pregnancy, it may cause irregularities of placental blood flow, abruptio placentae, and premature labor. Reported effects on fetal and infant development include low birth weight, malformations of the urogenital system, cerebral infarction, seizures, and sudden death syndrome.

Amphetamines

These stimulant drugs include d-amphetamine (Dexedrine), dl-amphetamine (Benzedrine—withdrawn from the market), and methamphetamine (Desoxyn, Methedrine). Amphetamines may be taken orally, smoked, or injected intravenously. Their effects include elevated mood, increased energy and alertness, decreased appetite, and slight improvement in task performance. Since their introduction into general use in the early 1930s, amphetamines have been prescribed by physicians for a variety of conditions, including depression, obesity, and narcolepsy. They were originally promoted as safe and effective medications without liability to addiction.

Drug-induced psychosis is common among individuals taking large doses of amphetamines (>50 mg per day). This psychosis may resemble schizophrenia with persecutory delusions, except that they occur with a clear sensorium. Hallucinations are common. Usually the psychosis subsides 1 or 2 weeks after cessation of drug use. When an apparent amphetamine psychosis persists, a hidden source of drugs or the diagnosis of schizophrenia should be considered.

Tolerance to amphetamines may be striking. Habitual users sometimes take as much as 1 or 2 g per day (compared to usual therapeutic doses of 5–30 mg per day). Users withdrawing from amphetamines experience fatigue and depression.

Methamphetamine, an amphetamine derivative, was first synthesized in 1919 in Japan using ephedrine as a precursor. Also known as "meth" and "speed," methamphetamine has a more rapid onset of action than other amphetamines. It exerts its effects through multiple neurotransmitter systems, predominantly dopamine, but also through the serotonergic, noradrenergic, and glutamatergic systems.

Methamphetamine was widely used for legal medicinal purposes in the 1940s and 1950s (99). It was provided to military troops in World War II and later wars to increase their stamina in battle. Methamphetamine came into common use by industrial workers to enhance productivity and assist shift work and by students and professionals to promote wakefulness, improve concentration and mood, and lose weight. Habitual users developed tolerance to amphetamines, leading them to increase the doses they used.

Increasing awareness of the highly addictive nature of methamphetamine and its toxicity to every organ system in the body led to its restriction to prescription use for established medical indications (99). General use of methamphetamine decreased dramatically over the next two decades, partly because of physicians' reluctance to prescribe the drug, and partly because of its displacement by the growing popularity of cocaine being used for similar desired effects. In some countries, amphetamines were removed from the market altogether despite strong evidence of their potential therapeutic benefits for treating patients with narcolepsy, attention-deficit disorders, and depression.

In the 1960s, San Francisco's Haight-Asbury neighborhood became a center for illicit methamphetamine use. At that time, most street methamphetamine was being manufactured in clandestine laboratories rather than diverted from legal sources. The moniker "speed freak" came into use to refer to compulsive, high-dose users. Methamphetamine's popularity spread from there to include a demographic consisting predominantly of white males, especially truck drivers, construction workers, and blue-collar workers. In the 1960s and 1970s, methamphetamine came to be associated with motorcycle gangs, earning the nickname "crank," because the drug was carried in motorcycle crankcases (99).

In the 1980s, a new hydrochloride form of methamphetamine, also known as "crystal meth," or "Ice," appeared in Hawaii (99). Its popularity spread to the West Coast and across the United States, reaching the Midwest in the 1990s and the East Coast in the following decade. Ice can be smoked, thus delivering the drug to the brain even faster than when injected. It also has a long duration of action—up to 18 hours. It stimulates the brain to a greater degree than regular methamphetamine, but with less stimulation of the heart, blood vessels, and lungs.

Efforts to stem the production of this easily synthesized and inexpensive-to-produce (in bulk) substance were made through an attempt to gain legal control of the availability of the precursor substances, ephedrine and pseudoephedrine (99). By the time that most states had restrictions placed on these substances and their precursors in the late-1980s, Mexican drug cartels began to smuggle large amounts of methamphetamine and its precursors into the country. Since then, most illicit methamphetamine in the United States is manufactured in Mexico. Neither the US nor the Mexican governments have been able to stem the rising production of il- licit methamphetamine (99). Meth labs proliferated in the United States in the 1990s, especially in rural areas where the strong odor associated with methamphetamine production is less likely to be noticed. Unfortunately, meth labs are sometimes housed in residential buildings, posing significant explosive hazard risks associated with methamphetamine manufacturing.

Use of Ice can produce states of severe psychosis and intense depres- sion as the drug wears off. Users may become paranoid. Suicidal ideation is common, as are suicide attempts. Acute hypertensive crisis and violence may occur. Haloperidol can usually control the psychotic symptoms, and antidepressants can usually control the depressive effects.

Because Ice does not require the use of needles, it does not contribute to risk of HIV infection through injection; however, the drug impairs judg- ment regarding safe sexual practices, increasing the risk of acquiring HIV. This drug is associated with significant medical morbidity and mortality (42, 86), including cerebrovascular accidents, liver failure, hyponatremia (and cerebral edema), serotonin syndrome, and exertional hyperpyrexia leading to rhabdomyolysis along with multi-organ failure.

Methamphetamine abuse poses serious and costly public health problems. Besides the direct effects of methamphetamine on the users' medical and mental health, social problems associated with chronic use in- clude crime and violence associated with obtaining the drug and aggressive drug-induced behaviors, as well as burdens on families, social networks, the criminal justice system, educational aspirations, workplace environ- ment, and treatment systems (67, 99).

The substituted amphetamine derivative 3, 4-methylenedioxymeth- amphetamine (MDMA), also known as "Ecstasy," can be classified both as a stimulant and as a hallucinogen (2). This drug works predominantly through the serotonin neurotransmitter system rather than predomi- nantly through the dopamine system that is characteristic of methamphet- amine. Ecstasy offers the special quality of experiencing strong empathy and closeness to others (18). MDMA was first synthesized "by accident" in 1912 by the German pharmaceutical company Merck (10), as part of a quest to develop a drug to stop abnormal bleeding (10). During the Cold War, the U.S. Central Intelligence Agency (CIA) experimented with

MDMA on non-human subjects as part of its fabled "mind control program" in attempts to develop drug weaponry (10, 74).

MDMA was not used in humans until 1970, when it was briefly explored for its potential as a psychotherapeutic agent. The drug developed an underground popularity in the 1970s and 1980s. In 1984, the *San Francisco Examiner* described MDMA as "the yuppie psychedelic" (p. A28) (63). The following year, the U.S. Drug Enforcement Agency (DEA) added MDMA to its Schedule I drug list. Subsequently, MDMA was widely adopted as a "club drug" at house parties and music clubs and concerts featuring music that fuses disco and electronic music styles, creating a new phenomenon known as a "rave scene" (p. 207) (10). Eventually, law enforcement moved to shut down rave parties, but regardless, MDMA continued to move into mainstream use, becoming caught up in gang activities and leaving fatalities in its wake.

Hallucinogens

Perceptual distortions are the primary effect of hallucinogenic drugs, which include LSD, mescaline, psilocybin, and a family of compounds chemically resembling either LSD or the amphetamines (e.g., DMT, STP [2,5-dimethoxy-4-methylamphetamine], and MDMA). This discussion of hallucinogens will focus on LSD because it has been the most widely used and studied drug of this type. (MDMA was previously discussed in the "Amphetamines" section of this chapter.) LSD became popular during the 1960s "drug culture" (27). Its use peaked in the 1970s and declined steadily thereafter, except for a brief increase in popularity in the mid-1990s.

Together with perceptual distortions, including illusions and hallucinations, LSD "trips" produce altered time sense, disturbed judgment, and sometimes confusion and disorientation (27). Some LSD trips are unpleasant. Users of LSD may be brought to emergency rooms for bad trips characterized by panic and sometimes persecutory delusions. There are reports of prolonged or flashback effects (a resurgence of the drug effect days, weeks, months, or even years subsequent to the end of a trip). Flashbacks have not been studied systematically, but they are reported so commonly that some authorities believe people do experience them. A number of deaths have been attributed to LSD, primarily from suicide or homicide, although causal connections remain unclear (66).

Repeated use of LSD results in marked tolerance. No withdrawal syndrome has been reported. The drug usually produces euphoria, but dysphoria may occur. No deaths have been reported from LSD overdose.

Treatment for acute adverse reactions to LSD consists of reassurance and, if this fails, tranquilizers. Benzodiazepines appear to be as effective as antipsychotic medications and are somewhat safer because they are less likely to produce hypotension.

Hallucinogens have complicated the problem of diagnosing psychiatric disorders among young drug users. Prolonged psychotic episodes are probably more often attributable to schizophrenia or other psychiatric illness than to LSD toxicity. To determine whether a patient has a psychiatric illness that is not associated with drug abuse, the patient must be drug-free for a lengthy period.

Inhalants

Inhalants represent an important category of substance abuse that has been understudied for a variety of reasons, including transient use (predominantly by young people), rareness as a drug of choice, use based on availability (or lack of availability of more desirable substances), poorly understood chemistry (not originally developed as a medication), and difficulty conducting this type of research. Nonetheless, inhalant abuse has been found to be second only to marijuana abuse in eighth graders (95). From the 1970s to the early 1990s, inhalant abuse in the United States increased steadily, but its popularity has since declined to the present. These substances have potential for serious acute complications, including central nervous system toxicity, hematological derangements, renal toxicity, cardiomyopathy, and death (95).

Inhalants are commonly divided into three types: nitrous oxide, nitrites, and volatile solvents. Nitrous oxide, commonly known as "laughing gas," is used in anesthesia. Nitrites (amyl, butyl, and isobutyl nitrite) are available in room odorizers and over-the-counter preparations. The largest group, volatile solvents, includes gasoline, solvents (e.g., correction fluid, paint thinner, and nail polish remover), fuel (butane), lighter fluid, commercial cleaning agents, adhesives (rubber cement, airplane glue, and PVC cement), and aerosols (spray paint, hair spray, deodorants, room freshener, analgesic spray, and asthma sprays) (95).

Designer Drugs

The popularity of drugs tends to wax and wane, and this is especially true for "designer drugs." These are substances that are developed synthetically by manipulating the molecular structure to avoid classification as illicit drugs (hence circumventing prosecution) while retaining the psychoactive properties of illicit drugs (33, 104). Also known as "new psychoactive substances" (NPS), these drugs fall into four major categories: 1) amphetamine-like stimulants including derivatives of cathinones (extracted from khat) and piperazines which are used as proxies for Ecstasy, 2) synthetic cannabinoids ("Spice" and "K2"), 3) hallucinogenic/dissociative agents, and 4) opioid-like compounds (104).

Designer drugs are chemically synthesized or structurally modified from other compounds. These drugs, especially cathinones, are sometimes marketed under the name "bath salts" (31, 76). Many of these drugs can be manufactured in basements by people who possess a modicum of technical knowledge. The recent rapid proliferation of these drugs has been attributed to mail-order sales through Internet sources (68). Most of these drugs have emerged only since 2010 (104); by the end of 2015, more than 600 of these substances had been discovered (31).

Use of these drugs, singly and in combination, and especially by young people, has produced a spectrum of bizarre reactions as confusing to physicians as to worried parents. The recent explosion of designer drugs represents a rapidly increasing public health problem, because these new drugs are being produced faster than regulations can be established to restrict their legal use, because there are not yet laboratory tests for their detection, and because increasing numbers of patients are presenting to poison centers and emergency medical systems with novel toxicities for which there are not yet established treatment protocols (31, 73, 76, 104).

Ketamine, phencyclidine (PCP), and gamma-hydroxybutyrate (GHB), also considered designer drugs, are members of the "dissociative" class of anesthetic drugs. These drugs are NMDA receptor antagonists with psychotomimetic properties, ostensibly through dopaminergic augmentation (62). PCP has been used as a veterinary anesthetic and ketamine as a human anesthetic agent. PCP is classified as a Schedule II substance and ketamine as Schedule III (62). GHB has been used for assisted sexual assault, earning it the name "date rape drug" and a Schedule I classification (10).

PCP is available in many forms—tablet, powder, leaf, rock crystal—and can be ingested, snorted, smoked, or injected. PCP has been called the "universal adulterant" because it has often been used to lace marijuana and other street drugs (19). It has been the most common drug of deception, being sold as LSD, cocaine, THC, and other street drugs (68). Known as "Angel Dust" on the street, PCP was discovered in 1956 and first appeared on the West Coast in 1965 (62, 68). Within a decade, its use reached epidemic proportions such that in Washington, DC, more patients were psychiatrically hospitalized for PCP toxicity than for alcoholism and schizophrenia combined (62). PCP toxicity is easily mistaken for schizophrenia and its symptoms can persist for weeks. PCP is known to induce cataleptic states in which pain is not perceived; the eyes are wide open, but the individual is unconscious and amnestic for the experience. Behavioral dyscontrol during PCP intoxication can progress to bizarre activities and violence, leading to encounters with police, unusual accidents, strange suicides, impulsive homicides, and lawsuits. The user is often amnestic about these events and may remember only the pleasant, floaty euphoria the drug produces at low doses.

The benefit of antipsychotic medications for psychotic disorders does not appear to extend to PCP psychosis, because of potential for severe postural hypotension and seizures with increased muscle rigidity during PCP intoxication. Intramuscular benzodiazepines may be a better choice. Trying to "talk down" a patient intoxicated with PCP may have the paradoxical effect of overstimulating the patient (19).

Fortunately, the popularity of PCP quickly waned. However, illicit use of ketamine, beginning in the mid-1960s, has increased in popularity, especially at rave parties and music venues (62). Ketamine has many of the properties of PCP, but its potency is lower and its duration of action is shorter. Recently, ketamine has received considerable notoriety and research interest for its potential use as a rapidly acting but incomplete treatment for refractory depression (8).

Tobacco

For the last 50 years, tobacco and nicotine addiction specifically have been the focus of intense scientific research, scientific argument, public health proclamations, regulation, public debate, and extensive litigation. Until the 1988 Surgeon General's conclusion that tobacco is an addictive drug is indisputably proven scientifically *and* fully accepted by society, it is unlikely that controversy over the addictive nature of this substance can be fully resolved. Further discussion of addiction and related issues are beyond the scope of this book, but the reader should be aware of various pathways to addiction and interventions to promote cessation after nicotine dependence is established.

Epidemiological studies have demonstrated that the majority of successful attempts to quit smoking occur without medical or pharmacological assistance (34, 85). Advising patients to quit has been demonstrated to double the quit rates (80). Generally, addressing motivational issues and using motivational techniques with education regarding associated risks can be helpful. A number of other nonpharmacological interventions have been found to be efficacious, including self-help materials, proactive telephone counseling, group counseling, individual counseling, social support, and recently developed technology-based interventions such as mobile apps and web-based interventions that are easily accessed 24/7 to support outpatient treatment (28, 32, 57, 58). Acupuncture, mesotherapy, hypnosis, and auriculotherapy have not been found to have positive smoking cessation results (32, 60). Pharmacological interventions include various forms of nicotine replacement therapy, bupropion, nortriptyline, and varenicline. A recent Cochrane review concluded that all of these interventions are effective at reducing smoking, and that combining nicotine replacement therapy with bupropion or varenicline is not more effective (14).

REFERENCES

1. [No authors listed]. Position statement on psychoactive substance use and dependence: up-date on marijuana and cocaine. Am. J. Psychiatry, *144*:5, 1987.
2. [No authors listed]. MDMA (Ecstasy) abuse. Bethesda, MD: National Institutes of Health, National Institute on Drug Abuse, 2017. Last accessed 12/22/17. https://d14rmgtrwzf5a.cloudfront.net/sites/default/files/1763-mdma-ecstasy-abuse.pdf.
3. Alberg, A. J., Shopland, D. R., and Cummings, K. M. The 2014 Surgeon General's report: commemorating the 50th Anniversary of the 1964 Report of the Advisory Committee to the US Surgeon General and updating the evidence on the health consequences of cigarette smoking. Am. J. Epidemiol., *179*:403–412, 2014.
4. Altman, I., Kroeger, H. H., Clark, D. A., Johnson, A. C., and Sheps, C. G. Dependence on barbiturates and other sedative drugs. JAMA, *193*:673–677, 1965.
5. American Psychiatric Association. *Diagnostic and Statistical Manual of Mental Disorders,* 4th edition, text revision. Washington, DC: Author, 2000.
6. American Psychiatric Association. *Diagnostic and Statistical Manual for Mental Disorders,* 5th edition. Washington, DC: Author, 2013.
7. Andrade, C. Cannabis and neuropsychiatry, 1: benefits and risks. J. Clin. Psychiatry, 77:e551–e554, 2016.
8. Andrade, C. Ketamine for depression, 1: clinical summary of issues related to efficacy, adverse effects, and mechanism of action. J. Clin. Psychiatry, 78:e415–e419, 2017.
9. Anthony, J. C., and Echeagaray-Wagner, F. Epidemiologic analysis of alcohol and tobacco use. Alcohol Res. Health, *24*:201–208, 2000.
10. Bearn, J., and O'Brien, M. "Addicted to euphoria": the history, clinical presentation, and management of party drug misuse. Int. Rev. Neurobiol., *120*:205–233, 2015.
11. Blachly, P. H. Management of the opiate abstinence syndrome. Am. J. Psychiatry, *122*:742–744, 1966.
12. Blanco, C., Hasin, D. S., Wall, M. M., Florez-Salamanca, L., Hoertel, N., Wang, S., Kerridge, B. T., and Olfson, M. Cannabis use and risk of psychiatric

disorders: prospective evidence from a US national longitudinal study. JAMA Psychiatry, 73:388–395, 2016.

13. Bloomquist, E. R. *Marijuana*. Toronto: Glencoe Press, 1968.

14. Cahill, K., Stevens, S., Perera, R., and Lancaster, T. Pharmacological interventions for smoking cessation: an overview and network meta-analysis. Cochrane Database Syst. Rev., 5:CD009329, 2013.

15. Childress, A. R., McLellan, A. T., and O'Brien, C. P. Abstinent opiate abusers exhibit conditioned craving, conditioned withdrawal and reductions in both through extinction. Br. J. Addict., 81:655–660, 1986.

16. Cicero, T. J., Ellis, M. S., and Kasper, Z. A. Increased use of heroin as an initiating opioid of abuse. Addict. Behav., 74:63–66, 2017.

17. Cicero, T. J., Ellis, M. S., Surratt, H. L., and Kurtz, S. P. The changing face of heroin use in the United States: a retrospective analysis of the past 50 years. JAMA Psychiatry, 71:821–826, 2014.

18. Clemens, K. J., McGregor, I. S., Hunt, G. E., and Cornish, J. L. MDMA, methamphetamine and their combination: possible lessons for party drug users from recent preclinical research. Drug Alcohol Rev., 26:9–15, 2007.

19. Cohen, S. Angel dust. JAMA, 238:515–516, 1977.

20. Compton, W. M., and Baler, R. The epidemiology of DSM-5 cannabis use disorders among U.S. adults: science to inform clinicians working in a shifting social landscape. Am. J. Psychiatry, 173:551–553, 2016.

21. Compton, W. M., Grant, B. F., Colliver, J. D., Glantz, M. D., and Stinson, F. S. Prevalence of marijuana use disorders in the United States: 1991-1992 and 2001-2002. JAMA, 291:2114–2121, 2004.

22. Compton, W. M., and Volkow, N. D. Improving outcomes for persons with opioid use disorders: buprenorphine implants to improve adherence and access to care. JAMA, 316:277–279, 2016.

23. Cooke, A., Fergeson, J., Bulkhi, A., and Casale, T. B. The electronic cigarette: the good, the bad, and the ugly. J. Allergy Clin. Immunol. Pract., 3:498–505, 2015.

24. Coop, C. E. The health consequences of smoking: nicotine addiction, a report by the Surgeon General. Rockville, MD: US Department of Health and Human Services, 1988. https://profiles.nlm.nih.gov/ps/access/nnbbzd.pdf.

25. Cottler, L. B., Ajinkya, S., Merlo, L. J., Nixon, S. J., Ben, A. A., and Gold, M. S. Lifetime psychiatric and substance use disorders among impaired physicians in a physicians health program: comparison to a general treatment population: psychopathology of impaired physicians. J. Addict. Med., 7:108–112, 2013.

26. Crits-Christoph, P., and Siqueland, L. Psychosocial treatment for drug abuse. Selected review and recommendations for national health care. Arch. Gen. Psychiatry, 53:749–756, 1996.

27. Das, S., Barnwal, P., Ramasamy, A., Sen, S., and Mondal, S. Lysergic acid diethylamide: a drug of 'use'? Ther. Adv. Psychopharmacol., 6:214–228, 2016.

28. Das, S., Tonelli, M., and Ziedonis, D. Update on smoking cessation: e-cigarettes, emerging tobacco products trends, and new technology-based interventions. Curr. Psychiatry Rep., 18:51, 2016.

29. Dutra, L., Stathopoulou, G., Basden, S. L., Leyro, T. M., Powers, M. B., and Otto, M. W. A meta-analytic review of psychosocial interventions for substance use disorders. Am. J. Psychiatry, 165:179–187, 2008.

30. Dwarakananth, S. C. Use of opium and cannabis in traditional systems of medicine in India. Bull. Narcotics, 17:15–19, 1965.

31. Feng, L. Y., Battulga, A., Han, E., Chung, H., and Li, J. H. New psychoactive substances of natural origin: a brief review. J. Food Drug Anal., 25:461–471, 2017.

32. Fiore, M., Bailey, W., Cohen, S., Dorfman, S. F. Goldstein, M. G., Gritz, E. R., Heyman, R. B., Holbrook, J., Jaen, C. R., Kottke, T. E., Lando, H. A., Mecklenburg, R. E., Mullen, P. D., Nett, L. M., Robinson, L., Stitzer, M. L., Tommasello, A. C., Villejo, L., and Vewers, M. E. Treating tobacco use and dependence. Clinical practice guideline. Rockville, MD: US Department of Health and Human Services, Public Health Service, 2000.

33. German, C. L., Fleckenstein, A. E., and Hanson, G. R. Bath salts and synthetic cathinones: an emerging designer drug phenomenon. Life Sci., 97:2–8, 2014.

34. Giovino, G. A. Epidemiology of tobacco use in the United States. Oncogene, 21:7326–7340, 2002.

35. Gold, M. S., Galanter, M., and Stimmel, B. Cocaine: a new epidemic (editorial). In *Cocaine: Pharmacology, Addiction and Therapy*, Gold, M. S., Galanter, M., Stimmel, B. (eds.). New York: Haworth Press, pp. 1–7, 1987.

36. Goldstein, R. A., DesLauriers, C., and Burda, A. M. Cocaine: history, social implications, and toxicity—a review. Dis. Mon., 55:6–38, 2009.

37. Goodwin, D. W. *Anxiety.* New York: Ballantine Books, 1986.

38. Grant, B. F. Comorbidity between DSM-IV drug use disorders and major depression: results of a national survey of adults. J. Subst. Abuse, 7:481–497, 1995.

39. Grant, B. F., Hasin, D. S., Stinson, F. S., Dawson, D. A., Patricia, C. S., June, R. W., and Huang, B. Co-occurrence of 12-month mood and anxiety disorders and personality disorders in the US: results from the national epidemiologic survey on alcohol and related conditions. J. Psychiatr. Res., 39:1–9, 2005.

40. Grant, B. F., Saha, T. D., Ruan, W. J., Goldstein, R. B., Chou, S. P., Jung, J., Zhang, H., Smith, S. M., Pickering, R. P., Huang, B., and Hasin, D. S. Epidemiology of DSM-5 drug use disorder: results from the National Epidemiologic Survey on Alcohol and Related Conditions-III. JAMA Psychiatry, 73:39–47, 2016.

41. Grucza, R. A., Agrawal, A., Krauss, M. J., Cavazos-Rehg, P. A., and Bierut, L. J. Recent trends in the prevalence of marijuana use and associated disorders in the United States. JAMA Psychiatry, 73:300–301, 2016.

42. Hall, A. P., and Henry, J. A. Acute toxic effects of 'Ecstasy' (MDMA) and related compounds: overview of pathophysiology and clinical management. Br. J. Anaesth., 96:678–685, 2006.

43. Hall, W., and Lynskey, M. Evaluating the public health impacts of legalizing recreational cannabis use in the United States. Addiction, 111:1764–1773, 2016.

44. Hamilton, G. R., and Baskett, T. F. In the arms of Morpheus: the development of morphine for postoperative pain relief. Can. J. Anaesth., 47:367–374, 2000.

45. Hardman, J. G., Lindbird, L. E., and Goodman, G. A. (eds.). *Goodman & Gilman's The Pharmacological Basis of Therapeutics*, 10th edition. New York: McGraw-Hill, 2001.

46. Henningfield, J. E., Cohen, C., and Slade, J. D. Is nicotine more addictive than cocaine? Br. J. Addict., 86:565–569, 1991.

47. Hoffman, D., Brunnermann, D. K., Gori, G. B., and Wynder, E. L. Carcinogenicity of marihuana smoke. In *Recent Advances of Phytochemistry*, Runeckles, V. C. (ed.). New York: Plenum, 1975.

48. Hughes, P. H., and Rieche, O. Heroin epidemics revisited. Epidemiol. Rev., 17:66–73, 1995.

49. Jamal, A., King, B. A., Neff, L. J., Whitmill, J., Babb, S. D., and Graffunder, C. M. Current cigarette smoking among adults—United States, 2005-2015. MMWR Morb. Mortal. Wkly. Rep., 65:1205–1211, 2016.

50. Johnston, L. D., O'Malley, P. M., and Bachman, J. C. Monitoring the Future. National survey results on drug use, 1975–2001. Volume 1. Secondary school students. NIH Publ. No. 01-5106. Bethesda, MD: National Institute on Drug Abuse, National Institutes of Health, 2002. Last accessed 12/23/17. http://monitoringthefuture. org/pubs/monographs/vol1_2001.pdf.

51. Johnston, L. D., O'Malley, P. M., Bachman, J. G., Schulenberg, J. E., and Miech, R. A. Monitoring the Future. National survey results on drug use, 1975–2015. Volume 2. College students and adults ages 19-55. Bethesda, MD: National Institute on Drug Abuse, National Institute on Drug Abuse, 2016. Last accessed 12/23/17. http://monitoringthefuture.org/pubs/monographs/mtf-vol2_2015. pdf.

52. Kalant, H. Adverse effects of cannabis on health: an update of the literature since 1996. Prog. Neuropsychopharmacol. Biol. Psychiatry, *28*:849–863, 2004.

53. Kaplan, L. Medical marijuana: legal and regulatory considerations. Nurse Pract., *40*:46–54, 2015.

54. Kessler, R. C., Aguilar-Gaxiola, S., Andrade, L., Bijl, R., Borges, G., Caraveo-Anduaga, J. J., Dewitt, D. J., Kolody, B., Merikangas, K. R., Molnar, B. E., Vega, W. A., Walters, E. D., Wittchen, H.-U., and Ustun, T. B. Mental substance comorbidities in the ICPE surveys. Psychiatr. Fenn., *32*:62–79, 2001.

55. Klein, T. W., Friedman, H., and Specter, S. Marijuana, immunity and infection. J. Neuroimmunol., *83*:102–115, 1998.

56. Koob, G. F., and Volkow, N. D. Neurobiology of addiction: a neurocircuitry analysis. Lancet Psychiatry, *3*:760–773, 2016.

57. Lancaster, T., and Stead, L. Individual behavioural counselling for smoking cessation. Cochrane Database Syst. Rev., *3*:CD001292, 2017.

58. Lancaster, T., Stead, L., Silagy, C., and Sowden, A. Effectiveness of interventions to help people stop smoking: findings from the Cochrane Library. BMJ, *321*:355–358, 2000.

59. Latimer, W., and Zur, J. Epidemiologic trends of adolescent use of alcohol, tobacco, and other drugs. Child Adolesc. Psychiatr. Clin. N. Am., *19*:451–464, 2010.

60. Le Foll, B., Melihan-Cheinin, P., Rostoker, G., and Lagrue, G. Smoking cessation guidelines: evidence-based recommendations of the French Health Products Safety Agency. Eur. Psychiatry, *20*:431–441, 2005.

61. Linszen, D., and van Amelsvoort, T. Cannabis and psychosis: an update on course and biological plausible mechanisms. Curr. Opin. Psychiatry, *20*:116–120, 2007.

62. Lodge, D., and Mercier, M. S. Ketamine and phencyclidine: the good, the bad and the unexpected. Br. J. Pharmacol., *172*:4254–4276, 2015.

63. Mandel W. The yuppie psychedelic. San Francisco Examiner, p. A2, June 10, 1984.

64. Maxwell, J. C., and Mendelson, B. What do we know now about the impact of the laws related to marijuana? J. Addict. Med., *10*:3–12, 2016.

65. McGlothlin, W. H., and Arnold, D. O. LSD revisited. A 10 year follow-up of medical LSD use. Arch. Gen. Psychiatry, *24*:35–49, 1971.

66. Mellman, T. A., and Uhde, T. W. Withdrawal syndrome with gradual tapering of alprazolam. Am. J. Psychiatry, *143*:1464–1466, 1986.

67. Meredith, C. W., Jaffe, C., Ang-Lee, K., and Saxon, A. J. Implications of chronic methamphetamine use: a literature review. Harv. Rev. Psychiatry, *13*:141–154, 2005.

68. Morris, H., and Wallach, J. From PCP to MXE: a comprehensive review of the non-medical use of dissociative drugs. Drug Test. Anal., *6*:614–632, 2014.

69. Muggli, M. E., Hurt, R. D., and Repace, J. The tobacco industry's political efforts to derail the EPA report on ETS. Am. J. Prev. Med., *26*:167–177, 2004.

70. Musto, D. F. *The American Disease: Origins of Narcotic Control*, 3rd edition. New York: Oxford University Press, 1999.

71. North, C. S., Eyrich, K. M., Pollio, D. E., and Spitznagel, E. L. Are rates of psychiatric disorders in the homeless population changing? Am. J. Publ. Health, *94*:103–108, 2004.

72. O'Toole, T. P., Conde-Martel, A., Gibbon, J. L., Hanusa, B. H., Freyder, P. J., and Fine, M. J. Substance-abusing urban homeless in the late 1990s: how do they differ from non-substance-abusing homeless persons? J. Urban Health, *81*:606–617, 2004.

73. Papaseit, E., Farre, M., Schifano, F., and Torrens, M. Emerging drugs in Europe. Curr. Opin. Psychiatry, 27:243–250, 2014.

74. Passie, T., and Benzenhofer, U. MDA, MDMA, and other "mescaline-like" substances in the US military's search for a truth drug (1940s to 1960s). Drug Test. Anal., *10*:72–80, 2018.

75. Patidar, K. A., Parwani, R., Wanjari, S. P., and Patidar, A. P. Various terminologies associated with areca nut and tobacco chewing: a review. J. Oral Maxillofac. Pathol., *19*:69–76, 2015.

76. Pourmand, A., Armstrong, P., Mazer-Amirshahi, M., and Shokoohi, H. The evolving high: new designer drugs of abuse. Hum. Exp. Toxicol., *33*:993–999, 2014.

77. Preskorn, S. H. A way of conceptualizing benzodiazepines to guide clinical use. J. Psychiatr. Pract., *21*:436–441, 2015.

78. Public Health Service. The health consequences of smoking: nicotine addiction. A report of the Surgeon General. DHHS publication no. (CDC) 88-8406. Washington, DC: U.S. Department of Health and Human Services, Public Health Service, 1988.

79. Regier, D. A., Farmer, M. E., Rae, D. S., Locke, B. Z., Keith, S. J., Judd, L. L., and Goodwin, F. K. Comorbidity of mental-disorders with alcohol and other drug abuse. Results from the Epidemiologic Catchment Area (ECA) study. JAMA, *264*:2511–2518, 1990.

80. Rigotti, N. A. Clinical practice. Treatment of tobacco use and dependence. N. Engl. J. Med., *346*:506–512, 2002.

81. Robins, L. N. *Follow-up of Vietnam Drug Users*. Washington, DC: National Institute of Drug Abuse, Special Action Office, 1973.

82. Roueché, B. *Alcohol*. New York: Grove Press, 1962.

83. Rubin, V., and Comitas, L. *Ganja in Jamaica*. The Hague and Paris: Mouton, 1975.

84. Sachdev, G., Gesin, G., Christmas, A. B., and Sing, R. F. Failure of lorazepam to treat alprazolam withdrawal in a critically ill patient. World J. Crit. Care Med., *3*:42–44, 2014.

85. Satcher, D. Reducing tobacco use: a report of the Surgeon General. Atlanta, GA: U.S. Department of Health and Human Services, US Centers for Disease Control and Prevention, National Center for Chronic Disease Prevention and Health Promotion, Office on Smoking and Health, 2000. Last accessed 5/22/18. https://www.cdc.gov/tobacco/data_statistics/sgr/2000/index.htm.

86. Schifano, F. A bitter pill. Overview of ecstasy (MDMA, MDA) related fatalities. Psychopharmacol. (Berl)., *173*:242–248, 2004.

87. Schneider, S., and Diehl, K. Vaping as a catalyst for smoking? An initial model on the initiation of electronic cigarette use and the transition to tobacco smoking among adolescents. Nicotine Tob. Res., *18*:647–653, 2016.

88. Schuckit, M. A. Treatment of opioid-use disorders. N. Engl. J. Med., 375:357–368, 2016.
89. Schwartz, R. H. LSD. Its rise, fall, and renewed popularity among high school students. Pediatr. Clin. North Am., 42:403–413, 1995.
90. Sertürner, F. W. Apotheker und Chemisten. Trommsdorff"s Journal der Pharmazie fur Aerzte, 14:47–93, 1806.
91. Sharma, B., Bruner, A., Barnett, G., and Fishman, M. Opioid use disorders. Child Adolesc. Psychiatr. Clin. N. Am., 25:473–487, 2016.
92. Sharma, T. D. Clinical observations of patients who used tetrahydrocannabinol (THC) intravenously. Behav. Neuropsychiatry, 4:17–19, 1972.
93. Soyka, M. Treatment of benzodiazepine dependence. N. Engl. J. Med., 376:1147–1157, 2017.
94. Spitzer, R. L., Endicott, J., and Gibbon, M. Crossing the border into borderline personality and borderline schizophrenia. The development of criteria. Arch. Gen. Psychiatry, 36:17–24, 1979.
95. Storck, M., Black, L., and Liddell, M. Inhalant abuse and dextromethorphan. Child Adolesc. Psychiatr. Clin. N. Am., 25:497–508, 2016.
96. Thomas, G., Kloner, R. A., and Rezkalla, S. Adverse cardiovascular, cerebrovascular, and peripheral vascular effects of marijuana inhalation: what cardiologists need to know. Am. J. Cardiol., 113:187–190, 2014.
97. U.S. Department of Health and Human Services. The health consequences of smoking: nicotine addiction. A report of the Surgeon General. DHHS Publication No. (CDC) 88-8406. Washington, DC: U.S. Department of Health and Human Services, Public Health Services, 1988.
98. Vaillant, G. E. A 12-year follow-up of New York narcotic addicts. Arch. Gen. Psychiatry, 15:599–609, 1966.
99. Vearrier, D., Greenberg, M. I., Miller, S. N., Okaneku, J. T., and Haggerty, D. A. Methamphetamine: history, pathophysiology, adverse health effects, current trends, and hazards associated with the clandestine manufacture of methamphetamine. Dis. Mon., 58:38–89, 2012.
100. Volkow, N. D., Baler, R. D., Compton, W. M., and Weiss, S. R. Adverse health effects of marijuana use. N. Engl. J. Med, 370:2219–2227, 2014.
101. Volkow, N. D., Frieden, T. R., Hyde, P. S., and Cha, S. S. Medication-assisted therapies—tackling the opioid-overdose epidemic. N. Engl. J. Med., 370:2063–2066, 2014.
102. Warner, L. A., Kessler, R. C., Hughes, M., Anthony, J. C., and Nelson, C. B. Prevalence and correlates of drug use and dependence in the United States. Results from the National Comorbidity Survey. Arch. Gen. Psychiatry, 52:219–229, 1995.
103. Washton, A. M., and Gold, M. S. Cocaine: A Clinician's Handbook. New York: Guilford Press, 1987.
104. Weinstein, A. M., Rosca, P., Fattore, L., and London, E. D. Synthetic cathinone and cannabinoid designer drugs pose a major risk for public health. Front. Psychiatry, 8:156, 2017.
105. Weinstein, S. P., Gottheil, E., Smith, R. H., and Migrala, K. A. Cocaine users seen in medical practice. Am. J. Drug Alcohol Abuse, 12:341–354, 1986.
106. Wilson, D. P., and Zhang, L. Characteristics of HIV epidemics driven by men who have sex with men and people who inject drugs. Curr. Opin. HIV AIDS, 6:94–101, 2011.

107. Wonderlich, S. A., Lilenfeld, L. R., Riso, L. P., Engel, S., and Mitchell, J. E. Personality and anorexia nervosa. Int. J. Eat. Disord., 37 *Suppl*:S68–S71, 2005.
108. World Health Organization. *WHO Framework Convention on Tobacco Control.* Geneva: WHO Document Production Services, 2005.
109. Zhang, M. W., and Ho, R. C. The cannabis dilemma: a review of its associated risks and clinical efficacy. J. Addict., *2015*:707596, 2015.

CHAPTER 13

ↄⱱↄ

Delirium and Dementia
(Neurocognitive Disorders)

Delirium, amnestic disorders, and dementia have often been referred to as "organic brain syndromes," or historically, simply as "brain syndromes." The clinical diagnosis is based primarily on the mental status examination and usually is applied to patients with recognizable medical and neurological disorders affecting function and/or brain structure. The older, very broad term, "brain syndrome," can still be found in the literature, and "acute brain syndrome" and "chronic brain syndrome" are still utilized by many outside psychiatry. They are used in this introduction for historical accuracy and as points of reference. Currently, in psychiatry, an acute brain syndrome is known as a delirium, and it is usually brief and presumably reversible. Delirium can be associated with excitement and agitation, and it is also frequently associated with hallucinations and delusions. Amnestic disorders are uncommon and are characterized by a disturbance of memory. Chronic brain syndrome, or dementia, is frequently progressive and chances of recovery are often limited. *DSM-5* introduced the term "neurocognitive disorders" to broadly encompass these organic disorders along with various specifiers (6). Time will tell if it gains acceptance.

The diagnoses depend on finding impairment of consciousness/inattention, orientation, memory, and other intellectual or cognitive functions. Additional psychiatric symptoms may occur, including delusions, hallucinations, depression, obsessions, and personality change. Judgment is impaired. Patients may or may not be aware of experiencing the disorder.

HISTORICAL BACKGROUND

It is not known with any certainty when the clinical picture of brain syndrome was first recognized as distinct from other psychiatric disorders. On this subject, extensive interesting material is presented in an annotated anthology of selected medical texts (64).

One of the earliest descriptions in English was provided in 1615 by a clergyman, Thomas Adams, in his treatise *Mystical Bedlam, the World of Mad-Men* (4). He referred to "some mad, that can rightly judge of the things they see, as touching imagination and phantasie: but for cogitation and reason, they swarve from naturale judgment" (p. 35). In 1694 William Salmon (99) described in detail a case of dementia and noted that the patient was "not mad, or distracted like a man in Bedlam [but] decayed in his Intellectuals" (p. 778).

In 1761 Giovanni Battista Morgagni, the great Italian pioneer in morphologic pathology, who first systematically correlated clinical features and course with postmortem findings, described certain areas of "hardness" in the brains of former mental patients (83). He emphasized, however, that the correlation between clinical picture and anatomical findings was not consistent. Morgagni's work set the stage for Antoine Laurant Jesse Bayle who, in 1822, published the first systematic clinicopathological study of paresis. In this study the clinical symptoms, including progressive dementia, were correlated with changes in brain parenchyma and meninges (13). Bayle's findings were confirmed in 1826 by Louis Florentin Calmeil (26).

Another milestone in the understanding of brain syndrome was Korsakoff's investigation of the disorder that bears his name (117). His observations, reported between 1887 and 1891, correlated to a particular form of dementia manifested by extreme amnesia with lesions of the brainstem.

Years of accumulation of case reports and clinical experience indicated that inattention to surroundings, disorientation, and memory impairment were the hallmarks of a clinical syndrome seen frequently in the presence of intoxications, systemic infections, or demonstrable brain damage. Early systematic investigations were infrequent. However, modern necropsy studies have consistently found that brain syndromes, particularly the chronic forms, are associated with organic brain pathology.

EPIDEMIOLOGY

There have been a number of relatively narrow epidemiological studies of delirium. It occurs commonly in the presence of pneumonia, systemic infections, AIDS, congestive heart failure, high fever, fluid and electrolyte imbalance, burns, dialysis, transplant, stroke, postoperative state (particularly cardiac and hip), post-injury state, advanced age, and intoxication or withdrawal with alcohol or other drugs. Reports of prevalence in hospitalized general medical patients range from 11% to 42% (105) and in the hospitalized elderly with dementia from 24% to 89% (100). Up to 51% of postoperative patients (115) and 80% of terminal patients near death (80) develop delirium. Seven screening instruments developed to aid assessment can be located in the literature as of 2014 (72), but concerns about ascertainment, definition of delirium, wide range of estimates, and generalizability abound. One issue endorsed by almost all experts is the concern that prevalence numbers significantly underestimate the problem.

The prevalence of the amnestic syndrome known as Wernicke-Korsakoff syndrome has been estimated through postmortem studies at between 0.8% and 2.8% (16, 57, 104). The upper range estimate is based on an epidemic of cases in Australia in the 1970s and 1980s. Concerns have been raised that the disorder is both under-identified and poorly treated (65, 104).

Early epidemiological studies of dementia had serious flaws related to a number of factors, such as extrapolation from hospitalization rates (78). It is now known that dementia of the Alzheimer's type (late-onset dementia) and vascular disease of the brain are two of the most common and perhaps best understood of the illnesses manifesting as dementia. Other causes of dementia, including Parkinson disease with dementia, dementia with Lewy bodies, and the frontotemporal dementias (17, 33, 43, 62), are described but are much less well understood. The prevalence of Alzheimer's disease (AD) and vascular disease increases with age. Alzheimer's disease is the most common, affecting an estimated 24 million people globally and accounts for 60%–80% of the dementia cases (81, 90, 108). Incidence (and prevalence) of AD remains rare in individuals under the age of 50 (90) (see "Biological Findings" section later in this chapter), but yearly risk after 65 (to 69) appears to be about 0.5% (66, 81). Subsequently, the prevalence of the illness is thought to double every 5 years, and one-third of people over the age of 85 manifest symptoms of AD (22).

CLINICAL PICTURE

Delirium is nearly always associated with medical, surgical, or neurological disorders or with drug intoxication or withdrawal. This association is so consistent that an unexplained delirium should alert the physician to the likelihood that such a disorder exists or is developing. A patient with pneumonia, for example, will sometimes present with a delirium hours before the other clinical findings appear.

A delirium may vary clinically, but two features are of special diagnostic importance: disorder of consciousness (i.e., reduced awareness of the environment) and change in cognition (i.e., impairment of recent memory and/or orientation). Without at least one of these, the diagnosis can only be suspected.

Patients may complain that they do not understand where they are and that they cannot find the bathroom; or they may bitterly insist that no one has fed them, even though the remains of the last meal are on the tray next to their bed. Other common clinical features include a depressed or fearful mood; apathy; irritability; impaired judgment; suspiciousness; delusions; hallucinations; and combative, uncooperative, or frightened behavior.

Examples of clinical features of delirium are a labile, shifting affect with sudden crying spells; an argumentative, demanding manner ("I've called and called and no one pays any attention to me"); visual hallucinations of frightening or threatening faces ("They're grinning at me all the time, . . .they know something bad will happen"); unreasonable pressure for changes in room, personnel, or food; and inappropriate efforts to get dressed and leave the hospital or to "escape" other patients who "want to hurt me."

The combination of impairment of consciousness/inattention, disorientation, impaired memory, suspiciousness, hallucinations, and combative or frightened behavior constitutes delirium. This can be the most dramatic, clinically severe form of delirium. It may develop rapidly without any preceding manifestations or gradually in a patient who has been quietly confused and apathetic for many hours or days. Frequently it can be superimposed on a chronic state of dementia.

A delirium may fluctuate strikingly from day to day and even from hour to hour. Some patients show a diurnal pattern with the most obvious and severe manifestations at night. They may appear normal in the morning except for haziness about the night before and yet be frankly disoriented, confused, and hallucinating at night. In some cases, the patient's mental status must be checked repeatedly to elicit disorientation or recent memory difficulty.

Disorientation may relate to time, place, or person. The first is the most common, the last the least common. Minor errors by patients who have been sick or hospitalized for some time should not receive undue emphasis. But persistent inability to recall the month or year correctly, especially if the correct answers have been offered recently, recurrent failure to identify where the patient is, or repeated inability to recall recent events correctly can be diagnostic. Because the manifestations are often more definite at night, the first indication of delirium may be recorded in the nurse's notes. A report of the patient mistaking the nurse for someone else—such as a neighbor or relative ("What is my sister doing here?") or experiencing hallucinations—is sometimes ignored until the patient is frankly disoriented and combative.

Delirium seen in a general hospital usually indicates that the patient is seriously ill physically (86). Available evidence suggests that when the condition interferes with nursing care or treatment or when it disturbs other patients, the prognosis is poorer than is the case for patients with similar medical illnesses matched for age, sex, and race who do not have delirium (28, 44).

Wernicke-Korsakoff syndrome (amnestic disorder) is associated with a long history of alcohol use along with the thiamine deficiency that results in a delirium (Wernicke encephalopathy). It can be caused by malnourishment related to other illnesses, including marasmus, gastric cancer, and HIV (71). Wernicke encephalopathy may also be seen following bariatric surgery (3, 107, 121), in anorexia nervosa (40), long-term total parental nutrition (TPN) (53), acute pancreatitis (8, 12, 31, 111), and thyrotoxicosis (18, 42). Patients presenting with the delirium may clear or they may develop Korsakoff syndrome, a permanent memory impairment. Patients with the memory impairment cannot recall (anterograde) newly learned information (e.g., nurse's name, ward number, etc.) or remember (retrograde) information after the Wernicke encephalopathy began (e.g., how they got to the hospital, who came with them, etc.). Individuals with the severe memory disturbance have significant functional disturbance of everyday living characterized by not being able to meet their basic needs.

Unfortunately, the diagnosis of Wernicke-Korsakoff is frequently missed, with autopsy studies (55, 56, 76) revealing more than 80% of confirmed cases had not been diagnosed while alive (65).

The diagnostic criteria for dementia are available in the *DSM-5*. Many patients with dementia may present with depressive symptoms (74) or somatic complaints such as headache, abdominal pain, and constipation. Others are brought to physicians by relatives because of temper outbursts, socially embarrassing behavior, or suspiciousness. The cognitive and memory impairment may become evident only as the patient's history is elicited.

Patients with depression may complain of poor memory, and some studies have revealed impairment of short-term memory in many such patients. The memory difficulty improves with remission of the depression (109).

Sometimes, however, it is important to distinguish between complaints of memory difficulty (pseudodementia) and actual impairment of memory. Some have argued that the term "pseudodementia" can be misleading because depression may also include significant cognitive impairment as part of the clinical picture, especially in older patients.

It has therefore been suggested that a more appropriate name for this condition might be "cognitive impairment of depression." In some middle-aged and older patients suffering from depression, the complaint of memory impairment is disproportionately greater than the degree of memory impairment noted on systematic testing, and the perceived memory difficulty subsides as the depression improves (27, 68, 82, 119). Clearly the relationship between depression and cognitive impairment may sometimes be puzzling. It is important to recognize that some patients with depression, especially older ones, may present with enough cognitive difficulty to raise differential diagnostic problems. In such cases, physicians should be cautious about making a firm diagnosis and be prepared to change their diagnosis as the clinical picture unfolds.

In dementia, the patient's insight may vary greatly. Sometimes, especially earlier in the illness, the patient may volunteer, "I keep losing things. I don't know where I left them. I occasionally can't remember the directions when I drive home." Often, however, and especially as the illness progresses, the patient may deny any memory difficulty and insist that he or she was preoccupied or distracted by worries or interruptions. Inability to follow directions and confusion about what others intend may lead to irritability and anger: "Nobody tries to explain things to me. Nobody cares about how I feel—I'll show them." Frustration at being unable to accomplish specific tasks, including specific cognitive tests, frequently leads to suspicion and resistance: "That's a silly thing to do. I could do it if I really wanted to, but I don't see a good reason for it. You're trying to trip me up and fool me." Inattention to cleanliness and grooming, deterioration in table manners, the use of abusive and foul language, social withdrawal and a generally inconsiderate manner, sudden and seemingly unprovoked outbursts of anger, and even physical violence present increasingly heavy burdens to the family as the disorder worsens; they may necessitate institutionalization.

The most important point about dementia is that in some cases the underlying illness is treatable (59). These cases should be recognized as early as possible because recovery may be related to the duration of the dementia. Drug intoxication (14, 89, 103, 114, 116), liver failure (101), hypothyroidism (39, 106), pernicious anemia (110), paresis (50), subdural hematomas, benign brain tumors (9), and normal-pressure hydrocephalus

(1, 91) are infrequent but recognizable causes of reversible dementia, though debate continues about the diagnosis and validity of the last entity (7). Recurrent hypoglycemia arising from insulin treatment of diabetes, pancreatic islet-cell tumors, or the too-rapid alimentary absorption of glucose in patients who have undergone subtotal gastric resection may also lead to severe dementia (10, 11, 25). All these disorders may be correctable. Chronic alcohol abuse has been associated with a memory impairment (77, 79, 96) that is distinct from the Wernicke-Korsakoff syndrome and, if recognized early, often can be reversed by abstention from further drinking; however, debate continues about the validity of an alcohol-induced dementia separate from Wernicke encephalopathy or hepatic encephalopathy (113). Dementia caused by aluminum intoxication from the water used in such great quantities during chronic renal dialysis is now avoided through modern water purification techniques in use since 1980 (2, 92).

Most cases of dementia are the result of intrinsic brain disease or arteriosclerotic changes in the blood vessels supplying the brain. The term "vascular dementia" is preferred over the older term "arteriosclerotic dementia," reflecting the recognition that the dementia results from loss of brain tissue. Other causes of dementia include a variety of previously mentioned presenile brain degenerations (mostly untreatable), central nervous system (CNS) disease (some treatable), systemic disease (mostly treatable), and medications or substances (some correctable). Of particular interest is the dementia associated with the CNS involving the acquired immune deficiency syndrome (AIDS). Indeed, dementia may be the first clinical manifestation of human immunodeficiency virus (HIV) infection (51). Finally, dementia may arise from more than one etiology and sometimes from multiple etiologies, making it difficult for clinicians to address the source of the problem (Box 13.1).

NATURAL HISTORY

As noted, delirium may occur in the course of various medical illnesses. Often it is impossible to determine the most crucial factor in a patient with simultaneous heart failure, infection, fever, and dehydration who is also receiving a variety of medications. Generally, the delirium subsides as the underlying abnormalities are corrected. Sometimes, when patients have been very sick and have had a prolonged delirium, many days pass after medical abnormalities are controlled before the mental picture clears. Acute delirium resulting from drug intoxication or drug withdrawal (e.g., alcohol,

BOX 13.1
CAUSES OF DEMENTIA

Primary central nervous system degenerative disorders (not including Alzheimer's disease/vascular dementia)

1. Frontotemporal dementias (including Pick disease)
2. Dementia with Lewy bodies
3. Parkinson disease with dementia
4. Huntington disease

Central nervous system disease

1. Brain injury (concussion/damage)
2. Neoplasms
3. Vascular disease
4. Normal pressure hydrocephalus
5. Viral/bacterial infections
6. Subdural hematoma
7. Chronic seizures

Systemic disease

1. Nutritional deficits (niacin, B-12)
2. Hepatic disease
3. Renal disease
4. Wilson disease
5. Endocrine (hypothyroidism, hypoparathyroidism)
6. Multiple sclerosis
7. Chronic metabolic dysregulation (hypocalcemia, hypoglycemia)
8. Autoimmune disease
9. Immune system disease
10. Cardiovascular disease

Medication(s)/substance(s)

1. Alcohol dementia

Adapted from diagnostic criteria in the Diagnostic and Statistical Manual of Mental Disorders, fourth edition, text revision. Washington, DC: American Psychiatric Association, 2000.

barbiturates, or benzodiazepines) nearly always subsides within a few days after discontinuing the drug.

Wernicke-Korsakoff syndrome develops after many years of heavy alcohol use and poor nutrition. Patients usually present in a marked delirious state without other classic signs of delirium tremens (autonomic instability and tremulousness). Patients may demonstrate ataxia. As the confusion clears, significant anterograde and retrograde amnesia become prominent. Interestingly, remote memory and intellectual function is spared. The deficit can be permanent (71), although in one series of patients, 20% did resolve (98).

Dementia usually develops insidiously. The early manifestations may be subtle, and only in retrospect does their significance become evident. Fatigability, moodiness, distractibility, depression, irritability, and carelessness may be present long before memory difficulty, intellectual deterioration, and disorientation can be clearly and easily detected. Depending on the underlying brain disease, the dementia may either stabilize for long periods or progress to total incapacity and death (17, 78, 97, 118). Both delirium and dementia appear to be associated with an excess mortality (15).

BIOLOGICAL FINDINGS

Delirium is a perturbation in the function of the brain caused by extrinsic factors. Certain vulnerabilities to this alteration, including age, illness, brain disease, or medication(s), may all play a part in this disorder. Genetic factors are not considered to play an active role. Although rarely used, the electroencephalogram (EEG) has historically been identified as the most reliable marker of integrated brain function (21). In their seminal work on delirium, published in 1959, Engel and Romano (41) reviewed signs of delirium and described "overall slowing of posterior background rhythm" (p. 530). They reported the electrical changes as reversible and associated with the level of the disturbance.

Wernicke-Korsakoff syndrome is widely accepted to be produced also by an extrinsic factor, namely thiamine deficiency. Because other causes of thiamine deficiency produce the same type of disorder, genetic factors have not generally been considered to actively contribute to the illness. However, a more recent review (104) has suggested some possible genetic contribution in thiamine-inadequate diets. The generally agreed-upon pathological lesions are located bilaterally in the temporal lobes and involve the associated hippocampus and mammillary body (57, 67).

For many years, a distinction was made between presenile dementia (onset in the fourth or fifth decade of life) and late-onset dementia-AD. Over time, the anatomical findings (senile plaques, neurofibrillary tangles, and granulovacuolar degenerative changes) of the two groups of patients have been found to be similar (97, 118), as are the clinical presentations. (See also "Family and Genetic Studies" section later in this chapter.)

As a direct result of the population's aging and the cost of caring for these individuals (estimated at $172 billion in 2010) (5), there has been an extraordinary effort expended to clearly understand the pathological process (and develop treatments). Space limitation does not permit detailed review of these evolving efforts (literally thousands of references) proffered to assist the field. Fortunately, there is now widespread agreement that the central pathological changes in brain tissue are increased levels of amyloid-β (Aβ) peptide found extracellularly in neuritic plaques and microtubule assembly protein found in the cell and described as a neurofibrillary tangle composed of hyperphosphorylated tau (p-tau) (90). As these downstream neuropathological changes are being further defined, the upstream genetics, initiation, evolution, risk factors, and potential treatments are coming more into focus.

Vascular dementia is generally thought to result from cerebrovascular disease or trauma. The course is usually associated with the underlying cause and may be rapid, stepwise progressive, or plateau without advance. The association between large strokes and detectable changes in cognition is understandable, but the precise correspondence of slow loss of neurons to progression of formal dementia is less clear.

Computerized tomography (CT), magnetic resonance imaging (MRI), and positron emission testing (PET) may contribute valuable information for the diagnosis of dementia, but it is important to appreciate that the correlation between cognitive impairment and the radiological findings is sometimes poor. It is likely, however, that refinements in all techniques will improve such correlations in the future.

COMPLICATIONS

Faulty judgment in important decisions, inability to care for oneself, accidents, aggression, and suicide are the principal complications of delirium and dementia. One of the more difficult decisions physicians must make concerns patients with delirium or dementia whose behavior raises questions about their mental capacity. At some point in the course of many chronic brain illnesses, the patients' confusion, forgetfulness, temper outbursts, and questionable financial dealings will lead relatives and friends to question whether they are still competent to handle their affairs and care for themselves properly. Losing or giving away large sums of money, writing bad checks, extreme carelessness of dress, unprecedented sexual behavior (e.g., displaying genitals or molesting children), wandering away from home, getting lost, and unpredictable temper displays may require legal action to protect patients from their own acts and permit extended placement in a safe environment. In some cases of delirium, it is not possible to tell whether the patient jumped from a window with the intention of committing suicide or fell because of confusion and fear.

Dementia complicated by secondary depression is one of the psychiatric disorders associated with suicide risk, though it accounts for only a small portion of suicides (93). The role of dementia—especially that of Alzheimer disease—as an important risk factor for serious falls has also been recognized (84).

FAMILY AND GENETIC STUDIES

Investigations of the familial prevalence of dementia have primarily focused on the most frequent form of late-onset dementia-AD. Of note, however, substantial numbers of family (19, 20) and linkage (47, 48) studies over the last 30 years have shown that less than 5% of dementia cases occur with early onset (prior to age 65), follow an autosomal dominate pattern of transmission, and are linked to three chromosomes (1, 14, and 21) (47, 54). Each gene was located by studying multiple generations of families with early dementia and identifying the mutations (chromosome 1—presenilin-2, chromosome 14—presenilin-1, and chromosome 21—amyloid precursor protein) (49, 58, 61, 75, 102), which alter the production of proteins responsible for AD. This autosomal dominant theory has become widely accepted (73). Careful elucidation of these mechanisms also led to the finding that late-onset dementia (AD) follows a sporadic and non-Mendelian form of inheritance (73). This disorder is associated with Apolipoprotein E (APOE) (85), which has three variants and is not a mutation but is considered a susceptibility gene, meaning that it is neither necessary nor sufficient to cause AD. However, presence of the APOE-4 allele increases the risk of the disorder. Calculations of the risk of AD in a multitude of studies (while there is some variance) have revealed that one APOE-4 allele increases chances three-fold to five-fold, and having two APOE-4 alleles renders an eight-fold risk (29, 88). Although APOE is the most significant known genetic risk, it does not explain all the genetic risk (88).

Genome-wide association studies have begun to suggest a contribution by other potential risk factors, including cholesterol, inflammatory, and endosomal synaptic vesicle recycling mechanisms (69).

Additional support for the genetic theory in late-onset AD is drawn from findings that first-degree relatives of those with AD have doubled lifetime risk (52) and AD occurs more frequently in monozygotic twins than in dizygotes (46). Finally, in the largest twin study of dementia conducted on Swedish twins, heritability was estimated at 58%–79% depending on the model applied (46).

Much work remains in order to fully understand the genetic (and environmental) contributions to this disorder.

DIFFERENTIAL DIAGNOSIS

Other psychiatric conditions may be mimicked by delirium or dementia: patients' anxiety attacks may suggest a primary anxiety disorder; low mood and apathy, an affective disorder; hallucinations and delusions, schizophrenia. The crucial question in each case is whether the patient exhibits definite inattention, disorientation, or memory impairment. These mental status abnormalities, when clearly present, are pathognomonic of a neurocognitive disorder; they are not manifestations of an uncomplicated, so-called functional disorder. If a patient with another psychiatric illness develops inattention, disorientation, or memory impairment, one should suspect that something else has developed: a drug reaction or medical or neurological illness.

When a patient is unable or unwilling to cooperate in the mental status examination, a delirium may be suspected. If there has been a sudden change in behavior, speech, or manner, and if the behavioral change develops in a clinical situation that frequently predisposes to a delirium, the diagnosis should be considered. A definitive diagnosis must await evidence of inattention, disorientation, or memory impairment; these will usually become apparent as the patient is observed carefully.

CLINICAL MANAGEMENT

Correction of the underlying medical or neurological condition, whenever possible, is the principal aim of therapy for patients with delirium or dementia. At the same time, certain measures often help in the management of the neurocognitive disorder itself. Good nursing care is very important (86, 87). A calm, sympathetic, reassuring approach can turn a frightened, combative patient into a quiet, cooperative one. Patients with a delirium often misinterpret stimuli and have unpredictable emotional responses. It is important, therefore, to provide a familiar, stable, unambiguous environment for such patients. Repeated simple explanations and frequent reassurance from familiar nurses, attendants, or relatives may be helpful (86). Patients do better with constant light; shadows or the dark easily frightens them.

Only the smallest effective doses of drugs acting on the CNS (including antipsychotics) should be used (86, 87) because patients with delirium are frequently sensitive to these agents. Delirium is, in fact, often precipitated by sedatives or hypnotics and may subside when such drugs are discontinued. No CNS-active medicine is entirely safe (86). Careful attention to dosage and mental status is most important.

Patients may need to be kept from harming themselves. Usually a relative, friend, or nurse who is able to be with the patient constantly—talking to the patient, explaining things, reassuring him or her—can calm the patient enough to permit appropriate care without restraints on a general hospital service (86, 87).

For patients with agitated delirium, physical restraint may be necessary (63), for example, to prevent the confused or frightened patient from pulling out intravenous lines and urinary catheters or striking caregivers, and to avoid falls. Obviously, a restrained patient should be watched carefully, and the previously described measures should be continued with the hope of calming the person quickly, making any period of restraint brief (86, 87).

The specific treatment for Wernicke-Korsakoff syndrome is initially parental thiamine followed by oral administration. Abstinence from further use of alcohol and good nutrition are the goals (71). A substantial number of these individuals require careful monitoring in the home or institution.

Organized groups (e.g., Alzheimer's Association and others) for relatives of patients with dementia patients can be very helpful in providing emotional support and practical suggestions for handling the wide range of problems that dementia presents to families (45). Too often the impact on family members is overwhelming, and this must be considered by the physician so that appropriate steps can be taken to reduce the burden, at least intermittently (36–38).

Currently, no pharmacological agent(s) has been developed that changes the pathology or alters the course of AD. It should be noted that a number of medications have been developed to ameliorate and/or minimize effects of progression of Alzheimer dementia (35). Potent, centrally active, reversible acetylcholinesterase inhibitors—tacrine, donepezil, rivastigmine, galantamine, and memantine—have been reported to have efficacy in clinical trials (23, 24, 34, 70, 95, 120) and are standard therapy (35, 60), but are not without risks. All have been associated with improvements in global functioning and cognition (30, 94, 112, 120). The result of these improvements has been a reduction in impaired behavior, stabilization (albeit temporary) of daily living activities, delay of placement in the nursing home setting, and decreased caregiver burden (32).

REFERENCES

1. [No authors listed]. Communicating hydrocephalus. Lancet, 2:1011–1012, 1977.
2. [No authors listed]. Dialysis dementia in Europe. Report from the Registration Committee of the European Dialysis and Transplant Association. Lancet, 2:190–192, 1980.
3. Aasheim, E. T. Wernicke encephalopathy after bariatric surgery: a systematic review. Ann. Surg., 248:714–720, 2008.
4. Adams, T. *Mystical Bedlam, the World of Mad-Men.* London: George Purslowe for Clement Knight, 1615.
5. Alzheimer's Association. 2010 Alzheimer's disease facts and figures. Alzheimers Dement., 6:158–194, 2010.
6. American Psychiatric Association. *Diagnostic and Statistical Manual for Mental Disorders,* 5th edition. Washington, DC: Author, 2013.
7. Anderson, M. Normal pressure hydrocephalus. Br. Med. J., 293:837–838, 1986.
8. Arana-Guajardo, A. C., Camara-Lemarroy, C. R., Rendon-Ramirez, E. J., Jaquez-Quintana, J. O., Gongora-Rivera, J. F., and Galarza-Delgado, D. A. Wernicke encephalopathy presenting in a patient with severe acute pancreatitis. J. Pancreas, 13:104–107, 2012.
9. Avery, T. L. Seven cases of frontal tumour with psychiatric presentation. Br. J. Psychiatry, 119:19–23, 1971.
10. Bale, R. N. Brain damage in diabetes mellitus. Br. J. Psychiatry, 122:337–341, 1973.
11. Banerji, N. K., and Hurwitz, L. J. Nervous system manifestations after gastric surgery. Acta Neurol. Scand., 47:485–513, 1971.
12. Basit, S., Elsas, T., Kvistad, K. A., and Hosoien, L. S. Wernicke's encephalopathy because of pancreatitis in a young boy. Acta Ophthalmol., 89:e656–e657, 2011.
13. Bayle, A. L. J. *Reserches sur l'arachnitis chronique.* Paris: Gabon, 1822.
14. Bergman, H., Borg, S., and Holm, L. Neuropsychological impairment and exclusive abuse of sedatives or hypnotics. Am. J. Psychiatry, 137:215–217, 1980.
15. Black, D. W., Warrack, G., and Winokur, G. The Iowa Record-Linkage Study. I. Excess mortality among patients with organic mental disorders. Arch. Gen. Psychiatry, 42:78–81, 1985.
16. Blansjaar, B. A., Horjus, M. C., and Nijhuis, H. G. Prevalence of the Korsakoff syndrome in The Hague, The Netherlands. Acta Psychiatr. Scand., 75:604–1607, 1987.

17. Bolla, L. R., Filley, C. M., and Palmer, R. M. Dementia DDx. Office diagnosis of the four major types of dementia. Geriatrics, 55:34–46, 2000.
18. Bonucchi, J., Hassan, I., Policeni, B., and Kaboli, P. Thyrotoxicosis associated Wernicke's encephalopathy. J. Gen. Intern. Med., 23:106–109, 2008.
19. Breitner, J. C., Folstein, M. F., and Murphy, E. A. Familial aggregation in Alzheimer dementia—I. A model for the age-dependent expression of an autosomal dominant gene. J. Psychiatr. Res., 20:31–43, 1986.
20. Breitner, J. C., Murphy, E. A., and Folstein, M. F. Familial aggregation in Alzheimer dementia—II. Clinical genetic implications of age-dependent onset. J. Psychiatr. Res., 20:45–55, 1986.
21. Brenner, R. P. Utility of EEG in delirium: past views and current practice. Int. Psychogeriatr., 3:211–229, 1991.
22. Brookmeyer, R., Gray, S., and Kawas, C. Projections of Alzheimer's disease in the United States and the public health impact of delaying disease onset. Am. J. Publ. Health, 88:1337–1342, 1998.
23. Bullock, R. New drugs for Alzheimer's disease and other dementias. Br. J. Psychiatry, 180:135–139, 2002.
24. Bullock, R. Galantamine: use in Alzheimer's disease and related disorders. Expert Rev. Neurother., 4:153–163, 2004.
25. Burton, R. A., and Raskin, N. H. Alimentary (post gastrectomy) hypoglycemia. Arch. Neurol., 23:14–17, 1970.
26. Calmiel, L. F. De la paralysie considérée chez les aliénés. Paris: Bailliere, 1826.
27. Cavenar, J. O., Maltbie, A. A., and Austin, L. Depression simulating organic brain disease. Am. J. Psychiatry, 136:521–523, 1979.
28. Cole, M. G., and Primeau, F. J. Prognosis of delirium in elderly hospital patients. Can. Med. Assoc. J., 141:41–46, 1991.
29. Corder, E. H., Saunders, A. M., Strittmatter, W. J., Schmechel, D. E., Gaskell, P. C., Small, G. W., Roses, A. D., Haines, J. L., and Pericak-Vance, M. A. Gene dose of apolipoprotein E type 4 allele and the risk of Alzheimer's disease in late onset families. Science, 261:921–923, 1993.
30. Corey-Bloom, J., Anand, R., and Veach, J. A randomized trial evaluating the efficacy and safety of ENA 713 (rivastigmine tartrate), a new acetylcholinesterase inhibitor, in patients with mild to moderately severe Alzheimer's disease. Int. J. Geriatr. Psychopharmacol., 1:55–65, 1998.
31. Cui, H. W., Zhang, B. A., Peng, T., Liu, Y., and Liu, Y. R. Wernicke's encephalopathy in a patient with acute pancreatitis: unusual cortical involvement and marvelous prognosis. Neurol. Sci., 33:615–618, 2012.
32. Cummings, J. L. Cholinesterase inhibitors: a new class of psychotropic compounds. Am. J. Psychiatry, 157:4–15, 2000.
33. Cummings, J. L., Vinters, H. V., and Felix, J. The Neuropsychiatry of Alzheimer's Disease and Related Dementias. London: Martin Dunitz, 2003.
34. Davis, K. L., Thal, L. J., Gamzu, E. R., Davis, C. S., Woolson, R., Gracon, S. I., Drachman, D. A., Schneider, L. S., Whitehouse, P. J., Hoover, T. M., et al. A double-blind, placebo-controlled multicenter study of tacrine for Alzheimer's disease. The Tacrine Collaborative Study Group. N. Engl. J. Med., 327:1253–1259, 1992.
35. Doody, R. S., Stevens, J. C., Beck, C., Dubinsky, R. M., Kaye, J. A., Gwyther, L., Mohs, R. C., Thal, L. J., Whitehouse, P. J., DeKosky, S. T., and Cummings, J. L. Practice parameter: management of dementia (an evidence-based review). Report of the Quality Standards Subcommittee of the American Academy of Neurology. Neurology, 56:1154–1166, 2001.

36. Eagles, J. M., Beattie, J. A., Blackwood, G. W., Restall, D. B., and Ashcroft, G. W. The mental health of elderly couples: I. The effects of a cognitively impaired spouse. Br. J. Psychiatry, 150:299–303, 1987.

37. Eagles, J. M., Craig, A., Rawlinson, F., Restall, D. B., Beattie, J. A., and Besson, J. A. The psychological well-being of supporters of the demented elderly. Br. J. Psychiatry, 150:293–298, 1987.

38. Eagles, J. M., Walker, L. G., Blackwood, G. W., Beattie, J. A., and Restall, D. B. The mental health of elderly couples: II. Concordance for psychiatric morbidity in spouses. Br. J. Psychiatry, 150:303–308, 1987.

39. Easson, W. Myxedema with psychosis. Arch. Gen. Psychiatry, 14:277–283, 1966.

40. Elmer, J., Tiamfook-Morgan, T., Brown, D. F., and Nadel, E. S. A 25-year-old woman with progressive neurological decline. J. Emerg. Med., 40:432–435, 2011.

41. Engel, G. L., and Romano, J. Delirium, a syndrome of cerebral insufficiency. 1959. J. Neuropsychiatry Clin. Neurosci., 16:526–538, 2004.

42. Enoch, B. A., and Williams, D. M. An association between Wernicke's encephalopathy and thyrotoxicosis. Postgrad. Med. J., 44:923–924, 1968.

43. Erkkinen, M. G., Kim, M. O., and Geschwind, M. D. Clinical neurology and epidemiology of the major neurodegenerative diseases. Cold Spring Harb. Perspect. Biol., 2017.

44. Francis, J., Martin, D., and Kapoor, W. N. A prospective study of delirium in hospitalized elderly. JAMA, 263:1097–1101, 1990.

45. Fuller, J., Ward, E., Evans, A., Massam, K., and Gardner, A. Dementia: supportive groups for relatives. Br. Med. J., 1:1684–1685, 1979.

46. Gatz, M., Reynolds, C. A., Fratiglioni, L., Johansson, B., Mortimer, J. A., Berg, S., Fiske, A., and Pedersen, N. L. Role of genes and environments for explaining Alzheimer disease. Arch Gen. Psychiatry, 63:168–174, 2006.

47. George-Hyslop, P. H. Molecular genetics of Alzheimer's disease. Biol. Psychiatry, 47:183–199, 2000.

48. George-Hyslop, P. H., Myers, R. H., Haines, J. L., Farrer, L. A., Tanzi, R. E., Abe, K., James, M. F., Conneally, P. M., Polinsky, R. J., and Gusella, J. F. Familial Alzheimer's disease: progress and problems. Neurobiol. Aging, 10:417–425, 1989.

49. George-Hyslop, P. H., Tanzi, R. E., Polinsky, R. J., Haines, J. L., Nee, L., Watkins, P. C., Myers, R. H., Feldman, R. G., Pollen, D., and Drachman, D. The genetic defect causing familial Alzheimer's disease maps on chromosome 21. Science, 235:885–890, 1987.

50. Gjestland, T. The Oslo study of untreated syphilis; an epidemiologic investigation of the natural course of the syphilitic infection based upon a re-study of the Boeck-Bruusgaard material. Acta Dermatol. Venereol., 35:3–368, 1955.

51. Grant, I., and Martin, A. *Neuropsychology of HIV Infection*. New York: Oxford University Press, 1994.

52. Green, R. C., Cupples, L. A., Go, R., Benke, K. S., Edeki, T., Griffith, P. A., Williams, M., Hipps, Y., Graff-Radford, N., Bachman, D., and Farrer, L. A. Risk of dementia among white and African American relatives of patients with Alzheimer disease. JAMA, 287:329–336, 2002.

53. Hahn, J. S., Berquist, W., Alcorn, D. M., Chamberlain, L., and Bass, D. Wernicke encephalopathy and beriberi during total parenteral nutrition attributable to multivitamin infusion shortage. Pediatrics, 101:E10, 1998.

54. Hardy, J. Amyloid, the presenilins and Alzheimer's disease. Trends Neurosci., 20:154–159, 1997.

55. Harper, C. Wernicke's encephalopathy: a more common disease than realised. A neuropathological study of 51 cases. J. Neurol. Neurosurg. Psychiatry, 42:226–231, 1979.

56. Harper, C. The incidence of Wernicke's encephalopathy in Australia—a neuropathological study of 131 cases. J. Neurol. Neurosurg. Psychiatry, 46:593–598, 1983.

57. Harper, C., Rodriguez, M., Gold, J., and Perdices, M. The Wernicke-Korsakoff syndrome in Sydney—a prospective necropsy study. Med. J. Aust., 149:718, 720, 1988.

58. Harrison, P. Alzheimer's disease and chromosome 14. Different gene, same process? Br. J. Psychiatry, 163:2–5, 1993.

59. Hendrie, H. C., Unverzagt, F. W., and Austrom, M. G. The dementing disorders. Psychiatr. Q., 68:261–279, 1997.

60. Herrmann, N., Chau, S. A., Kircanski, I., and Lanctot, K. L. Current and emerging drug treatment options for Alzheimer's disease: a systematic review. Drugs, 71:2031–2065, 2011.

61. Heston, L. L., Orr, H. T., Rich, S. S., and White, J. A. Linkage of an Alzheimer disease susceptibility locus to markers on human chromosome 21. Am. J. Med. Genet., 40:449–453, 1991.

62. Holmes, C., Cairns, N., Lantos, P., and Mann, A. Validity of current clinical criteria for Alzheimer's disease, vascular dementia and dementia with Lewy bodies. Br. J. Psychiatry, 174:45–50, 1999.

63. Hui, D., Frisbee-Hume, S., Wilson, A., Dibaj, S. S., Nguyen, T., De La Cruz, M., Walker, P., Zhukovsky, D. S., Delgado-Guay, M., Vidal, M., Epner, D., Reddy, A., Tanco, K., Williams, J., Hall, S., Liu, D., Hess, K., Amin, S., Breitbart, W., and Bruera, E. Effect of lorazepam with haloperidol vs haloperidol alone on agitated delirium in patients with advanced cancer receiving palliative care: a randomized clinical trial. JAMA, 318:1047–1056, 2017.

64. Hunter, R., and Macalpine, I. *Three Hundred Years of Psychiatry. 1535-1860.* London: Oxford University Press, 1963.

65. Isenberg-Grzeda, E., Kutner, H. E., and Nicolson, S. E. Wernicke-Korsakoff-syndrome: under-recognized and under-treated. Psychosomatics, 53:507–516, 2012.

66. Jorm, A. F., and Jolley, D. The incidence of dementia: a meta-analysis. Neurology, 51:728–733, 1998.

67. Jung, Y. C., Chanraud, S., and Sullivan, E. V. Neuroimaging of Wernicke's encephalopathy and Korsakoff's syndrome. Neuropsychol. Rev, 22:170–180, 2012.

68. Kahn, R. L., Zarit, S. H., Hilbert, N. M., and Niederehe, G. Memory complaint and impairment in the aged. The effect of depression and altered brain function. Arch. Gen. Psychiatry, 32:1569–1573, 1975.

69. Karch, C. M., and Goate, A. M. Alzheimer's disease risk genes and mechanisms of disease pathogenesis. Biol. Psychiatry, 77:43–51, 2015.

70. Knapp, M. J., Knopman, D. S., Solomon, P. R., Pendlebury, W. W., Davis, C. S., and Gracon, S. I. A 30-week randomized controlled trial of high-dose tacrine in patients with Alzheimer's disease. JAMA, 271:985–991, 1994.

71. Kopelman, M. D. The Korsakoff syndrome. Br. J. Psychiatry, 166:154–173, 1995.

72. LaMantia, M. A., Messina, F. C., Hobgood, C. D., and Miller, D. K. Screening for delirium in the emergency department: a systematic review. Ann. Emerg. Med., 63:551–560, 2013.

73. Lane, C. A., Hardy, J., and Schott, J. M. Alzheimer's disease. Eur. J. Neurol., 2017.

74. Lazarus, L. W., Newton, H., Cohler, B., Lesser, J., and Schweon, C. Frequency and presentation of depressive symptoms in patients with primary degenerative dementia. Am. J. Psychiatry, *144*:41–45, 1987.

75. Levy-Lahad, E., Wasco, W., Poorkaj, P., Romano, D. M., Oshima, J., Pettingell, W. H., Yu, C. E., Jondro, P. D., Schmidt, S. D., Wang, K., et al. Candidate gene for the chromosome 1 familial Alzheimer's disease locus. Science, *269*:973–977, 1995.

76. Lindboe, C. F., and Loberg, E. M. Wernicke's encephalopathy in non-alcoholics. An autopsy study. J. Neurol Sci., *90*:125–129, 1989.

77. Lishman, W. A. Cerebral disorder in alcoholism. Syndromes of impairment. Brain, *104*:1–20, 1981.

78. Liston, E. H. The clinical phenomenology of presenile dementia. A critical review of the literature. J. Nerv. Ment. Dis., *167*:329–336, 1979.

79. Martin, P. R., McCool, B. A., and Singleton, C. K. Genetic sensitivity to thiamine deficiency and development of alcoholic organic brain disease. Alcohol. Clin. Exp. Res., *17*:31–37, 1993.

80. Massie, M. J., Holland, J., and Glass, E. Delirium in terminally ill cancer patients. Am. J. Psychiatry, *140*:1048–1050, 1983.

81. Mayeux, R., and Stern, Y. Epidemiology of Alzheimer disease. Cold Spring Harb. Perspect. Med., *2*, 2012.

82. McAllister, R. W., and Price, T. R. Severe depressive pseudodementia with and without dementia. Am. J. Psychiatry, *139*:626–629, 1982.

83. Morgagni, G. B. *The Seats and Causes of Diseases Investigated by Anatomy*, Alexander, B. (trans.). London: Millar, Cadell, Johnson and Payne, 1769.

84. Morris, J. C., Rubin, E. H., Morris, E. J., and Mandel, S. A. Senile dementia of the Alzheimer's type: an important risk factor for serious falls. J. Gerontol., *42*:412–417, 1987.

85. Myers, R. H., Schaefer, E. J., Wilson, P. W., D'Agostino, R., Ordovas, J. M., Espino, A., Au, R., White, R. F., Knoefel, J. E., Cobb, J. L., McNulty, K. A., Beiser, A., and Wolf, P. A. Apolipoprotein E epsilon4 association with dementia in a population-based study: the Framingham study. Neurology, *46*:673–677, 1996.

86. Oh, E. S., Fong, T. G., Hshieh, T. T., and Inouye, S. K. Delirium in older persons: advances in diagnosis and treatment. JAMA, *318*:1161–1174, 2017.

87. Pandharipande, P. P., and Ely, E. W. Humanizing the treatment of hyperactive delirium in the last days of life. JAMA, *318*:1014–1015, 2017.

88. Plassman, B. L., and Breitner, J. C. The genetics of dementia in late life. Psychiatr. Clin. North Am., *20*:59–76, 1997.

89. Preskorn, S. H., and Simpson, S. Tricyclic-antidepressant-induced delirium and plasma drug concentration. Am. J. Psychiatry, *139*:822–823, 1982.

90. Reitz, C., Brayne, C., and Mayeux, R. Epidemiology of Alzheimer disease. Nat. Rev. Neurol., *7*:137–152, 2011.

91. Rice, E., and Gendelman, S. Psychiatric aspects of normal pressure hydrocephalus. JAMA, *223*:409–412, 1973.

92. Rob, P. M., Niederstadt, C., and Reusche, E. Dementia in patients undergoing long-term dialysis: aetiology, differential diagnoses, epidemiology and management. CNS Drugs, *15*:691–699, 2001.

93. Robins, E., Gassner, S., Kayes, J., Wilkinson, R. H., Jr., and Murphy, G. E. The communication of suicidal intent: a study of 134 cases of successful (completed) suicide. Am. J. Psychiatry, *115*:724–733, 1959.

94. Rogers, S. L., Farlow, M. R., Doody, R. S., Mohs, R., and Friedhoff, L. T. A 24-week, double-blind, placebo-controlled trial of donepezil in patients with Alzheimer's disease. Donepezil Study Group. Neurology, *50*:136–145, 1998.

95. Rogers, S. L., Friedhoff, L. T., and the Donepezil Study Group. The efficacy and safety of donepezil in patients with Alzheimer's disease: results of a US multicentre, randomized, double-blind, placebo-controlled trial. Dementia, 7:293–303, 1996.

96. Ron, M. A. Brain damage in chronic alcoholism: a neuropathological, neuroradiological and psychological review. Psychol. Med., 7:103–112, 1977.

97. Ron, M. A., Toone, B. K., Garralda, M. E., and Lishman, W. A. Diagnostic accuracy in presenile dementia. Br. J. Psychiatry, 134:161–168, 1979.

98. Ropper, A. H., and Brown, R. H. Adams and Victor's Principles of Neurology, 8th edition. New York: McGraw-Hill, 2005.

99. Salmon, W. Iatrica: Sen Praxis Medendi. The Practice of Curing Disease, 3rd edition. London: Rolls, 1694.

100. Sampson, E. L., Blanchard, M. R., Jones, L., Tookman, A., and King, M. Dementia in the acute hospital: prospective cohort study of prevalence and mortality. Br. J. Psychiatry, 195:61–66, 2009.

101. Schafer, D. F., and Jones, E. A. Hepatic encephalopathy and the gamma amino-butyric-acid neurotransmitter system. Lancet, 1:18–20, 1982.

102. Schellenberg, G. D., Bird, T. D., Wijsman, E. M., Orr, H. T., Anderson, L., Nemens, E., White, J. A., Bonnycastle, L., Weber, J. L., Alonso, M. E., Potter, H. P., Heston, L. L., and Martin, G. M. Genetic linkage evidence for a familial Alzheimer's disease locus on chromosome 14. Science, 258:668–671, 1992.

103. Schentag, J. J., Cerra, F. B., Calleri, G., DeGlopper, E., Rose, J. Q., and Bernhard, H. Pharmacokinetic and clinical studies in patients with cimetidine-associated mental confusion. Lancet, 1:177–181, 1979.

104. Sechi, G., and Serra, A. Wernicke's encephalopathy: new clinical settings and recent advances in diagnosis and management. Lancet Neurol., 6:442–455, 2007.

105. Siddiqi, N., House, A. O., and Holmes, J. D. Occurrence and outcome of delirium in medical in-patients: a systematic literature review. Age Ageing, 35:350–364, 2006.

106. Smith, C. K., Barish, J., Correa, J., and Williams, R. H. Psychiatric disturbance in endocrinologic disease. Psychosom. Med., 34:69–86, 1972.

107. Sola, E., Morillas, C., Garzon, S., Ferrer, J. M., Martin, J., and Hernandez-Mijares, A. Rapid onset of Wernicke's encephalopathy following gastric restrictive surgery. Obes. Surg., 13:661–662, 2003.

108. Sosa-Ortiz, A. L., Acosta-Castillo, I., and Prince, M. J. Epidemiology of dementias and Alzheimer's disease. Arch. Med. Res., 43:600–608, 2012.

109. Sternberg, D. E., and Jarvik, M. E. Memory functions in depression. Arch. Gen. Psychiatry, 33:219–224, 1976.

110. Strachan, R., and Henderson, J. Psychiatric syndromes due to avitaminosis B12 with normal blood and marrow. Q. J. Med., 34:303–317, 1965.

111. Sun, G. H., Yang, Y. S., Liu, Q. S., Cheng, L. F., and Huang, X. S. Pancreatic encephalopathy and Wernicke encephalopathy in association with acute pancreatitis: a clinical study. World J. Gastroenterol., 12:4224–4227, 2006.

112. Tariot, P. N., Solomon, P. R., Morris, J. C., Kershaw, P., Lilienfeld, S., and Ding, C. A 5-month, randomized, placebo-controlled trial of galantamine in AD. The Galantamine USA-10 Study Group. Neurology, 54:2269–2276, 2000.

113. Thomas, P. K. Brain atrophy and alcoholism. Br. Med. J., 292:787, 1986.

114. Trimble, M. R., and Reynolds, E. H. Anticonvulsant drugs and mental symptoms: a review. Psychol. Med., 6:169–178, 1976.

115. Tune, L. E. Postoperative delirium. Int. Psychogeriatr., 3:325–332, 1991.

116. Tune, L. E., Damlouji, H. F., Holland, A., Gardner, T. J., Folstein, M. F., and Coyle, J. T. Association of postoperative delirium with raised serum levels of anticholinergic drugs. Lancet, 2:651–653, 1981.

117. Victor, M., Adams, R. D., and Collins, G. H. *The Wernicke-Korsakoff Syndrome*. Philadelphia: F.A. Davis, 1971.

118. Wells, C. E. Chronic brain disease: an overview. Am. J. Psychiatry, 135:1–12, 1978.

119. Wells, C. E. Pseudodementia. Am. J. Psychiatry, 136:895–900, 1979.

120. Winblad, B., Jones, R. W., Wirth, Y., Stoffler, A., and Mobius, H. J. Memantine in moderate to severe Alzheimer's disease: a meta-analysis of randomised clinical trials. Dement. Geriatr. Cogn. Disord., 24:20–27, 2007.

121. Worden, R. W., and Allen, H. M. Wernicke's encephalopathy after gastric bypass that masqueraded as acute psychosis: a case report. Curr. Surg., 63:114–116, 2006.

CHAPTER 14

The Psychiatric Evaluation

Such is man that if he has the name for something, it ceases to be a riddle.
Isaac Bashevis Singer

The purpose of a psychiatric evaluation is to examine psychological function and to diagnose a psychiatric disorder or disorders if present. To elicit enough information about the disorder(s) to make a diagnosis, one must know the signs, symptoms, course, and complications. This is the primary reason this chapter concludes the book.

Eliciting clinical information is an art. It can be only partially learned in a formal manner. Establishing rapport and trust between the doctor and patient facilitates accurate history gathering, communicates empathy, and allows logical arrival at reasoned conclusions regarding clinical status and diagnosis or diagnoses. This ability is essential, and it cannot be learned from textbooks. In this chapter we offer advice on interviewing, provide a logical framework for organizing observations, and suggest how case histories should be presented. We begin with just a few words about terminology and time.

The *mental status examination* is the part of the physical examination that deals with the patient's thoughts, feelings, and behavior at a particular point in time. This term is often used as a synonym for a *psychiatric examination*, but "mental status" refers to one part of the psychiatric examination: the current thoughts, feelings, and behavior of the patient. *Psychiatric evaluation* includes the past history (medical, social, family, records, collateral information) of the patient as well. The distinction between the two terms is somewhat artificial. Similar to *liver status* or *cardiac status*, what exists now is inseparable from what came before; a certain amount of historical background is unavoidable in describing the current mental status of a patient. Nonetheless, the term "mental status" is used when the *primary* focus of the questioning is on current functioning.

Internists, family practitioners, and other nonpsychiatrists generally have little time to spend with patients—often no more than 15 minutes to review the file, check laboratory results, interview the patient, and conduct a physical assessment. If the examination is "complete," it will include some attention to the mental status of the patient. This may be limited to a few minutes. Although managed care may put extra time pressure on the clinician, the expenditure of at least a few moments will broaden the perspective about the patient (whether the answers are positive or negative) and may save substantial time during the course of treatment. For example, learning that an obviously depressed individual also has a history of one or more manic episodes will not only change the diagnosis from major depressive disorder to bipolar disorder but also the treatment that may have otherwise switched the patient from a depressive episode into a manic phase.

Later we will provide some screening questions that will help nonpsychiatrists quickly ascertain whether the mental state of the patient is abnormal. For now, we will assume the mental status examination is being conducted by a psychiatrist, a student, or a resident in psychiatry who has the luxury of being able to spend a fair amount of time with the patient, observing him or her and asking questions.

ADVICE ON INTERVIEWING

Following are four rules for conducting a psychiatric evaluation:

1. *Start open-ended.* After exchanging friendly greetings with the patient and attempting to set a relaxed tone, the interviewer should ask an open-ended question, such as "What is the problem that brings you here?" "What can I do for you?" Unless the patient is uncooperative or incapable of free expression (perhaps because of physical disability), let the patient tell his or her story with little or no interruption during the first 2–5 minutes.

   The patient is often anxious early in the interview and this tension may indeed stimulate the information flow. A patient with a *formal thought disorder* (where the thoughts do not connect coherently) will reveal this quickly. Much of the information needed for the diagnosis is often provided in the first few minutes if the patient proceeds without interruption. Early steering of the interview through certain question lines may result in missing important material.

On the other hand, for a particularly tense patient, more structure at the beginning of the interview may lead to easier communication. The interviewer can ask specific questions that are emotionally neutral. Questions about the patient's background, including where the patient grew up and attended school, marital status, employment history, and other physicians seen, can provide a comfortable transition into asking about a presenting problem.

2. *Ask specific questions later.* One purpose of the mental status examination is to make a diagnosis, if possible. This requires specific questions if merely to rule out remote possibilities. For example, patients are likely to avoid volunteering information about hallucinations. "Do you hear voices or see things that others do not hear or see?" or some variation on this query is often necessary to determine whether the patient is psychotic. "Do you feel in danger?" may elicit persecutory delusions. "Do you have a special mission in life?" may bring out grandiose delusions. "What are your plans after leaving the hospital?" may bring out unrealistic thinking, raising questions about judgment.

Even with the advantage of a long interview, the psychiatric examiner must ask specific questions bearing on a reasonable differential diagnosis. There is usually no point, for example, in going through a complete review of systems if the patient experiences excellent health and presents with symptoms of a psychiatric condition in which physical symptoms do not usually play a role.

Details about positive early life experiences rarely bear on the problem of making a differential diagnosis in adults. School and social history are often important, but not always, particularly with elderly people.

3. *Establish the chronology of the illness.* Kraepelin (3) noted that the course of a psychiatric illness is as important as the symptoms. Sydenham (5) said that "true" illnesses should have common symptoms and a common course. Few, if any, pathognomonic symptoms exist in psychiatry. We agree with Kraepelin that establishing the course of an illness is as important as recognizing current symptoms.

When did the symptoms begin? Was the patient ever free of psychiatric symptoms? When? Age of onset is an important clue to diagnosis, as many conditions typically begin at particular times in life. Has the illness been continual, always present with fluctuations, or episodic in the sense that symptoms sometimes go away entirely?

How rapid was the onset? (Psychotic illnesses with abrupt onsets generally have a better prognosis than those with a gradual onset.) Have professional interventions (medications, psychotherapy) altered the course of illness? In general, has the patient tended to improve or get worse?

"Diagnosis is prognosis" is an old saying in medicine, and knowledge of the course of illness as well as the symptoms forms the basis for determining prognosis.

4. *Be friendly, sympathetic, respectful.* Establish good eye contact and listen attentively. Encourage the patient to tell his or her history through noninterfering encouragement (e.g., smiling, nodding, reflecting the patient's expressed feelings). Adult patients should be called "Mr." or "Mrs." or "Ms.," at least until the clinician knows them well. Clinicians should never insult patients. They should never make fun of them. This may seem obvious, but there are subtle ways of betraying disrespect.

Be sensitive to the emotional state of the patient. If certain questioning makes the patient angry, anxious, sad, or tearful, this may offer an opportunity to enhance the patient's ability to communicate, though sometimes a return to more neutral ground is indicated so that the patient is not overwhelmed by emotion.

A word about the uncooperative patient: to say, "I can't help you unless you help me" sometime works, but usually it does not. Asking specific questions such as "What led to your coming here?" or "Whose idea was it that you come here?" may help lower resistance. Sometimes the interview must be postponed until another time when the patient may be more helpful. Anger toward the uncooperative patient is never appropriate.

Psychiatry, probably more than any other specialty, benefits greatly from informants—friends and family who will tell what the patient will not (or cannot). Although caution should be exercised in judging the merit of such information, it can be very helpful in making a diagnosis. One should also remember to obtain permission from the patient before seeking outside or collateral information.

THE DECISION TREE

Except for open-ended questions at the beginning and specific questions toward the end, history taking should flow easily and casually, as in a conversation. Initially, patients should be permitted to talk about what they want to talk about, but eventually they should be gently guided back into channels that provide information the examiner requires for a diagnosis. From the moment a patient walks into the examination room, however, the examiner's mental "computer" starts making relevant observations. How is the patient dressed and groomed? Does the patient have a normal gait and range of motion? Is the patient hostile or friendly? How old does the patient appear to be?

Based on early impressions, the interviewer starts constructing the differential diagnosis. Over the course of the interview, the examiner's choices about *probable* diagnoses will determine which areas to emphasize and which to skip over lightly or omit entirely. The examiner's mind, indeed, functions as a computer. By the end of the interview—if it is successful—the choices will have narrowed to one or a few.

A highly simplified branching process for approaching the diagnosis of psychiatric disorders begins by addressing the potential for psychosis and memory impairment. The first important decision concerns psychosis. Is the patient psychotic or nonpsychotic? Psychosis generally refers to the presence of persistent hallucinations and/or delusions and/or disordered thoughts.

The diagnostic possibilities for a nonpsychotic person would include the anxiety disorders (in *DSM-5* there are six main anxiety disorder diagnoses plus "other specified" and "unspecified" anxiety disorder) (1), major depression, bipolar disorder, substance use disorder, antisocial personality disorder, other personality disorder, obsessive-compulsive disorder, eating disorders, and somatization disorder. Thus, in some conditions such as mood disorders and substance use disorders, the patient may or may not be psychotic. An individual with psychosis may suffer from schizophrenia, a mood disorder, or drug intoxication. Hallucinogens, amphetamines, and phencyclidine (PCP) are commonly associated with psychosis. Earlier chapters in this text provide fuller discussion of the various diagnoses and their many presentations in these specific types of disorders.

The second early decision concerns memory. Memory problems can usually be sorted into acute or chronic conditions. The nomenclature and presentations were reviewed in detail in Chapter 13. Several issues warrant review. First, poor intellectual functioning is associated with, and often indistinguishable from, bad memory. Impaired memory *produces* impaired intellectual functioning. Intelligence encompasses more than memory, but even those skills not normally associated with memory (e.g., reasoning ability) often suffer when memory is impaired. Second, patients with major depressive disorder sometimes have difficulty with memory, and this is called "pseudodementia." Their memory improves as their depression improves. Finally, patients with gross memory impairment (as distinguished from absentmindedness, normal forgetting, or "not paying attention") may display any psychiatric symptom associated with any of the disorders not classified as disorders primarily involving memory. Although symptoms of disorders not classified as disorders primarily involving memory may temporally correspond to or antedate onset of memory impairment, identification of a new organic impairment is *of paramount importance*. Diagnosis of a new onset of a neurocognitive disorder is one of the most important things a psychiatrist can do because it initiates a search for the *cause* of the disorder that may be *treatable*. Physicians are uniquely qualified among mental health professionals to identify the neurocognitive disorder. Trained in anatomy, physiology, and biochemistry, and aided by modern imaging and laboratory techniques, physicians can evaluate the entire range of sources of organic disorders, including brain tumors, endocrine disorders, metabolic illness, and infections.

In most hospitals, about one-fifth of the patients who clearly have psychiatric abnormalities do not meet criteria for any specific psychiatric diagnosis. The suitable label for these people is "undiagnosed." One advantage of this term is that physicians who deal with the patient in the future will not be biased by having a poorly grounded diagnosis in the chart. Another advantage is the sense of modesty it correctly implies. In particular, there is no diagnostic test to conclusively establish a psychiatric diagnosis other than delirium and dementia.

Unfortunately, many insurance companies *require* a diagnosis. One can include the most likely diagnosis or diagnoses prefaced by the term "rule out." Many insurance companies will accept this practice. Alternatively, use of the "unspecified" diagnostic category (e.g., unspecified anxiety disorder) may suffice and be clinically useful because it conveys the core symptom or symptoms without overstating certitude.

Outside of hospitals, many patients who consult psychiatrists do not have a diagnosable illness. They even lack symptoms of sufficient severity to justify being called "undiagnosed." One label for these more or less normal people who see psychiatrists is "problem of living," which suggests, if nothing else, that no conventional diagnosis seems to fit them.

THE MENTAL STATUS FORMAT

The purpose of the mental status format is to help the interviewer organize and communicate his or her observations about a patient. Minor deviations occur in the format from expert to expert, but some framework for observations is necessary to facilitate thinking and communication. The format presented here is commonly used and includes the following categories:

Appearance and behavior
Form and content of thought
Affect and mood
Memory and intellectual functioning
Insight and judgment

Appearance and Behavior

The patient's appearance is generally relevant to the psychiatric diagnosis. Patients with schizophrenia, for example, may sometimes appear poorly groomed or even dirty. Patients with major depression can be negligent about their dress and grooming. Patients with mania may wear odd or unusual clothing. Sunglasses worn indoors may suggest paranoia; a puffy face and red palms are suggestive, but not diagnostic, of alcohol dependence.

A physical appearance older than the patient's stated age may suggest depression or long-term substance abuse. If this is the case, a more youthful appearance may be restored as the patient recovers.

The patient's attitude toward the interviewer may be informative. Patients with paranoia are often suspicious, guarded, or hostile. Patients with somatization disorder sometimes try to flatter interviewers by comparing them favorably with previous doctors; they are often dramatic, friendly, and sometimes seductive. During manic episodes, patients may crack jokes and occasionally are quite funny—when they are not irritable or unpleasant. Patients with antisocial personality disorder may seem like con men—and sometimes are.

The patient may be agitated—unable to sit still, moving constantly. Patients who are retarded may slump in their seats, with slow movements and speech. Talking may seem an effort. Disturbance of motor function may have several causes. Antipsychotic medications may produce a restlessness called "akathisia," in which the patient cannot sit still and may feel compelled to walk. Antipsychotics also may produce Parkinson-type symptoms, including tremor and an expressionless face. Pacing and hand-wringing may be expressions of agitated depression; joviality and volubility may portray mania.

Antipsychotics are given so commonly that it is often impossible to determine whether abnormal movements are drug induced or represent catatonic symptoms. In fact, similar involuntary movements were observed in schizophrenia years ago before medications were introduced. It is said that catatonic symptoms (cataplexy, stupor, hyperkinesia) are disappearing, but what previously was called catatonic may now be interpreted as drug induced without knowing whether medications are responsible.

Schizophrenia also may involve psychomotor disturbances such as mannerisms, posturing, stereotypical movements, and negativism (doing the opposite of what is requested). Also seen is *echopraxia*, in which movements of another person are imitated, and *catalepsy*, in which awkward positions are maintained for long periods without apparent discomfort. Some patients say nothing. Called "mutism," this behavior may be seen in schizophrenia, depression, delirium or dementia, and drug intoxication.

Form and Content of Thought

Form refers to intelligibility related to associations: Does the patient have "loose associations" in the sense of being circumstantial, tangential, or incoherent? Older people may be circumstantial. They return to the subject but only after providing excessive detail. Tangentiality is a flow of thought directed away from the subject being inquired about, with no return to the point of departure. Patients with schizophrenia are often tangential. Pressure of speech and flight of ideas are seen in mania and in drug intoxication. The patient with pressured speech seems to be compelled to talk. Manic speech flits from idea to idea, sometimes linked by only the most tenuous connections. Unlike tangentiality, however, manic speech frequently has connections that can be surmised. Patients in manic episodes often rhyme or pun and make "clang" associations, using one word after another because they sound similar. They tend to be overinclusive, including irrelevant and extraneous details.

Derailment, often seen in schizophrenia, is a form of speech lacking coherent logical connections between associations. Patients with schizophrenia may invent new words (neologisms) that presumably have a private meaning. Patients with schizophrenia may display poverty of thought, conveying little information with their words. *Echolalia* refers to repetition of the interviewer's words by the patient. Other abnormal speech patterns associated with schizophrenia (as well as dementia) are *perseveration*, in which the patient seems incapable of changing topics, and *blocking*, in which the flow of thought is suddenly stopped, often followed by a new and unrelated thought.

Patients who persistently display any of these symptoms (excluding poverty of thought) are said to have a *formal thought disorder*, meaning that the structure or form of thinking is disordered. Patients with somatization disorder or borderline personality disorder can be extremely circumstantial (providing excessive detail of little clinical importance) yet at the same time being quite vague (lacking specific information being sought). When severe, this "nonpsychotic thought disorder" pattern (4) can be mistaken for the tangentiality of formal thought disorder observed in patients with psychosis.

Content of thought refers to what the patient thinks and talks about. This category comprises hallucinations, delusions, obsessions, compulsions, phobias, suicidal or homicidal thoughts, and preoccupations deemed relevant to the psychiatric problem.

Delusions are fixed false beliefs neither amenable to logic or social pressure nor congruent with the patient's culture. They should be distinguished from *overvalued* ideas—fixed notions that most people consider false but that are not entirely unreasonable or that cannot be disproved, such as certain superstitions. Delusions occur in delirium or dementia, schizophrenia, mood disorders, and various intoxications.

Jaspers (2) believed the *subject* of the delusion has diagnostic significance. If the delusional ideas are "understandable," they more likely occur in depressed patients. Understandable delusions include those in which persons are convinced they have a serious life-threatening illness such as cancer, are impoverished, or are being persecuted because they are bad persons. Jaspers pointed out that healthy, prosperous, and likable people often worry about their health, finances, and approval by others. Such concerns are thus understandable.

Delusions that are *not* understandable are seen in schizophrenia, according to Jaspers. Schizophrenic delusions tend to be bizarre; for example, the patient's acts are controlled by outside forces (delusions of control or influence) or the patient believes that he is Jesus or Napoleon. Schizophrenia-like delusions occur often in amphetamine psychosis and, less commonly, in other intoxicated states (e.g., from cocaine or cannabis). The delusions of schizophrenia fall outside the ordinary person's experience: the examiner finds it difficult to identify with the schizophrenic's private world; hence, the term "autistic," derived from "auto," is often applied to schizophrenic thinking.

Religious delusions are sometimes hard to interpret. Religious beliefs may seem delusional to those who do not accept the beliefs but normal to those who do. Truly pathological religious delusions are usually identified without difficulty by members of the patient's congregation.

Content also encompasses perceptual disturbances. In *illusions*, real stimuli are mistaken for something else (e.g., a belt for a snake).

Hallucinations are perceptions without an external stimulus. *Auditory hallucinations* may consist of voices or noises. They are associated primarily with schizophrenia but occur in other conditions such as alcoholic hallucinosis and affective disorders. Visual hallucinations are most characteristic of organic disorders, especially delirious states. They also occur with psychedelic drug use and in schizophrenia. (Certain hallucinations are more common in some conditions, but no type of hallucination is found exclusively in any illness.) *Hypnagogic hallucinations* arise in the period between sleep and wakefulness, especially when falling asleep. *Hypnopompic hallucinations* occur when awakening from sleep. These sleep-cycle hallucinations are normal except when they are a symptom of narcolepsy.

Olfactory hallucinations are sometimes associated with complex partial seizures that involve the temporal lobes. *Haptic* (tactile) *hallucinations* occur in schizophrenia and also in cocaine intoxication and delirium tremens. The sensation of insects crawling in or under one's skin (formication) is particularly common in cocaine intoxication, but it also occurs in delirium tremens.

In *extracampine hallucinations*, the patient sees objects outside the sensory field (e.g., behind his or her head). In *autoscopic hallucinations*, patients visualize themselves projected into space. The patient occasionally has a *doppelgänger* (sees his or her double). Other perceptual distortions include *depersonalization* (the feeling that one has changed in some bizarre way) and *derealization* (the feeling that the environment has changed).

It is not uncommon for nonpsychiatric patients to report hallucinations, particularly seeing dead relatives. They have no other psychiatric symptoms and the hallucinations are not judged to be clinically important. Thus, a history of transient hallucinations or other perceptual disturbances, which occur occasionally during exhaustion or grief, does not necessarily signify the presence of psychosis. Such disturbances must be interpreted in the context of the overall clinical picture.

Affect and Mood

Affect refers to a patient's outwardly (externally) expressed emotion, which may or may not be appropriate to his or her reported mood and content of thought. For example, if a person smiles happily while telling of people trying to poison her, the affect would be described as inappropriate. If a person describes unbearable pain but looks as if she were discussing the weather, the affect again would be inappropriate.

Affect is sometimes referred to as "flat," meaning that the usual modulation in facial expression is absent. Patients with schizophrenia sometimes have a flat affect, but so do patients taking antipsychotic medications, and depressed patients may show little change of expression while speaking.

"Flat affect" is probably the most overused and misused term in the psychiatric examination. It should be used only if the affect is extremely "flat" or "blunted." Inappropriate and flat affects are especially associated with schizophrenia.

Some patients with somatization disorder display an inappropriate affect in that they describe excruciating pain and other extreme distress with the same indifference or good cheer with which they would describe a morning of shopping. (The French call this *la belle indifférence*.)

Mood refers to what the patient says about his or her internal emotional state. "I am sad," "I am happy," and "I am angry" are examples. Mood and affect are sometimes labile, meaning there is rapid fluctuation between manifestations of happiness, sadness, anger, and so on. *Labile* affect is often seen in patients with mania, somatization disorder, and delirium or dementia.

Memory and Intellectual Functioning

Subsumed under memory is *orientation*, meaning orientation for person, place, and time. To be disoriented for time, the patient should be more than 1 day off the correct day of the week and more than several days off the current date. Misidentifying people (e.g., thinking the nurse is one's aunt) is a clear case of disorientation, as is giving the wrong year or the wrong city and wrong hospital where one is currently. This part of the mental status is exceedingly important because, if a patient has a gross memory impairment (and is not malingering), he or she almost always has a neurocognitive disorder and all other psychiatric symptoms may be explainable in this context. (The exceptions are substance dependence and memory impairments arising from severe depression.)

There are many tests for memory and intellectual functioning. Memory can be subdivided into immediate, short-term, recent, and remote memory. *Immediate memory* can be tested by asking the patient to repeat a series of digits. Serially subtracting 7 from 100 is a test of immediate memory (assuming the person's arithmetic was ever adequate for the task), as are tests of attention and concentration. Short-term memory loss can be tested by asking patients to remember three easy words you have spoken or showing them three objects and then, 5 to 15 minutes later, asking them to repeat what they heard or saw. A short-term memory deficit is the *sine qua non* of Korsakoff's syndrome (see also Chapter 13). *Recent memory* refers to recall of events occurring in recent days, weeks, or months; *remote memory* involves recall of events occurring many years before, such as the winner of a long-ago presidential election. In early dementia, recent memory is usually more severely impaired than remote memory.

As noted earlier, tests of intellectual functioning should be interpreted with the patient's background, education, cooperativeness, and mood state in mind. A history major should be able to name the last seven presidents, but a "normal" person with a third-grade education may not be able to do so. Depressed patients may be too slowed down or distractible to concentrate. One approach would be to ask questions that are crafted to the particular situation that the examiner believes the patient should be able to answer. Another approach might be to ask the patient about his or her interests and then test the patient's fund of information in those areas.

Insight and Judgment

A person who has insight will know whether he is (or was) psychiatrically ill. If the person says, for example, that the voices are "real," he lacks insight. If he says it was simply his imagination playing tricks on him, he has insight. If he says there is nothing wrong with him but that his evil uncle has arranged for his hospitalization because of a Communist conspiracy, he may or may not have insight. (Even paranoids, as the saying goes, sometimes have real enemies.) Psychosis and delirium or dementia are associated with lack of insight.

The term "judgment" is used here in the same sense as "competence" is used in a court of law: a competent person is able to understand the nature of the charges and to cooperate with counsel. It implies that a person is realistic about his or her limitations and life circumstances. A good question to ask is "What are your plans when you leave the hospital?" If the patient with no money describes a plan to start a chain of restaurants, this displays impaired judgment. Severe impairment of judgment is seen most often in dementia and psychotic disorders.

EXCLUDING PSYCHIATRIC DISORDERS

Sometimes for all physicians and often for nonpsychiatric physicians, examination of the "mind" must be accomplished quickly, lest the liver, lungs, heart, and deep tendon reflexes be slighted. For the major disorders described in this book (and the less valid ones), a single question may suffice to strongly suggest ruling out the possibility that the patient has the disorder. Some disorders will be missed, but one or two questions will identify the great majority of patients who do *not* have a particular psychiatric illness:

Depression: Although it seems obvious, just ask the patient if he or she has periods of feeling down or depressed for days on end. Rare is the seriously depressed individual who will deny these feelings.

Mania: Ask if the patient has ever had elevated mood or felt too good for days at a time. People with a history of mania love to reflect on past times when they felt "really good."

Schizophrenia: Ask if the patient has ever heard or seen things that other people did not hear or see. Ask if he has ever been afraid of being poisoned or controlled by external forces. Hallucinations sometimes occur in normal people, but the presence of both hallucinations and delusions in a person with more or less normal mood suggests schizophrenia.

Panic disorder: Has the patient ever thought she was having a heart attack that did not occur? Does she ever become intensely apprehensive for no apparent reason? Patients with panic disorder report both. At church, does she find a seat on the aisle close to the back? Patients with panic disorder almost always do. They feel the need to make a quick exit if a panic attack seems impending.

Posttraumatic stress disorder: Was the patient involved in, or eyewitness to, a violent or physically traumatic event? After such an experience, did the patient develop new problems with jumpiness or sleeplessness, or intrusive memories of the experience? Are reminders of the event so upsetting that the patient will go to great lengths to avoid them?

Somatization disorder: Mostly women. Inquire in a neutral manner roughly how many doctors the patient has consulted for various symptoms and what surgical procedures she has had. If the patient has consulted few physicians and has all of her abdominal and pelvic structures intact, it is unlikely that the patient has somatization disorder.

Obsessive-compulsive disorder: Does the patient compulsively count things, such as the number of tiles on the floor? Does the patient repeatedly check a door to see if it is locked or an oven to see if it is turned off? Counting and checking are so common in this disorder that, if absent, the diagnosis should be questioned.

Phobic disorders: Does the patient avoid certain situations or things because they frighten him or her? Is the fear unreasonable?

Alcohol use disorder: Has the patient ever stopped drinking for a period of time (or tried unsuccessfully to do so)? If so, and the reason is not medical or a desire to lose weight, the patient probably stopped because he was worried about his drinking. At this point, the clinician can ask why he was worried, and this may break down the denial that is characteristic of alcoholism. Almost every patient with alcohol dependence has stopped, or tried to stop, at some time in their life. This is a better approach than asking, "Do you drink too much?"

Drug use disorder: "Have you ever worried about a drug habit?" is probably as good an opener as any.

Antisocial personality disorder: Ask if the patient was frequently truant in grade and high school. Rare is the adult with antisocial personality disorder who did not cut classes and get in trouble with school authorities as a teenager.

Borderline personality disorder: Ask if the patient suffers from reactive mood swings characterized by brief intense episodes of dysphoria, or irritability or anxiety lasting a few minutes, hours, or days. If not, the chance of the disorder is unlikely.

Dementia: Ask if the patient forgets where she parks her car. If this happens often, there should be some concern about her memory. Or simply ask, "How is your memory?" Many people with memory problems are relieved to have the chance to talk about them.

Anorexia nervosa: If the person is intelligent, ask her (and it is usually a her) if she has ever been told she had anorexia nervosa. Patients with this disorder usually know their diagnosis; the disorder is well described in popular media. Does the patient stuff herself (or himself) with food and then induce vomiting? This practice, called "bulimia," commonly occurs with eating disorders in both sexes.

Another question: "Are you the right weight?" If the patient is 5 foot 7 inches, weighs 92 pounds, is not a model, and says, "I'm too fat," a diagnosis of anorexia is strongly suggested.

Sexual problems: "Do you have any sexual issues?" is usually sufficient. This is a neutral approach to sexual problems.

These questions, when answered in the negative, will eliminate most people who have the disorders listed here. There will be few false negatives. There will be many false positives. (Some people who do not have depression or anxiety disorders sleep poorly and sit at the back of churches.) But for the physician trying to rule out disorders, false positives are much less important. They simply mean probing is required. Probing takes time, and referral to a psychiatrist may be in order.

SUGGESTIONS FOR PRESENTING CASES

There is obviously a good deal of latitude in presenting case histories for teaching purposes. Different institutions and different teachers within the institutions will have their own advice on the subject. However, discussions with these teachers reveal some agreement about certain points. Following are some general rules for presenting patients:

1. Do not read the history.
2. Do not exceed 10 to 15 minutes (allowing for interruptions).
3. Start with *identifying data*: name, age, race, marital status, vocation.
4. Provide a clue to the problem you will highlight, for example, "This patient presents a diagnostic problem," "He has not responded to standard treatments," "She comes from an unusual family." Such clues offer a framework for your audience into which the rest of the presentation will fit.
5. Avoid dates. Open with "Patient was admitted to [hospital] _____ (days, weeks, months) ago. Do not refer to events occurring on December 3, 1997, but say, "At the age of 15, the patient _____." Instead of saying, "Between November and January of 1995 and 1996," say, "For a 3-month period when the patient was 20 years old, he _____." It may be easier for patients to remember events by dates, but the listener has to translate dates into ages and, for the non-mathematically inclined, this may be difficult while concentrating on the presentation.
6. Begin with the *psychiatric history*. A good way to begin is, "The patient had no psychiatric problems until age _____ (or _____ days, weeks, or months ago) when he (slowly or rapidly) developed the following symptoms: _____," then list the symptoms in order of severity. Tell how long the symptoms persisted (for weeks, months, years, or to the present) and what happened as a result (hospitalization, other treatment, full or partial recovery).

Often, of course, establishing time of onset is difficult or impossible, particularly when dealing with a poor historian or a complicated case. The onset of illness in a person with intellectual disability would be "from birth," which does not help much. But an attempt to establish onset can be of considerable help because different illnesses characteristically begin at different ages.

7. It is important to know whether the illness has been chronic, perhaps with fluctuations, or episodic with full remissions between episodes. If the patient has had more than one episode, describe subsequent episodes, briefly giving the same information that was given for the first episode. Symptoms and life events obviously are interrelated, but emphasize the symptoms rather than the life events unless the life events appear to be causally related to the symptoms.

8. A brief *family history* should include the following: whether a close blood relative of the patient had a serious psychiatric illness requiring treatment (and what the treatment was, if known), pertinent medical illnesses, history of suicide, and alcohol or drug problems.

9. *Social history* should include (very briefly) circumstances of upbringing, particularly whether the parents were divorced or separated or whether the patient was brought up by both parents; parental vocation; siblings; years of education and how well the patient did in school from the standpoint of grades and adjustment; military and employment history; marital history; and number and ages of children.

10. Review the *medical history* only as it is pertinent to the psychiatric problems. The same applies to the review of systems, physical findings, and laboratory results.

11. Give the *mental status* as it was obtained at the first opportunity to fully examine the patient. The mental status findings should be presented in the order provided in the previous section.

12. End the presentation with *course in treatment*. Tell how the patient has been doing, whether he or she has improved, and what treatment the patient is receiving. In other words, bring the patient up to the present moment.

13. With rare exceptions, all of this can be presented in 10 to 15 minutes. The trick is to keep in mind at all times the goal of the presentation. If it is diagnostic, the differential diagnosis and the points for and against each of the reasonably likely diagnoses should be given. If you start out by saying the patient was psychiatrically well until the age of 60, dwelling on such diagnoses as intellectual disability, schizophrenia, somatization disorder, or panic disorder is unlikely to be

useful. Assuming the history is correct (though, granted, this is often a dubious assumption), people who are well until the age of 60 and then develop major psychiatric problems generally have either a mood disorder or delirium or dementia.

14. The reasons for presenting the history and mental status according to this sequence are to avoid leaving out important information and to make it easier for the listeners to follow the narration. There are many variations on this format, and none is perfect. (People's lives are much more complicated than formats.) Unlike written psychiatric histories, however, oral presentations should not attempt to be comprehensive. They should touch on the following categories, but not all with equal emphasis.

HISTORY

Identifying data
Focus of the presentation
Psychiatric history
Family history
Social history
Medical history
Review of systems
Physical findings
Laboratory results

MENTAL STATUS

Appearance and behavior
Form and content of thought
Affect and mood
Memory and intellectual functioning
Insight and judgment

REFERENCES

1. American Psychiatric Association. *Diagnostic and Statistical Manual for Mental Disorders,* 5th edition. Washington, DC: Author, 2013.
2. Jaspers, K. *General Psychopathology.* Chicago: University of Chicago Press, 1963.

3. Kraepelin, E. *Dementia Praecox and Paraphrenia*, Barclay, R. M., Robertson, G. M. (trans.). Edinburgh: E. & S. Livingstone, 1919.
4. North, C. S., Kienstra, D. M., Osborne, V. A., Dokucu, M. E., Vassilenko, M., Hong, B., Wetzel, R. D., and Spitznagel, E. L. Interrater reliability and coding guide for nonpsychotic formal thought disorder. Percept. Mot. Skills, *103*:395–411, 2006.
5. Sydenham, T. *Selected Works of Thomas Sydenham, M.D.* London: John Bales & Sons, Danielson, 1922.

INDEX

References to boxes and tables are indicated with an italicized *b* and *t* respectively.

CPSIA information can be obtained
at www.ICGtesting.com
Printed in the USA
BVHW031834200722
642213BV00002B/4

9 780190 215460